THE IOC MANUAL OF EMERGENCY SPORTS MEDICINE

June 2016.

To Eoin,

Wishing you every success & happiness for your future career in Physiotherapy.

With Best Wishes

Marie-Elaine

THE IOC MANUAL OF EMERGENCY SPORTS MEDICINE

EDITED BY

David McDonagh

and

David Zideman

WILEY Blackwell

Wiley-Blackwell is an imprint of John Wiley & Sons, formed by the merger of Wiley's global Scientific, Technical and Medical business with Blackwell Publishing.

Registered office: John Wiley & Sons, Ltd, The Atrium, Southern Gate, Chichester, West Sussex, PO19 8SQ, UK

Editorial offices: 9600 Garsington Road, Oxford, OX4 2DQ, UK
The Atrium, Southern Gate, Chichester, West Sussex, PO19 8SQ, UK
111 River Street, Hoboken, NJ 07030-5774, USA

For details of our global editorial offices, for customer services and for information about how to apply for permission to reuse the copyright material in this book please see our website at www.wiley.com/wiley-blackwell

Library of Congress Cataloging-in-Publication Data
The IOC Manual of Emergency Sports Medicine / edited by David McDonagh and David Zideman.
p. ; cm.
International Olympic Committee manual of emergency medical care in sports
Includes bibliographical references and index.
ISBN 978-1-118-91368-0 (pbk.)
I. McDonagh, David O'Sullivan, editor. II. Zideman, David A., editor. III. International Olympic Committee, issuing body. IV. Title: The International Olympic Committee manual of emergency sports medicine.
[DNLM: 1. Olympic Games. 2. Athletic Injuries--therapy. 3. Emergency Treatment. QT 261]
RD97
617.1'027--dc23

2014041849

A catalogue record for this book is available from the British Library.

Wiley also publishes its books in a variety of electronic formats. Some content that appears in print may not be available in electronic books.

Typeset in 9.5/12pt Plantin Std by Laserwords Private Limited, Chennai, India
Printed and bound in Singapore by Markono Print Media Pte Ltd

1 2015

The editors would like to thank Lesley Zideman for her efforts and the many hours she has contributed to this project.

Contents

List of Contributors

Kathryn E. Ackerman
USA Rowing, Boston, MA, USA
Female Athlete Program, Division of Sports Medicine Boston Children's Hospital, Boston, MA, USA
Sports Endocrine Research Lab, Neuroendocrine Unit Massachusetts General Hospital, Boston, MA, USA
Harvard Medical School, Boston, MA, USA

Glenn Brown
Supreme Court of Queensland, Brisbane, Australia
High Court of Australia, Kingston, ACT, Australia

Mark Brown
Sports Medicine Australia, Oceania National Olympic Committee Medical Commission, Griffith University Centre of Musculoskeletal Research, Southport, QLD, Australia

Richard Budgett
International Olympic Committee, Lausanne, Switzerland

Brian Carlin
UCD Centre for Emergency Medical Science School of Medicine, University College, Dublin, Ireland

Michael R. Carmont
Gloucester Rugby, Gloucester, England
Princess Royal Hospital, Telford, Shropshire, England
Orthopedic Department, Shrewsbury and Telford, Shrewsbury, UK

Anthony Clough
Eastman Dental Institute, University of London, London, UK

Joseph Cummiskey
Faculty of Sports and Exercise Medicine, Royal College of Surgeons and Royal College of Physicians of Ireland, Dublin, Ireland

Lars Engebretsen
Oslo Sports Trauma Research Center, Department of Sports Medicine, Norwegian School of Sport Sciences, Oslo, Norway
Medical & Scientific Department, IOC, Lausanne, Switzerland

Uğur Erdener
Department of Ophtalmology, Hacettepe University Faculty of Medicine, Ankara, Turkey
IOC Member, Chairman IOC Medical Commission

Éanna Falvey
Ireland Rugby Team, Dublin, Ireland
Sports Surgery Clinic, Dublin, Ireland

Mark Faulkner
Major Trauma and Legal Services, London Ambulance Service NHS Trust, London, UK

Geraint Fuller
Department of Neurology, Gloucester Royal Hospital, Gloucester, UK

Gordon Giesbrecht
Kinesiology and Recreation Management, Departments of Anaesthesia and Emergency Medicine, University of Manitoba, Winnipeg, Canada

Marie-Elaine Grant
IOC Medical Commission (Games Group)
Institute of Sport and Health, University College Dublin, Dublin, Ireland

Jonathan Hanson
Broadford Hospital, Skye, Scotland
Department of Sport and Exercise Medicine Musgrave Park Hospital, Belfast, UK
Scottish Rugby Football Union

Hiu Fai Ho
Accident and Emergency Department, Queen Elizabeth Hospital, Hong Kong, China

Michael Kenihan
Sports Medicine Australia, Albert Park, Victoria, Australia

Sibel Kocabeyoglu
Department of Ophtalmology, Hacettepe University Faculty of Medicine, Ankara, Turkey

Ruth Löllgen
Emergency Medicine, Children's Hospital at Westmead, Sydney, Australia

Herbert Löllgen
German Federation of Sports Medicine, Remscheid, Germany

Mike Loosemore
English Institute of Sport, The Institute of Sport, Exercise and Health, University College London, London, UK
Medical Committee International Bobsleigh and Skeleton Federation, Lausanne, Switzerland.

Dara Lundon
Surgical Laboratory, School of Medicine and Medical Sciences, University College Dublin, Dublin, Ireland

Saul Marks
Department of Psychiatry, University of Toronto, Toronto, ON, Canada

Paul McCrory
The Florey Institute of Neuroscience, Melbourne Brain Centre – Austin Campus, University of Melbourne, Parkville, Australia

David McDonagh
Emeregency Deptartment, St.Olavs Hospital, Trondheim, Norway
Faculty of Medicine, NTNU - National University of Science and Technology, Trondheim, Norway
Medical Commission, AIBA - International Boxing Association, Lausanne, Switzerland.

Lyle J. Micheli
Division of Sports Medicine, Boston Children's Hospital, Boston, MA, USA
Orthopaedic Surgery, Harvard Medical School, Boston, MA, USA

Fionna P. Moore
London Ambulance Service NHS Trust, London, UK
Emergency Medicine, Imperial Healthcare NHS Trust, London, UK

Margo Mountjoy
M.G. DeGroote School of Medicine, McMaster University, Kitchener, ON, Canada

João Grangeiro Neto
Brazilian Olympic Committee and Olympic Games Rio 2016, Brazil
Sports Medicine Department, INTO-MS, Rio de Janeiro, Brazil

Jerry Nolan
Anaesthesia and Intensive Care Medicine, Royal United Hospital, Bath, UK

Mike Nolan
Emergency Services, County of Renfrew, ON, Canada

Paul Piccinini
Dental Department, York University, Toronto, ON, Canada

Craig Roberts
South Africa Rugby Team, Cape Town, South Africa

Eduardo de Rose
Brazilian Olympic Committee, Rio de Janeiro, Brazil

Padraig B. Sheeran
Department of Paediatric Anaesthesia and Paediatric Critical Care, Our Lady's Children's Hospital Crumlin, Dublin, Ireland
Connacht Rugby, Ireland
Faculty of Sports & Exercise Medicine, Royal College of Surgeons in Ireland, Dublin, Ireland

Eunice M. Singletary
Department of Emergency Medicine, University of Virginia, Charlottesville, VA, USA

Andy Smith
Yorkshire Ambulance Services, Leeds Medical School, Leeds, UK

Torbjørn Soligard
Medical & Scientific Department, IOC, Lausanne, Switzerland

Kathrin Steffen
Oslo Sports Trauma Research Center, Department of Sports Medicine, Norwegian School of Sport Sciences, Oslo, Norway
Medical & Scientific Department, IOC, Lausanne, Switzerland

Michael Turner
British Horseracing Authority, London, United Kingdom

Alan Vernec
World Anti-Doping Agency, Montreal, Quebec, Canada

Peter Van de Vliet
International Paralympic Committee, Bonn, Germany

Lisa M. Vopat
Childrens Hospital, Harvard University, Boston, MA, USA

David Whitmore
London Ambulance Service NHS Trust, London, UK

Sally Whitmore
District Nursing, UK

Mike Wilkinson
Department of Sports Medicine, University of British Colombia, Vancouver, Canada
Sports Medicine and Human Performance, Vancouver Canucks, Vancouver, Canada
FISA Medical Commission, Canada

Kenneth Wing Cheung Wu
Accident and Emergency Department, Queen Elizabeth Hospital, Hong Kong, China

Ken Zafren
Emergency Programs, State of Alaska, Anchorage, Alaska, USA
Division of Emergency Medicine, Stanford University Medical Center, Stanford, CA, USA
Alaska Native Medical Center, Anchorage, Alaska, USA

David Zideman
Anaesthesia, Imperial College Healthcare NHS Trust, London, UK
London Ambulance Service NHS Trust, London, UK
Emergency Medical Services, London Organising Committee of the Olympic and Paralympic Games, London 2012, London, UK

Foreword

Sports-related injuries represent a significant health hazard worldwide. The aim of this book is to provide both medical students and clinicians with a substantial, evidence-based overview of the field of injuries, especially due to sport-related trauma, with clinical picture of the patients. The clinician's role in preventing the damage from sporting activities is multifaceted, and includes the appropriate evaluation of injuries when they occur, educating team physicians and trainers in the acute care of trauma, assessing the risk and mechanism of injuries, and designing and certifying appropriate protection.

We trust that this book will serve to illustrate the appropriate approaches for the evaluation and treatment of sport-related injuries and emergencies. This book should be available in every medical library and on the desk of all clinicians dealing with any trauma. The need to have rapid and accurate information immediately at hand is becoming essential to the practice of emergency medicine.

Prof. Dr. Uğur Erdener
President IOC Medical Committee
IOC Executive Committee Member
President World Archery (FITA)

May 2014

I would like to congratulate Drs. McDonagh and Zideman on the production of their latest work. Sport at all levels relies on experts to plan and execute efficient and effective services to ensure the safety of all athletes, particularly when serious injuries occur. As President of an International Sports Federation and SportAccord my primary concern is the safety and health of our athletes, thus allowing International Federations to conduct safe and entertaining sporting events around the world, in the knowledge that our athletes will be properly managed when most in need.

This manual is the first manual to address the on-field treatment of seriously injured or ill athletes. It offers a practical and methodical management approach to what can be extremely difficult and demanding situations. This manual will be an invaluable tool for medical professionals to provide the highest quality care at sporting events of all kinds.

The IJF and SportAccord are delighted to play a part in promoting excellence and best practices in the conduct of sporting events and in supporting projects that will advance the care of athletes within the International Federations.

Marius Vizer
President International Judo Federation
President SportAccord

Preface

The alternate biannual summer and winter Olympic and Paralympic Games provide regular and recurrent arenas for the world's elite athletes to perform to their utmost ability and skill. The same level of excellence should be demonstrated by venue medical staff requiring the provision of a high-class, efficient, and up-to-date athlete medical care system not only during the Games itself, but also in the pre- and post event periods.

This manual examines the medical provision both on the Field of Play and at the fieldside for all athletes participating in summer and winter Olympic and Paralympic sports. Although the manual has focused on the medical provision at an Olympic Games, the editors would recommend that its recommendations be extended to the Field of Play medical provision at all larger sporting events. The Field of Play is a high-performance arena not only for the athlete but also for the medical teams. In most sports, the venue medical team is the conduit between the active athlete, the athlete's own medical support, and the International Federations' medical experts. In addition, the Field of Play teams are under constant scrutiny from the many thousands of spectators and the ever-observant media and their audience. This is a complex and difficult situation that demands constant vigilance. The Field of Play team must immediately recognize injury and illness, then rapidly and safely retrieve and treat casualties efficiently and effectively, to the most current standards of medical care. This is no simple task and requires appropriate knowledge, experience, and skills that must be honed to the highest levels of efficiency by repeated training and practice.

Contributions to this manual have been gathered from experts in Field of Play medicine from around the world. The individual chapters present the current knowledge for the management medical emergencies and system injuries and, where appropriate, the editors have selected the primary recommended action in highlighted text. In addition, the international algorithms for life-threatening emergencies have been included as an appendix of the Manual for easy to find reference.

The editors have also supplied two more useful resources as appendices; The *Sport Specific Injury Profile* (outlining for each sport the most frequently encountered injuries, and the most relevant skills and equipment prescribed for treatment) and the *Healthcare Professional Skillbase* (as required for Field of Play responders). The full text of The Olympic Movement Medical Code has also been reproduced as an appendix for reference purposes.

Fundamental recommendations have been made as to how to medically lead teams of healthcare professionals both on the Field of Play and at the fieldside and to what equipment and drugs are needed. These recommendations have evolved from the real-time experience of the authors in both summer and winter Games.

The editors and contributors hope that this manual will be useful in establishing the base knowledge and fundamental skillset needed to ensure optimal athlete management on the Field of Play in future Olympics, Paralympics, and major sporting arenas.

David McDonagh
David Zideman

July 2014

About the Authors

Dr. David McDonagh,
MD, MB, BCh, BAO, FFSEM, RCSI, RCPI, FSSEMM, DTM

David is the Medical Director of the SportAccord medical section, MedAccord, which is based in Lausanne, Switzerland. He is the Director and consultant at the Accident and Emergency Department, University Hospital Trondheim, Norway. He is a senior lecturer at NTNU (the Norwegian University of Science and Technology), Trondheim. He was a founder member of the Norwegian Emergency Forum. He is currently the Secretary of the International Boxing Association Medical Commission and has been a member and then Chair of the International Bobsleigh and Skeleton Federation Medical Committee. He was the Association of Winter Olympic Federations representative to FIMS. He has also been the Head of the Scientific and Education Committee in the European Federation of Sports Medical Associations. He is the author of several publications and articles, including the FIMS Event Management and Emergency Care Manual. He has conducted courses in Emergency Sports Medicine in more than 15 countries and been an invited speaker at congresses around the world. David has been the team physician for the Norwegian Boxing, Nordic Combined, Bobsled and Luge team. He is the Senior Advisor to the Norwegian Rugby Union. He is the physician for the Olympic Athlete Program in central Norway. He is in his third term as Chair of the Norwegian Boxing Unions Medical Committee. He has also been a member of the Norwegian Antidoping Tribunal and the International Cricket Council (ICC) Antidoping Tribunal. David was Deputy CMO at the Lillehammer 1994 Olympic Winter Games, as well as CMO/Deputy CMO for World Ice Hockey Championships, World Nordic Skiing Championships and over one hundred other World Cup and World Championships events in various sports and countries. He has been an advisor to five Olympic Games organization committees.

Contact information: SportAccord, Maison du Sport International. Avenue de Rhodanie 54, CH – 1007, Lausanne, Switzerland email: mcdonagh@ntnu.no

Dr. David Anthony Zideman,
LVO, QHP(C), BSc, MBBS, FRCA, FRCP, FIMC, FERC

David Zideman has been a consultant anesthetist at Hammersmith Hospital, Imperial College Healthcare NHS Trust, London, since 1980 and an honorary senior lecturer in the University of London since 1981.

He was a founder member of the Resuscitation Council (United Kingdom) and was chair of the European Resuscitation Council (ERC) from 2003 to 2008. David was a founder member of the International Liaison Committee on Resuscitation (ILCOR) and cochaired the Paediatric Task Force in 2000 and 2005. In 2010, he cochaired the ILCOR Consensus on Science Meeting. In 2010, the American Heart Association named David as a "Resuscitation Great" for his International contribution to resuscitation medicine.

David chaired the British Association for Immediate Care (BASICS) from 2003 to 2007. He is an Honorary Medical Advisor to the London Ambulance Service NHS Trust and he has flown as a HEMS doctor on the London Air Ambulance. He recently held the post of Director of Clinical Operations for East Anglian Air Ambulance and now flies as a HEMS doctor with Thames Valley and Chiltern Air Ambulance. In 2012, he was awarded the esteemed Honorary Fellowship of the Royal College of Physicians and received the Gold Medal from the Royal College of Anaesthetists in recognition of his services to anesthesia and medicine.

David's services to the Royal Family, as a Queen's Honorary Physician, has been recognized by the highly prestigious award in Her Majesty's the Queen's 2009 Birthday Honours list as Lieutenant in the Royal Victorian Order (LVO).

In 2008, David was appointed as Clinical Lead – Emergency Medical Services for the 2012 London Olympic and Paralympic Games and is now the Scientific Director of the SportAccord medical section, MedAccord, which is based in Lausanne, Switzerland.

1 Emergency Care at the Olympic Games

Richard Budgett

International Olympic Committee, Lausanne, Switzerland

Introduction

The priority for medical care at any large multisport Games is to ensure the safety of all client groups. The larger the event the earlier the preparation has to start. In the case of the Olympics (the largest multisport event in the world), medical preparations start at least 5 years before the Games themselves. At an Olympic Games, the person with overall responsibility for preparation and delivery of medical services, including emergency care, is normally the Chief Medical Officer (CMO). This person is appointed early to develop a strategic plan for the treatment of all those attending the Games, in every venue, including the Olympic Villages. In addition to spectators, the client groups include athletes, their immediate support staff, International Federation (IF) staff, judges and technical officials, the Olympic Family (consisting of the IOC, senior members of the IFs, and sponsors), media, press, and workforce (contracted, volunteers, and members of the organizing committee staff).

An Olympic Games is a huge complex project of which the medical provision is a small part, requiring integration with all other functional areas from security to ceremonies to cleaning and waste management to accreditation. An Olympic Games is a mass gathering and requires both public health and disaster planning preparation. The CMO will need backup from an experienced project manager (the Medical Services Manager) at an early stage in planning.

Early Preparations

The CMO and the Medical Services Manager must review the data obtained from previous Games in order to set and plan the level of service in cooperation with the IOC and IFs. This team must ensure that relevant data and activities are recorded from the outset and provide a transfer of knowledge for future Games organizers. Details of all medical encounters, outcomes, and use of resources will facilitate better medical care planning at future Games and hopefully help prevent injury and illnesses in all client groups.

A high-level Medical Advisory Group (MAG) should be formed early, bringing both experts and important stakeholders into the project, ensuring essential support from government, national and regional health services, emergency, and hospital services. This advisory group also provides backup to the CMO and medical managers. Outline

The IOC Manual of Emergency Sports Medicine, First Edition. Edited by David McDonagh and David Zideman.

agreements or memoranda of understanding need to be formed with health authorities, relevant hospitals, and the ambulance service. The decision to use private or national public health services needs to be made, and also how these services are to be paid for (national funding, direct payment, personal medical insurance). It may be that a mixed provision is required for different client groups. The obligation to provide repatriation in case of severe injury or illness should not be forgotten. The Olympic Games organizing committee (OCOG) should plan to establish emergency services and thus minimize the strain on the local population healthcare services, which must also function at Games time.

Expert leaders in specific clinical areas should be recruited early. These may be experts in emergency care, dentistry, pharmacy, physiotherapy, imaging, sport medicine, and polyclinic (management) services. Equipment procurement should also be started at this stage. Thousands of medical service items need to be sourced from sponsors or from commercial suppliers, either on a sale or return or loan basis. Plans must also be put in place for the distribution and resale of purchased equipment after the Games.

Every sport should be reviewed individually as each has unique rules, risks, equipment, and culture. The emergency cover should be carefully planned to reflect these risks under IF rules and depending on the needs of the sport and athletes. The venues are the gold fish bowls in which medical teams operate most visibly so, despite the fact that in most sports, full Field of Play (FoP) evacuation by the medical team is infrequent, FoP extraction needs to be carefully practiced and prepared for.

The personnel and equipment put in place to provide Venue care must also be ready to be used in the event of a major disaster. Venue planning must include integration with a larger emergency response, and appropriate plans to utilize these significant resources should be put in place. The relevant authorities should be encouraged to hold Games-specific exercises in the lead up to the event incorporating all emergency services. Preparation for integration is important.

Final Preparations

After the initial recruitment and strategic planning, further detailed planning is needed including focus on patient flow, for instance, extraction from the FoP, using emergency transportation to either the Athlete Medical Centre, Games Polyclinic, or one of the local designated hospitals.

A full-time Workforce Manager will be needed for at least 2 years before the Games to manage the recruitment of medical volunteers. This work should also start 2 years prior to the Games and preferably be completed a year before the Games. This is a specialist workforce and individuals need to be appointed in a timely manner to allow them to participate in test events and be adequately trained. The Workforce Manager has a huge and complex task in organizing shifts and venue rosters. It is important to set realistic expectations for volunteers both in the lead up to recruitment and through training. Medical volunteers need time to plan their leave from their places of employment.

During the Games, the clinical load may not be great but the presence of competent and well-trained staff is essential to provide the safety net and the immediate expert response if needed. Many volunteers will not end up at the FoP or even attend a sports event. The Venue Medical Managers (VMMs), with the assistance of clinical experts, must organize and ensure the role-specific training of the volunteer workforce. The VMMs should be identified as early as possible and should be brought on full time several weeks before the Games actually start to enable them to prepare their venues properly. The task of a VMM is extremely important, covering all medical care in their venue, the integration of this care with all the other services at a venue, and coordination of any serious incidents with the medical headquarters. Venue preparations should include the locating of the Athlete Medical room, the positioning of all FoP teams and ambulances, and the identification of exit routes from both the FoP and the Venue.

For most sports, medical workforce training can normally be done in 2 days – one well before the Games and the other on a day just before the event starts. For more complicated rescue FoPs (alpine, bobsled, BMX), more time must be allocated. This should be complemented with daily onsite rehearsal and specific team building to ensure that the individuals work together to form a rapid and efficient extraction from the FoP. Each FoP team should have an appointed leader, preferably a doctor with leadership skills and with knowledge and experience of the sport/s they are covering. In most sports, at least one ambulance is needed at every Venue as per the IF regulations. In some winter sports, an air ambulance (helicopter) may be considered, if conditions allow. Paramedic staff with these ambulances should be incorporated into the Venue team. This provides for better and seamless care in the case of any accident.

The Memoranda of Understanding with ambulance services, health providers, and hospitals need to be converted into detailed contracts, so that provision is guaranteed. The Venue emergency services and the residential area clinic (Polyclinic in an Olympic Village) should protect the local hospitals from being overwhelmed or overstretched at Games time. In reality, hospitals are very rarely significantly affected by a major event (unless in the event of a mass injury incident). The agreement with the hospitals needs to include a liaison officer who can ensure that any accredited patients are guided efficiently through the admission system obtaining the medical advice, services, and treatment they need as efficiently as possible.

Owing to the large number of ambulances needed at the various venues, it is extremely important to ensure that the Games Ambulance Service does not in any way weaken the existing municipal ambulance service. This usually requires the provision of extra ambulances, either purchased or relocated from other parts of the country, with qualified staff, in a timely manner. It is also wise to delay the retirement of old ambulances and cancel the service training for the time of the Games so that those trainers and trainees can relieve the load. Other strategies may be to pool ambulances for use by Venues that are in close proximity and where the likelihood of severe injury is low. This pooling must be with the agreement of the IFs for the sports concerned. The need for backfilling (replacing an ambulance that has left the Venue) can be reduced using nonemergency vehicles where appropriate and agreeing a "fast-return" policy with the ambulance service for vehicles that have had to leave the venue.

Access to the FoP is restricted in most sports. Sports-specific rules may often determine when the team doctor, the team physiotherapist, the IF doctor, and the organizing committee staff are allowed on the FoP. Coordination of this response is very important, particularly as the incident may be viewed by both stadium spectators and millions of television viewers around the world. The FoP Team Leader and the VMM must work closely with both the IF doctors, the technical delegate, and the national team doctors to avoid any possibility of confusion. In reality, very little treatment takes place on or around the FoP. The majority of athlete care takes place in the Athlete Medical room (or by the team doctor and physiotherapist in their team spaces). The Athlete Medical room is normally manned by at least a doctor and physiotherapist and supported by the appropriate nursing staff. In order to facilitate team medical staff, it is recommended that space be allotted in the Athlete Medical room so that they can treat their own athletes. Nonathletes are normally treated in separate medical centers that are usually manned by a doctor and a nurse, providing emergency care and care for minor injuries and illnesses.

The impressive spread of experience and expertise in a venue (paramedics, sport doctors, Emergency doctors, physiotherapists, national team doctors, IF doctors, and VMMs) is a great resource but needs to be carefully coordinated with an agreed command structure. The VMM should be in charge, but should work in close cooperation with the IF-appointed medical officer and the national team doctors. On the FoP, authority is usually delegated to the local FoP medical Team Leader. This individual should ensure that the team members understand their role and rehearse extensively, thus gaining an appreciation of the challenges and variety of medical care in a specific sport's venue. Medical experts are not always intimately familiar with the equipment used and building the FoP medical team into an integrated unit is a high priority. The morale and work of the medical teams can be helped by rotating roles within the team, thus increasing learning opportunities and encouraging continuous professional development.

The VMM is responsible for coordinating transfers from the Venue to either the polyclinic or an appropriate designated hospital. The designated hospitals must be able to offer general care, relevant diagnostic facilities as well as specialist surgical units for major trauma, vascular trauma, neurotrauma, and orthopedics. Specific cardiac and stroke units needs to be identified. Agreements with hospitals, providing all these services, need to be in place in the year leading up to the major Games. There are normally a series of test events, which is a great opportunity to test systems, people, equipment, and partners. However, the time required to plan and deliver the medical care at these test events should not be underestimated. Extra resources are needed and must be negotiated. It is normally sensible to prioritize just a few test events, such as those where the organizing committee puts in place complete medical care. Other test events can be used as observation opportunities.

Team and IF Doctors

Visiting national team doctors also need to prepare well before an Olympic Games. This should involve medication checks, periodic health examinations of team members, checking that therapeutic use exemptions are valid and updated as well as preparing for traveling abroad. Visiting team doctors (who may not have a license to practice medicine in the host country) normally receive temporary registration to allow them to practice in a limited way. This should include the right to prescribe from a limited formulary and also to request laboratory sampling and imaging. The right to practice is normally restricted to the team doctor's own team. The visiting doctors should be encouraged to bring their own supplies of medication and this importation of drugs needs to be facilitated locally. There may be special rules and restrictions on the use and importation of medical equipment and needle policies may be in place, which must be communicated to all those who might be affected. It is inevitable that the level of expertise and experience of team doctors will vary and this may pose challenges for an organizing committee to ensure that the proper and specific level of medical competency is available in what can be an unpredictable and challenging environment. Thus, the organizing committee team and IF doctors must make every effort to cooperate to define the appropriate level of response and authority. In particular, it is necessary to be absolutely clear who has responsibility at every stage on the FoP, in the Athlete Medical room, during emergency transportation, and at the treating hospital.

Summary

The complexities in a multisport event are multiplied many times by the different venues and sports, so medical planning must start early.

Work with existing structures and institutions in an attempt to keep newly developed plans as simple as possible. Try and leave a legacy of enhanced services and skills in those existing structures. At an Olympic Games, the medical providers are usually already experts and professionals and their expertise must be respected. However, input from the IOC, IFs, and team physicians might fine-tune the sports-specific and venue-specific response in both the training phase and during the actual event.

During the years of preparation for the Games, plans and even venues may be changed, so all arrangements or decisions on medical provision must be constantly checked and updated.

Patient flows need to be carefully coordinated and will vary depending on the type of accreditation, the venue, and the ultimate patient destination. In addition to attempting to provide optimal and efficient medical care, the organizing committee medical services should avoid overloading the existing local healthcare services. Besides the training of sports-specific skills, test events should be used to ensure that medical staff become acquainted with the Venue. Management must use these events to identify and define problem areas that need to be resolved to ensure optimal staff performance when the Games finally commence.

Team and particularly IF doctors are often some of the most experienced and discerning of all Games time clients. Concerted interaction with these colleagues will likely lead to other client groups also being satisfied with the medical provision.

The protection of the health of all client groups is the central role of medical provision, and the care of athletes must take the highest priority.

2 Injury and Illness During the 2008 Summer and the 2010 Winter Olympic Games

Kathrin Steffen,[1,2] Torbjørn Soligard[2] and Lars Engebretsen[1,2]

[1]*Oslo Sports Trauma Research Center, Department of Sports Medicine, Norwegian School of Sport Sciences, Oslo, Norway*
[2]*Medical & Scientific Department, IOC, Lausanne, Switzerland*

During the XXIX Summer and XXI Winter Games, comprehensive injury and illness recording through the medical staff of the participating National Olympic Committees and the sports medicine clinics at the different Olympic venues revealed that between 7% and 11% of all athletes incurred an injury or suffered from at least one occurrence of illness during the Games. In the two Olympics, the overall injury rate was similar at around 10% of registered athletes sustaining at least one injury (Table 2.1) with the Vancouver injury incidence being slightly higher than reported from the Beijing Games (111.8 vs 96.1 injuries per 1000 athletes). The incidence of injuries and illnesses varied substantially between sports. Continuous injury and illness surveillance during major sporting events will build a foundation for providing evidence for the development of injury prevention programs.

An athlete was defined as injured or ill if he/she received medical attention regardless of the consequences with respect to absence from competition or training. Following the IOC injury surveillance system, an injury was reported if it fulfilled the following criteria:

1. Musculoskeletal complaint or concussion
2. Newly incurred (preexisting, not fully rehabilitated should not be reported) or reinjuries (if the athlete has returned to full participation after the previous injury)
3. Occurred in competition or training
4. Occurred during the XXIX Summer Olympic Games 2008 (August 9–24, 2008) or the XXI Winter Olympic Games 2010 (February 12–28, 2010)

An illness was defined as any physical complaint (not related to injury), which newly occurred during the Games and that received medical attention regardless of the consequences with respect to absence from competition or training.

The IOC Manual of Emergency Sports Medicine, First Edition. Edited by David McDonagh and David Zideman.
2015 International Olympic Committee. Published 2015 by John Wiley & Sons, Ltd.

	Beijing 2008	Vancouver 2010
Participating athletes	10,977	2567
Injuries (per 1000 athletes)	1055 (96.1)	287 (111.8)
Most common diagnosis	Ankle sprains (7%), thigh strains (7%)	Concussions (7%)
Most affected locations	Trunk (13%), thigh (13%), head/neck (12%), knee (12%)	Head/neck (16%), knee (14%), thigh (7%)
Most common mechanisms	Noncontact (20%) Overuse (22%) Contact with another athlete (33%)	Contact with another athlete (15%) Contact with a stagnant object (22%) Noncontact (23%)
Expected time-loss injuries	50%	23%[a]
Competition – training injuries	73% – 27%	46% – 54%
High-risk sports (injuries per 100 athletes)	Football, taekwondo, field hockey, handball, weightlifting	Snowboard cross, freestyle aerials and cross, bobsleigh, ice hockey
Low-risk sports (injuries per 100 athletes)	Canoeing/kayaking, diving, rowing, sailing, synchronized swimming, fencing	Nordic skiing disciplines, curling, speed skating

Table 2.1 Comparison of injury risk between the 2008 Beijing and 2010 Vancouver Olympic Games

Source: Data from Junge *et al.* ((2009)) and Engebretsen *et al.* ((2010)).

[a] This figure may underestimate the number of time-loss injuries as the response rate to this information was low and many of the injuries were of severe outcome, without estimated time-loss registered (more details in the Vancouver paper).[3]

Vancouver Winter Games 2010

More than 2500 athletes participated in the XXI Winter Olympic Games held in Vancouver in 2010. Throughout the 17 days of the Vancouver Olympics, the 33 participating National Olympic Committees (NOCs) (with more than 10 athletes) returned a total of 461 out of a maximum of 561 forms (82%).

For both genders, the face, head, and cervical spine (female 20%, male 21%) and knee (female 16%, male 11%) were the most prominent injury locations. In alpine, freestyle, and snowboarding, 22 out of 102 injuries (22%) affected the head/cervical spine and one-quarter of all injuries affected the knee (24%). Twenty concussions were reported, affecting 7% of the registered athletes. A death occurred in luge.

A major concern was that every fifth injury affected the head, neck, and cervical spine, which were mainly diagnosed as abrasion, skin lesion, contusion, fracture, or concussion. The figures for concussions were twice as high as reported from the Summer Olympic Games.

The injury risk was highest for bobsleigh, ice hockey, short track, alpine, and for freestyle and snowboard cross (15–35% of registered athletes were affected in each sort).

Ice hockey, bobsleigh, and the skiing and snowboard disciplines emerge as sports with high injury risk. The low injury risk for athletes competing in the Nordic Skiing disciplines compared to alpine, freestyle, and snowboard athletes is not surprising as they are not exposed to high speed on icy surfaces with minimal protection.

The three most common reported injury mechanisms were a noncontact trauma (23%), contact with a stationary object (22%), and contact with another athlete (15%) (Table 2.1). In addition to this, many winter sports also involve high speed.

In freestyle and snowboard cross, for example, athletes race while tackling challenges such as turns, jumps, and waves. Combined with the speed component, competition in heats may promote an additional risk-taking attitude for the athletes. Injuries were evenly distributed between official training (54%) and competition (46%). Of the 287 injuries, 65 (23%) were expected to result in a time-loss situation for the athlete (Table 2.2).

Olympic sport	Registered athletes	Number of injuries	Percentage of all injuries	Percentage of participating athletes
Alpine skiing	308	46	3.5	14.9
Archery	128	9	0.7	7.0
Athletics	2132	241	18.3	11.3
Badminton	172	8	0.6	4.7
Baseball	189	21	1.6	11.1
Basketball	287	38	2.9	13.2
Beach volleyball	96	8	0.6	8.3
Biathlon	202	3	0.2	1.5
Bobsleigh	159	32	2.4	20.0
Boxing	281	42	3.2	14.9
Canoeing/kayaking	324	4	0.3	1.2
Crosscountry skiing	292	9	0.7	3.1
Curling	100	4	0.3	4.0
Cycling	518	30	2.2	5.8
Diving	145	3	0.3	2.1
Equestrian	193	10	0.8	5.2
Fencing	206	5	0.4	2.4
Field hockey	382	78	5.9	20.4
Figure skating	146	21	1.6	14.3
Freestyle aerials	47	9	0.7	19.1
Freestyle cross	68	13	1.0	19.0
Freestyle moguls	57	1	0	1.8
Gymnastics	318	24	1.8	7.5
Handball	334	58	4.4	17.4
Ice hockey	444	82	6.2	18.5
Judo	385	53	4.0	11.2
Luge	108	2	0.1	1.9
Modern pentathlon	71	4	0.3	5.6
Nordic combined	52	1	0	1.9
Rowing	548	10	0.8	1.8
Sailing	400	3	0.2	0.8
Shooting	386	3	0.2	7.8
Short track	109	5	0.4	9.0
Skeleton	47	3	0.3	6.4
Ski jumping	67	3	0.3	4.5
Snowboard cross	57	20	1.5	35.0
Snowboard half pipe	69	9	0.7	13.0

Olympic sport	Registered athletes	Number of injuries	Percentage of all injuries	Percentage of participating athletes
Snowboard slalom	59	4	0.3	6.8
Soccer	496	156	11.8	31.5
Softball	119	16	1.2	13.4
Speed skating	176	5	0.4	2.8
Swimming	1046	36	2.7	3.4
Synchronized swimming	104	2	0.1	1.9
Table tennis	172	9	0.7	5.2
Taekwondo	126	34	2.6	27.0
Tennis	168	10	0.8	5.9
Triathlon	109	10	0.8	9.2
Volleyball	287	23	1.7	8.0
Water polo	259	25	1.9	9.7
Weightlifting	255	43	3.3	16.9
Wrestling	341	32	2.4	9.4
Total	13,544[a]	1320[b]	100.0	10.8

Table 2.2 Injury distribution of injuries from selected sports registered during the 2008 Summer Olympics (n = 1055 injuries) and 2010 Winter Olympics (n = 287 injuries)

[a] Sport is missing for 22 injuries.
[b] Sport is missing for 20 athletes.

Among 173 out of 2567 athletes (7%) in Vancouver, a total of 185 illnesses were reported, resulting in an incidence of 72.1 illnesses per 1000 athletes. Illnesses were reported from a variety of sports and they mostly affected the respiratory system (63%). The most frequent diagnosis was upper respiratory tract infection (pharyngitis, sinusitis, and tonsillitis) (54%).

The incidence of illnesses from Vancouver is comparable to data from athletics (7%), aquatics (7%)[12], and football (12%). Almost two-thirds of the illnesses affected the respiratory system, of which 62% are caused by infections, 64% which has a higher rate than reported in swimming (respiratory system 50%, infection 49%). Airway inflammation has been shown to often affect elite swimmers, ice hockey players, and cross-country skiers. It has been documented that good sanitation, early recognition, and isolation of ill players can successfully reduce infections and illness in a team setting.

Beijing Summer Olympic Games

In Beijing, the distribution of injuries was as follows:

1. About half of the diagnoses (54%) affected the lower extremity
2. 20% were related to the upper extremity
3. 13% to the trunk
4. 12% to the head/neck

The thigh (13%) and knee (12%) were most commonly injured, followed by the lower leg, ankle, and head injuries (9%).

In Beijing, one-third of the 1055 injuries were caused by contact with another athlete. Noncontact trauma (20%) and overuse, either gradual (9%) or sudden onset

(13%), were also frequent causes of injury. A total of 73% of the injuries occurred in competition. About half of the injuries were expected to prevent the athletes from further training or competition. Physicians estimated that one-third of the injuries would result in an absence from sport for up to 1 week.

Of those with expected time-loss, 11 injuries (17%) had an estimated absence from training or competition of more than 1 week (Table 2.1).

The incidence of injuries varied substantially among the different sports, where the risk of sustaining an injury was highest for football, taekwondo, field hockey, handball, weightlifting, and boxing (all ≥15% of the athletes). The lowest injury risk was observed for water sports such as sailing, canoeing/kayaking, rowing, synchronized swimming, diving, and swimming.

Bibliography

Alonso, J.M., Junge, A., Renström, P. *et al.* (2009) Sports injuries surveillance during the 2007 IAAF World Athletics Championships. *Clinical Journal of Sport Medicine*, **19**, 26–32.

Alonso, J.M., Tscholl, P.M., Engebretsen, L. *et al.* (2010) Occurrence of injuries and illnesses during the 2009 IAAF World Athletics Championships. *British Journal of Sports Medicine*, 44, 1100–1105.

Arnason, A., Andersen, T.E., Holme, I. *et al.* (2008) Prevention of hamstring strains in elite soccer: an intervention study. *Scandinavian Journal of Medicine and Science in Sports*, **18**, 40–48.

Bahr, R. (2009) No injuries, but plenty of pain? On the methodology for recording overuse symptoms in sports. *British Journal of Sports Medicine*, **43**, 966–972.

Bahr, R. & Reeser, J.C. (2003) Injuries among world-class professional beach volleyball players. The Federation Internationale de Volleyball beach volleyball injury study. *American Journal of Sports Medicine*, **31** (**1**), 119–125.

Bakken, A., Bere, T., Bahr, R. *et al.* (2011) Mechanisms of injuries in World Cup Snowboard Cross: a systematic video analysis of 19 cases. *British Journal of Sports Medicine*, **45**, 1315–1322.

Bere, T., Flørenes, T.W., Krosshaug, T. *et al.* (2011a) Mechanisms of anterior cruciate ligament injury in World Cup Alpine Skiing: a systematic video analysis of 20 cases. *American Journal of Sports Medicine*, **39**, 1421–1429.

Bere, T., Flørenes, T.W., Krosshaug, T. *et al.* (2011b) Events leading to anterior cruciate ligament injury in World Cup Alpine Skiing: a systematic video analysis of 20 cases. *British Journal of Sports Medicine*, **45**, 1294–1302.

Chumanov, E.S., Schache, A.G., Heiderscheit, B.C. *et al.* (2012) Hamstrings are most susceptible to injury during the late swing phase of sprinting. *British Journal of Sports Medicine*, **46**, 90.

Clarsen, B., Krosshaug, T. & Bahr, R. (2010) Overuse injuries in professional road cyclists. *American Journal of Sports Medicine*, **38**, 2494–2501.

Dvorak, J., Junge, A., Derman, W. *et al.* (2011) Injuries and illnesses of football players during the 2010 FIFA World Cup. *British Journal of Sports Medicine*, **45**, 626–630.

Engebretsen, L., Steffen, K., Alonso, J.M. *et al.* (2010) Sports injuries and illnesses during the Winter Olympic Games 2010. *British Journal of Sports Medicine*, **44**, 772–780.

Finch, C. (2006) A new framework for research leading to sports injury prevention. *Journal of Science and Medicine in Sport*, **9**, 3–9.

Fitch, K.D. (2012) An overview of asthma and airway hyper-responsiveness in Olympic athletes. *British Journal of Sports Medicine*, **46**, 413–416.

Flørenes, T.W., Bere, T., Nordsletten, L. *et al.* (2009) Injuries among male and female World Cup alpine skiers. *British Journal of Sports Medicine*, **43**, 973–978.

Flørenes, T.W., Heir, S., Nordsletten, L. *et al.* (2010a) Injuries among World Cup freestyle skiers. *British Journal of Sports Medicine*, **44**, 803–808.

Flørenes, T.W., Nordsletten, L., Heir, S. *et al.* (2010b) Injuries among World Cup ski and snowboard athletes. *Scandinavian Journal of Medicine and Science in Sports*, **22**, 58–66.

Fuller, C.W., Laborde, F., Leather, R.J. *et al.* (2008) International Rugby Board Rugby World Cup 2007 injury surveillance study. *British Journal of Sports Medicine*, **42**, 452–459.

Greene, J.J. & Bernhardt, D. (1997) Medical coverage analysis for Wisconsin's Olympics: the Badger State Games. *Wisconsin Medical Journal*, **96**, 41–44.

Hanstad, D.V., Rønsen, O., Andersen, S.S. *et al.* (2011) Fit for the fight? Illnesses in the Norwegian team in the Vancouver Olympic Games. *British Journal of Sports Medicine*, **45**, 571–575.

Junge, A., Dvorak, J. & Graf-Baumann, T. (2004a) Football injuries during the World Cup 2002. *American Journal of Sports Medicine*, 32 (1 Suppl), 23S–27S.

Junge, A., Dvorak, J., Graf-Baumann, T. *et al.* (2004b) Football Injuries During FIFA Tournaments and the Olympic Games, 1998–2001: development and implementation of an injury-reporting system. *American Journal of Sports Medicine*, 32 (1 Suppl), 80S–89S.
Junge, A. & Dvorak, J. (2007) Injuries in female football players in top-level international tournaments. *British Journal of Sports Medicine*, 41 (Suppl 1), i3–i7.
Junge, A. & Dvorak, J. (2010) Injury risk of playing football in Futsal World Cups. *British Journal of Sports Medicine*, **44**, 1089–1092.
Junge, A., Engebretsen, L., Alonso, J.M. *et al.* (2008) Injury surveillance in multi-sport events: the International Olympic Committee approach. *British Journal of Sports Medicine*, **42**, 413–421.
Junge, A., Engebretsen, L., Mountjoy, M.L. *et al.* (2009) Sports injuries during the Summer Olympic Games 2008. *American Journal of Sports Medicine*, **37**, 2165–2172.
Junge, A., Langevoort, G., Pipe, A. *et al.* (2006) Injuries in team sport tournaments during the 2004 Olympic Games. *American Journal of Sports Medicine*, **34**, 565–576.
Koga, H., Nakamae, A., Shima, Y. *et al.* (2010) Mechanisms for noncontact anterior cruciate ligament injuries: knee joint kinematics in 10 injury situations from female team handball and basketball. *American Journal of Sports Medicine*, **38**, 2218–2225.
Krosshaug, T., Nakamae, A., Boden, B. *et al.* (2007) Estimating 3D joint kinematics from video sequences of running and cutting maneuvers-assessing the accuracy of simple visual inspection. *Gait & Posture*, **26**, 378–385.
Langevoort, G., Myklebust, G., Dvorak, J. *et al.* (2007) Handball injuries during major international tournaments. *Scandinavian Journal of Medicine and Science in Sports*, **17**, 400–407.
Ljungqvist, A., Jenoure, P., Engebretsen, L. *et al.* (2009) The International Olympic Committee (IOC) Consensus Statement on periodic health evaluation of elite athletes March 2009. *British Journal of Sports Medicine*, **43**, 631–643.
Martin, R.K., Yesalis, C.E., Foster, D. *et al.* (1987) Sports injuries at the 1985 Junior Olympics: an epidemiologic analysis. *American Journal of Sports Medicine*, **15**, 603–608.
McClay, I.S., Robinson, J.R., Andriacchi, T.P. *et al.* (1994) A profile of ground reaction forces in professional basketball. *Journal of Applied Biomechanics*, 10, 222–236.
van Mechelen, W., Hlobil, H. & Kemper, H.C. (1992) Incidence, severity, aetiology and prevention of sports injuries. A review of concepts. *Sports Medicine*, 14, 82–99.
Mountjoy, M., Junge, A., Alonso, J.M. *et al.* (2010) Sports injuries and illnesses in the 2009 FINA World Championships (Aquatics). *British Journal of Sports Medicine*, 44, 522–527.
Olsen, O.E., Myklebust, G., Engebretsen, L. *et al.* (2004) Injury mechanisms for anterior cruciate ligament injuries in team handball: a systematic video analysis. *American Journal of Sports Medicine*, 32, 1002–1012.
Steffen, K. & Engebretsen, L. (2010) More data needed on injury risk among young elite athletes. *British Journal of Sports Medicine*, 44, 485–489.
Steffen, K., Soligard, T. & Engebretsen, L. (2011) The IOC's endeavour to protect the health of the athlete continues. *British Journal of Sports Medicine*, 45, 551–552.
Torjussen, J. & Bahr, R. (2006) Injuries among elite snowboarders (FIS Snowboard World Cup). *British Journal of Sports Medicine*, 40 (3), 230–234.
Yoon, Y.S., Chai, M. & Shin, D.W. (2004) Football injuries at Asian tournaments. *American Journal of Sports Medicine*, 32 (1 Suppl), 36S–42S.

3 The Medical Team Response

David McDonagh[1,2,3] and David Zideman[4,5,6]

[1]Emeregency Deptartment, St.Olavs Hospital, Trondheim, Norway
[2]Faculty of Medicine, NTNU - National University of Science and Technology, Trondheim, Norway
[3]Medical Commission, AIBA - International Boxing Association, Lausanne, Switzerland.
[4]Anaesthesia, Imperial College Healthcare NHS Trust, London, UK
[5]London Ambulance Service NHS Trust, London, UK
[6]Emergency Medical Services, London Organising Committee of the Olympic and Paralympic Games, London 2012, London

Serious injuries and illnesses are fortunately rare in sport and, in particular, at an Olympic Games (see Chapter 2). At the Olympic Games in London in 2012, there was a total of over 38,000 medical encounters for all client groups in all venues. The number of athlete encounters on the Field of Play (FoP) and in the venue athlete medical room totaled 2261 of which 389 (17%) were direct FoP encounters. A total of 15 (4%) athletes were transferred to hospital directly from the FoP, 11 by ambulance including 8 as a result of trauma. A total of 13 (3%) athletes were transferred to the Olympic Polyclinic from the FoP, 7 by ambulance. The most serious injuries were the following:

1. One fracture/dislocation (weightlifting)
2. Three closed fractures (two sailing, one football)
3. One open fracture (mountain bike)
4. One facial injury (hockey)
5. One head injury (sailing)
6. One suspected cervical spinal injury (BMX)

These figures reflect the relatively small number of FoP medical encounters and serious injuries at an Olympic Games. However, it is essential that the Olympic Games organizing committee (OCOG) medical planning includes the provision for a full FoP medical response at all venues.

All healthcare professionals (HCPs) on the FoP team would be expected to intervene and treat sick athletes, especially those with acute life-threatening injuries and illnesses (see Appendix 2). This is the event doctor's (ED) primary task and the ED and his team members must be prepared for all such eventualities by ensuring that they have sufficient skills and competencies in emergency medical diagnosis and treatment. These skills must be up-to-date and in accordance with relevant local and international guidelines and recommendations.

Different doctors have different professional skills and their reactions are often defined by their training. An anesthetist or emergency doctor with little experience of covering

The IOC Manual of Emergency Sports Medicine, First Edition. Edited by David McDonagh and David Zideman.

a sports event will often be more concerned with treating the symptom or finding (shortness of breath, chest pain, etc.) before transferring the patient to hospital for further investigation, whereas a team doctor may be more focused on an immediate diagnosis to allow a rapid return to play. The ED's role is somewhere in between the need to detect and treat serious injury or illness and to, if possible, return the athlete to the FoP with minimal delay. They need to prevent unnecessary hospital referrals in fit athletes but be aware of the long-term consequences of allowing a sick or injured athlete to continue to compete.

At a major sporting event such as an Olympic Games, there is usually a handpicked medical team of HCPs that encompass a wide variety of skills, available to assist athletes. This is a luxury that is not often present at minor weekend events where the ED may be the sole HCP present.

At most Olympic Games, the Chief Medical Officer (CMO) and his team, in conjunction with the International Federation (IF) medical officer, evaluate the need for medical staff at a particular venue several years before the actual event starts. It is important to staff a medical FoP response team with the correct number of HCPs in order to be able to treat many different athletes over a period of time or even several injured athletes at the same time. Similarly, one must ensure that the FoP team has the necessary medical competencies to treat the types of injuries that are prevalent in each sporting discipline See appendix 3.

At the London 2012 Olympics, sports that were defined as contact sports were staffed with teams comprising an anesthetist, a sports medical doctor, and two other HCPs (doctor, nurse, paramedic, or physiotherapist) with emergency training, selected to provide the best FoP service for that particular sport. A team of four HCPs was defined as minimal number required to be able to transfer an injured athlete from the FoP. The authors of this chapter support this team structure concept with the team, as a group, providing the relevant FoP medical skills. It is the authors' opinion that it is not essential to have an anesthetist present at most noncontact sports other than some equestrian events, open water swimming and gymnastics. An anesthetist may be substituted with a sports doctor, emergency nurse, or paramedic who should possess the requisite advanced airway management, trauma, and resuscitation skills. Whatever the choice of medical staff, the team must be trained and practiced to function as a unit with the equipment supplied and on the actual sport FoP.

Never underestimate the level of difficulty that the medical response team will encounter when evacuating an injured athlete – it is obviously much more difficult to immobilize and evacuate a crashed downhill skier, an equestrian athlete, or a bobsled pilot than, for example, a fallen tennis player. Each individual sport presents unique challenges to the FoP team and it is essential that these are formally assessed and evaluated before the event, and that the team members are aware of proposed solutions.

Direct FoP medical supervision must be maintained throughout the whole competition time, even when an athlete is being managed fieldside or being transferred to the athlete medical room. This will inevitably lead to temporarily downsizing the number of the available team members at the FoP while other team members are transferring and managing a sick or injured athlete. Medical teams should plan for such eventualities before the event but the final decision about allocation of resources must rest with the Team Leader. Temporary downsizing can be resolved by calling additional staff from other FoP teams, if there are several such teams at an event, or by temporarily moving medical staff from the athlete medical room to the FoP. If the medical staff is being overwhelmed by the number of casualties, the Team Leader should contact the venue competition organizer and discuss alternative arrangements – such as delaying training. Delaying a competition is a dramatic scenario for the Games organizers, so the Team Leader should contact the IF doctor and the CMO to discuss alternative options. If the venue medical team do not have the capacity to monitor several patients at the same time (e.g., after a multiple athlete BMX crash), then athletes will have to be transferred to the Olympic Village Polyclinic or a hospital for further monitoring. Finally, it is essential that the FoP medical team be supported by a fully equipped and appropriately skilled ambulance staff, not only for movements on or around the FoP but also for the transfer of the injured athlete to hospital.

ABC on the Field of Play

Most medical specialties are liberally endowed with mnemonics and emergency medicine is no exception. While wishing to keep the use of such mnemonics to a minimum, there is one which cannot be avoided – *ABC* (airway, breathing, circulation), which has now matured to become *S-ABCDE*: safety – airway, breathing, circulation, disability, environment (or exposure).

The S-ABCDE mnemonic has been designed to help HCPs structure their examination by prioritizing the most important body functions. If the professional adheres strictly to this progressive management regime, then the likelihood of overlooking important clinical "Red Flags" can be minimized even in these most stressful of situations. There are several emergency triage procedure variations in use around the world though the clinical evaluation parameters are almost universally the same – it is not this manual's intention to define which system is best, merely to emphasize the importance of strict adherence to the chosen model.

Preparation

Preparation and safety aspects should be primarily addressed in the period leading up to the commencement of the event and they should be continuously reevaluated during the event. Adequate preparation for minor sporting events should be initiated well before the event starts, ideally several weeks prior to an event. For larger events, such as the Olympic Games, preparations begin many years in advance (see Chapter 1).

There are many areas to prepare, the event doctor should do the following:

1. Know the dates of the event
2. Know the schedule of times for each day of the event
3. Confirm the FoP medical teams' role with the event organizer and define responsibilities (a contract may need to be signed)
4. Agree upon a time schedule for the medical staffs' arrival and departure
5. Agree upon payment/insurance issues
6. Know if the FoP doctor is to be alone or have assistance (HCPs, paramedics, and first aid providers)
7. Know what rules, if any, pertain to the organization of the sports event (are ambulances or specific FoP skills obligatory according to national or IF rules) (See Appendix 2)
8. Be familiar with relevant local, national, and international guidelines
9. Ensure that the roles of all HCPs are clearly defined
10. Know what kind of injuries to expect in the sport and ensure that he/she has appropriate equipment and sufficient medical staff with suitable skills to treat these injuries
11. Decide where medical staff and equipment are to be located during the event
12. Identify the Team Leader
13. Ensure that adequate access/accreditation to the appropriate zones/FoP is in place
14. Ensure that the FoP team members have adequate communications systems available to them (radios, phones, etc.) and that these are linked to the venue command structure

15. Be familiar with arena telecommunications systems and access telephone lists
16. Emphasize the importance of patient confidentiality in all communications regarding the FoP treatment of athletes
17. Be familiar with access/exit routes from the FoP and the medical facilities within the venue
18. Know which facilities are available at local hospitals and clinics
19. Have a predetermined agreement with the following:
    a. The EMS transport professional
    b. The local hospitals covering the event
20. Agree a plan in the case of a major incident

On the day, there are several things that must be in place:

1. Ensure all the team members know and understand their role
2. Confirm and support the appointed Team Leader
3. Ensure that all the team members have correct and appropriate FoP and emergency room accreditation and passes
4. Ensure that all the team members have correct and appropriate uniform, clothing, and accessories (warm and cold drinks, food, or snacks should be available – worst case, bring your own)
5. Ensure all the team members know and understand how to use their equipment
6. Check FoP/fieldside equipment is complete and fully functional
7. Check medical room equipment is complete and fully functional
8. Ensure that communication systems are fully operational (charge up mobile phones and radios)
9. Ensure that the FoP team communications is operational and fully functional in all FoP areas
10. Ensure that the team members understand and practice the procedures for FoP extrication, removal to the medical room, and direct transfer to hospital
11. Ensure that the team members undertake FoP scenario training and resolve any problems that arise
12. Emphasize the importance of patient dignity and confidentiality at all times during patient treatment
13. Check that appropriate emergency transport vehicles are in place and that staff do the following:
    a. Have appropriate accreditation and passes to access the FoP
    b. Understand their role
    c. Are appropriately equipped
    d. Have a fully functional communication system with the FoP team and the athlete medical room
    e. Know which hospitals are "on standby" for the event and the route to the hospital

Safety

The FoP Team Leader's primary task is to ensure the team's safety (S) if for no other reason than to ensure that there is medical care available to be able to assist the athlete.

Safety must be an established procedure using a predetermined protocol. It is important to remember that at major events, such as the Olympic Games, access to the FoP may be limited by accreditation and only open to the OCOG FoP medical team and not the injured athlete's team medical staff.

If the FoP team has observed an incident and it is clear that there has been a severe injury (e.g., head or neck injury, or if the patient is unconscious), then the Team Leader or the team's representative should enter the FoP as soon possible to attend to the injured athlete once it is safe to do so.

In normal circumstances, a referee will usually signal, using preagreed signals, that medical assistance is required and the FoP team is called to attend. In some sports, these signals have been described in the relevant sports manual.

However, if, for some reason, an incident occurs without the official having noticed it, the Team Leader may wish to consider entering the FoP uninvited if it is obvious that a serious incident has occurred and especially if the athlete's life may be in danger. A FoP HCP should always be reserved about entering the FoP uninvited, as there are different rules and regulations in different sports, and entering the FoP may compromise the competing athletes depending on the sport regulations.

Besides the issue of personal safety, there may be athlete disqualification issues that one must be aware of. In several sports, if a HCP enters the FoP, then the competition/bout/session is automatically abandoned (e.g. boxing) and this may result in the automatic disqualification of the competing athletes. In rugby, it is now accepted practice for medical staff to enter the FoP to treat injured athletes during active play and without necessarily receiving the referee's approval.

Different sports, different practices but beware, the rules are frequently changed and many are open to local interpretation. These are issues that should be discussed with the event organizer and the IF technical delegate in the preevent phase so that there is a formal understanding of what is expected and required from the FoP team. Therefore, it is essential to define with the event officials how and when the medical team can enter the FoP to assist an athlete with a life-threatening condition. The authors would advise each individual IF to adopt rule changes that facilitate the immediate treatment of athletes by medical staff in emergency situations.

Fieldside Observation

The FoP medical response begins with observation from the fieldside. Observing an injury may facilitate in making a diagnosis. This is relatively simple when the competition takes place on a pitch, court, or athletics track, but it is much more difficult where the track or course is spread out over a large area (skiing, some equestrian events, rowing, long-distance running events, etc). In these situations, it may be possible to follow the event on a television.

Some Sports Federations require a "clean FoP" with minimal personnel on the fieldside. The location of the FoP medical team and its line of sight must be agreed prior to the event. Should event officials decide not to allow fieldside medical observation, then they must also accept responsibility for any delay in medical response and treatment (usually this is an unacceptable risk when this delay in response and its consequences have been pointed out).

If the injury or incident has not been personally observed, quickly ask witnesses, referees, officials, or judges to describe the incident. This may easily happen when the incident occurs away from the focus of play. Much information can be gained from understanding the mechanism of injury:

1. Has the athlete been struck in the jaw or face by an elbow or shoulder?
2. Did the athlete hit his/her head before or after falling?
3. Did the athlete land on an uneven or dangerous object/surface?

The mechanism of injury may give valuable clues to both the anatomical location and the severity of injury present. Such information may guide the FoP team as to what is an appropriate medical response, what personnel and which equipment needs to be taken onto the FoP and what can probably be kept on the fieldside. If the immediate impression is that there is a critical injury or illness, immediately call other medical staff onto the FoP. If the FoP Team Leader has a radio, it may be appropriate to activate ambulance assistance and request the necessary appropriate medical equipment to be brought forward even before entering the FoP. Have mobile phones on loudspeaker mode (volume should have been set to maximum) and ensure that communication radios are fitted with earpieces.

If the medical team is required to enter the FoP, it is usually because the athlete is incapacitated or is in pain. When an athlete falls due to overbalancing or slipping on a surface, then it is not uncommon to find a joint sprain due to an exaggerated movement and/or a contact injury where the athlete has hit the ground or other object. If the athlete falls due to a tackle or collides with another athlete or object, then there is likely to be an injury at the anatomical site of collision and/or at the part of the body where the athlete hits the ground. There will often be a rotational injury to the ankle or knee, shoulder, elbow or wrist and, most importantly, some form of deceleration injury to the brain and neck.

If an athlete has collapsed without slipping or without having had any significant contact with another athlete or object, then there is a possibility of a sinister underlying cardiac or cerebral pathology. Healthy athletes do not normally faint or lose consciousness unless in extreme heat conditions. In these circumstances it is appropriate to bring an automated external defibrillator (AED), oxygen, and other resuscitation equipment when entering the FoP.

Avoid taking unnecessary staff or equipment onto the FoP as this may interfere with the continuity of the competition and may slow the extrication process to the detriment of the patient and the event. Pre-agreed protocols as to who enters the FoP, what they carry, and what tasks each team member has on reaching the athlete should be agreed prior to the event and practiced by the team-of-the-day with the equipment available on the event FoP in the preevent scenario drills.

Observations on approaching the Athlete

Important information may be gained while approaching the athlete. The HCP should look for details that may be readily apparent:

1. Is the athlete moving?
2. Are there any signs of life?
3. Is the athlete impaled upon an object?
4. Has the athlete a grossly deformed limb or a major bleed

The Medical Team Response

This process will vary from sport to sport but we will in this manual propose a standardized procedure, which can be adapted to the specific laws and requirements of individual sports. The response will also depend on the number, competency, and skillbase of the HCPs available on the FoP at the event (see Appendix 3).

The initial response should include the following steps:

1. *The team enters the FoP and conducts a primary survey* to rapidly identify, treat, and stabilize life-threatening conditions. This should be limited to the most essential forms of treatment:
   a. Airway management
   b. Cardiopulmonary resuscitation (CPR)

3. Supporting respiration
4. Pneumothorax decompression
5. Hemorrhage control
6. Spinal movement restriction

Possible treatment modalities include the following:

1. Head tilt/chin lift
2. Head tilt jaw thrust
3. Foreign body airway removal
4. Chest compressions
5. Assisted respiration and ventilation
6. Needle chest decompression
7. Digital compression of bleeding vessels
8. Intravenous infusion
9. Spinal or limb immobilization

When the patient's airway, breathing, and circulation are stable, secure and immobilize the patient before transporting to the fieldside, the athlete medical room, or ambulance for further assessment, treatment, or transfer. In the case of serious injury, rapid direct transfer to an appropriate definitive medical facility must be initiated immediately. For example, in alpine skiing, the athlete may be heli-lifted from the mountain directly to a trauma hospital. If the patient can stand and walk unassisted, it is often wise to remove the athlete from the FoP to make a fieldside evaluation (including SCAT Card (Sport Concussion Assessment Tool) evaluation) before allowing the athlete to return to play.

For a minor injury, depending on the sport, an evaluation on the FoP may be adequate and the player can either continue to compete or briefly be removed to the fieldside for further evaluation. Some IFs designate that a medical evaluation be conducted at the fieldside.

2. *Transfer the athlete from the FoP to the fieldside*: This extrication process will vary for individual sports and the FoP. It must be rapid, efficient, and safe for both medical team and athlete and will require specialist teams and equipment in complex FoP environments such as aquatics (see Chapter 21). In a serious injury, the athlete may need to be immobilized and transferred on a backboard, vacuum mattress, or in a basket but on most occasions, the athlete will self-extricate and walk assisted or unassisted, to the fieldside.
3. *Fieldside evaluation*: If the athlete is seriously injured but has been stabilized and immobilized, transfer directly to the ambulance and do not delay proceedings by taking the athlete to the athlete medical room. Immediately evacuate the injured casualty to an appropriate medical facility for ongoing care, ensuring that the facility has been prewarned and that adequate documentation accompanies the patient.

   If the athlete does not need immediate evacuation by ambulance or helicopter, then the athlete must be reevaluated at the fieldside. Remember that some sports have rules about time allowed for medical time-outs – injury assessment and treatment must be carried out within a specific time or the athlete will be disqualified (e.g. Taekwondo). These medical time-outs may have individual incident time restraints and may have a cumulative value that must not be exceeded or will result in a penalty for the competitor.

   The fieldside evaluation includes the following:

   a. A repeat of the primary survey
   b. Establishing basic monitoring and recording of vital signs
   c. Conduct a secondary survey (this should take no longer than 2–3 mins)
   d. Conduct a focused examination in the less seriously injured athletes

4. *Management plan*: The FoP medical Team Leader will make a decision regarding the athlete's need for hospitalization or further observation. Return to play decisions must also be made, but the HCP should never be pressurized into a rapid decision or to shorten treatment.

The FoP Primary Survey

The purpose of the primary survey is to rapidly evaluate the patient's condition and to detect if a patient is or is not critically ill or injured.

If the athlete is conscious, a focused history may help in guiding the ED to the source of the problem. If the athlete is unresponsive, it may be appropriate to immediately call for additional clinical assistance. This should be a predetermined standard operating procedure.

While kneeling on the ground by the patient's side, initiate the primary survey by immediately evaluating the *A*irway, continuing on to evaluate *B*reathing, the *C*irculation and review the neurological status (*D*isability). In a critical situation 'E' stands for *E*xposure – a reminder to the HCP to expose the patient in order to examine for otherwise unseen serious wounds, fracture deformities, or even petechia. In some countries, 'E' stands for Environmental Evaluation, a concept that has been introduced to remind the HCP to do the following:

1. Expose the chest, abdomen, and extremities
2. Exclude hypothermia as a cause of cardiac arrest
3. To consider hypoglycemia as a cause of coma or convulsions

In the confines of an Olympic Games, the vast majority of patients this exposure evaluation on can be conducted on reaching the fieldside.

> The primary survey is a diagnostic and treatment process that should only be interrupted by emergency interventions when a life-threatening condition is discovered. It should be treated effectively before continuing to the next stage.

In certain circumstances, a patient may have several life-threatening conditions simultaneously. All life-threatening conditions must be diagnosed and treated in a specific order as part of the primary survey so as not to overlook any one particular life-threatening situation.

Synopsis of the FoP primary survey:

1. Apply pressure to any significant bleeding. If this bleeding is potentially catastrophic, apply manual pressure to the bleeding site immediately on arriving at the patient's side – in exceptional circumstances, consider the need for tourniquet application (see Chapter 6).
2. Is the patient responsive? Ask if the patient is OK or in pain and conduct an alert, verbal stimuli response, pain response, or unresponsive (AVPU) assessment. Take a rapid focused history if possible.
3. Does the patient appear to be breathing normally through the mouth? Is there noisy breathing? Is the patient choking? The presence of abnormal or noisy breathing or difficulty talking may indicate the presence of a foreign body in the mouth or larynx, injury to the larynx or chest, or acute respiratory or cardiac disease. The doctor should immediately remove any mouthguard and if necessary perform a visual mouth sweep. If there is vomitus or fluid in the mouth use a suction device. If necessary, follow the choking algorithm (see Chapter 4).
4. Immediately and carefully, place the head in neutral alignment, support the head and neck, and perform a head tilt/chin lift (or jaw thrust with a potential spinal injury) if there is any suspicion of an impaired airway or breathing. Insert an oropharyngeal airway to maintain a patent airway in the unresponsive patient.
5. Continue on to evaluate the patient's breathing (B). If during the breathing (B) evaluation a tension pneumothorax is discovered, then this should be decompressed.
6. If the patient is unconscious and there is absent or pathological breathing that has not been corrected in A or B above, initiate CPR (see Chapter 4).

7. If the athlete is conscious or if the athlete is unconscious but breathing adequately, assess circulation (C) by checking the pulse, perfusion, and blood pressure (BP).
8. If circulation is found to be adequate in the conscious patient, continue on to evaluate (D) disability. On the FoP, this may include a simple gross evaluation of sensation and motor function. If the patient is unconscious, this is not performed and further neurological evaluation is usually of limited value.
9. If disability is found to be normal in the conscious and stable patient, a decision about exposing the patient (E) on the FoP must be made. Undressing the athlete on the FoP should only be done if absolutely necessary; this can usually be delayed until the athlete has been transferred to the fieldside. The ED must consider how undressing may compromise patient privacy and confidentiality and how this will add value to the clinical assessment.

Airway evaluation (A) If the airway is obstructed or damaged, the patient may not be receiving adequate oxygen and may suffer an altered level of consciousness, organ hypoxia, or even die. Ensuring the patency of the airway is the first step in ensuring that a patient survives a life-threatening injury or illness.

If the patient is conscious and appears to be choking – follow the Choking algorithm (see Chapter 4).

If the patient is unconscious, not breathing or not breathing adequately remove any mouthguard, perform a head tilt/chin lift or jaw thrust maneuver and observe if normal breathing returns. Should the mouth be full of vomitus, perform oral suctioning with a portable suctioning device and a large bore rigid (Yankauer) suction catheter.

> *Noisy breathing may be due to the presence of a foreign body in the airway but may also be due to the tongue obstructing the pharynx in an unconscious patient.*

If the athlete is unconscious and not breathing, commence chest compressions immediately.

Noisy breathing may also be caused by trauma to the pharynx, larynx, chest, or abdomen or acute asthma, pulmonary embolism, an acute collection of fluid in the lungs, or an acute myocardial condition. High-pitched noisy breathing sounds (stridor) in a conscious patient could indicate an injury to the larynx or trachea, particularly if these sounds are present in both inspiration and expiration. Low-pitched inspiratory snoring-like noises (stertor) are more typical of a "knockout" and usually disappear once the patient regains consciousness. However, stertor may also be present with more serious brain injuries. In an unconscious nontraumatized patient, the presence of deep snoring sounds may indicate the presence of cerebral hypoxia usually secondary to severe acute cardiac, cerebrovascular or pulmonary pathology, or even severe hypoglycemia.

Primary Survey

A – Airway evaluation

General inspection: Is the airway clear and the patient breathing normally? Does a simple airway maneuver establish a clear airway?
Inspection of the airway: Inspect the mouth for foreign bodies, bleeding, vomitus, and swelling. Remove foreign bodies and suction the upper airway if necessary.
Look for wounds, bleeding, bruising, swelling, impaled foreign bodies, and deformities/displacement of the throat. Is there stertor or stridor?
Palpation of the airway: Quickly but gently palpate the throat for swellings, deformity, and subcutaneous emphysema.

Auscultation of the airway: Rarely necessary but may be performed if abnormal breathing is found.
Treatment intervention:

1. Try a simple chin lift, head lift, or jaw thrust
2. Consider inserting an oropharyngeal airway in the unconscious or semiconscious patient, moving the inverted tip along the hard palate and then rotating 180° to place the tube in the hypopharynx behind the tongue
3. Check for the effectiveness of the airway intervention by looking for symmetrical chest movements, listening, and feeling over the mouth for air movement
4. If the simple airway maneuver is not effective, reposition the airway again or move to an advanced maneuver (see Chapter 4)

Throat injuries Tracheal deformity or deviation may indicate an upper airway structure fracture with dislocation. Tracheal deviation can also be found with a tension pneumothorax. If upper airway injury is suspected, then the degree of airway patency must be assessed. Air flow through the trachea is dependent on the radius of the airway to the power of four (r^4) – so small decreases in tube diameter will have significant effects on airway resistance and air entry. Reduced airway patency may lead to reduced oxygenation of the blood which may be characterized by central or peripheral cyanosis, dyspnea, reduced oxygen percentage saturation values on pulse oximetry (SpO_2) or more sinisterly, an altered level of consciousness.

Following the insertion of an oropharyngeal airway consider supporting oxygenation with supplemental oxygen administration if the SpO_2 reading is below 94%. A patient who continues to deteriorate may require advanced airway management (see Chapter 4). However, this is usually not necessary unless there is gross deformity of the upper airway. Performing endotracheal intubation, cricothyrotomy, or tracheostomy in throat injuries is a complex procedure that requires training and experience. If the airway is damaged, then only those HCPs with the required skills should perform advanced airway management.

Breathing evaluation (B) Once it has been established that the airway is patent, evaluate the patient's breathing – absent or present, normal, or abnormal? On the FoP, the patient's breathing can best be examined when the patient is in the supine position. If the athlete is not supine, make a rapid inspection of the patient's back before turning the patient supine (log roll – see Chapter 4) carefully supporting the patient's head and neck.

With the airway open, check for air movement by observing symmetrical chest movements, listening for breath sounds over the patient's mouth, and feeling for expired air on the cheek. If breath sounds are absent in the unconscious patient, then initiate CPR immediately (see Chapter 4). If respirations are absent but the patient is conscious, this is not a cardiac arrest and may be, for example, traumatic apnea from a severe head injury. Continue to maintain the airway and support the breathing with ventilation using bag, valve, and mask and supplemental oxygen if necessary while a fuller examination establishes the cause of the respiratory arrest.

In the organized sporting environment if an athlete is found with absent respiration, the most likely and potentially treatable causes are the following:

1. An obstructed airway
2. Unconscious (tongue)
3. Foreign body

4. Throat injury
5. Cardiac arrest
6. Secondary to commotio cordis or head injury

If trauma has been involved, then the doctor must also consider the following:

1. Reflex apnea from a sudden severe abdominal blow
2. Cardiac tamponade or tension pneumothorax (after severe chest trauma)
3. Hypovolemia (external bleeding from a wound, internal bleeding from a femur/pelvic fracture, or from a splenic rupture)

At a sports event, it is unlikely that the patient has ceased breathing due to hypothermia, hypokalemia, hyperkalemia, or toxin exposure but these conditions must be remembered and excluded, particularly if resuscitation is failing.

If the patient is breathing abnormally, ascertain the cause and correct if possible. When the patient is deteriorating and the breathing is becoming even more abnormal, consider supporting with carefully controlled assisted ventilation.

For the clinician, abnormal breathing parameters can be defined in the following way:

1. Resting respiratory rate of lower than 8 rpm or higher than 24 rpm (adult values).
2. Depth of respiration is either deep or superficial. Shallow respiration or hypoventilation (hypopnea) is often due to pain, chest wall damage, pneumothorax, hemothorax, or head injury, but may also occur if the patient is anxious or hysterical. In these conditions, the patient usually compensates for superficial breathing by breathing more rapidly, that is, there is also an increase in the respiratory rate and the patient hyperventilates. Similarly with asthma, not an uncommon medical condition in athletes, athletes compensate for decreased bronchial diameter with superficial breathing at a rapid respiratory rate.

   Deep respiration or hyperventilation (hyperpnea) may be due to pain, stress, asthma, or head injury. Deep respirations may be normally seen in athletes after a great expenditure of energy, for example, after a marathon race or during demanding events at high altitude. Deep respirations may also be seen as a response to metabolic acidosis, often associated with diabetic ketoacidosis, where rapid superficial breathing turns into rapid deep respiration (Kussmaul breathing) as the acidosis becomes more severe.
3. Asymmetric chest wall movement.

Primary Survey

B – Breathing evaluation

General inspection: Check for breathing by looking for chest movement, placing your cheek over the patient's mouth, and listening and feeling for air movement. Inspect the lips and face for cyanosis (cyanosis may be misleading especially in dark skinned patients or with poor or noncolor coded ambient light). Is the patient short of breath?

Inspection of the chest:

1. Expose the chest
2. Are there chest wounds or penetrating objects? If the patient has an open chest wound, place an ear over the wound and listen for air entry or escape

3. Rapidly evaluate chest movement for symmetry, deformity (flail chest, rib/sternal fractures), paradoxical, or reduced chest movement
4. Is respiration painful?
5. Evaluate the depth of respiration – (normal, shallow, and deep)
6. Count the respiratory rate

If working as a team, it may be appropriate for another HCP to attach a pulse oximeter at this time.

Palpation for:

1. Symmetry
2. Deformity (rib fractures and swelling)
3. Tenderness
4. Subcutaneous emphysema

Percussion for:

1. Hyperresonance (the tympanitic sounds of a pneumothorax)
2. Hyporesonance (the dull sounds of a hemothorax)

Auscultation of the chest: Auscultate over the lung apices and the upper, lower, and lateral chest walls for the symmetric distribution of breath sounds or the presence of pathological sounds. While auscultating the chest, count the respiratory rate. Decide if breath sounds are normal or abnormal

Treatment intervention:

1. Maintain oxygen saturation by administering high-flow (15 L/min) 100% oxygen via a nonrebreathing or trauma mask (masks with reservoirs ensure a higher concentration of supplemental oxygen)
2. Titrate the inspired O_2 to a saturation between 94% and 98%
3. If the patient is dyspneic and no pulse oximeter is available, administer 100% oxygen
4. Perform a needle or surgical thoracostomy if a tension/major pneumothorax is found (see Chapter 16)

Respiratory rate (RR): The number of chest movements is indicative of inspiration and expiration per minute. Measured in respirations per minute (rpm) values can be the following:

1. Normal (16–24 rpm)
2. Fast (tachypnea >24 rpm)
3. Slow (bradypnea <8 rpm)
4. Absent (apnea)

There is still no universal agreement on what normal RR values are. Rates under 8 or over 30 are considered to be indicative of serious pathology.

The RR increases with exercise but also when an athlete is in pain, distressed, or anxious.

If breathing is normal, continue the primary survey and evaluate (C) – circulation.

Circulation evaluation (C) The primary goal of this evaluation is to ensure that there is an effective and adequate circulation. Evidence has been published that shows that HCPs are poor at determining the presence of a pulse using simple palpation. Therefore, to avoid delay and false positive conclusions, if the patient is unconscious and not breathing commence chest compressions immediately.

If the patient is breathing, whatever the level of consciousness, carefully palpate a radial or carotid pulse to evaluate pulse frequency, quality, and regularity.

The pulse rate, quality, and regularity offer important information about the cardiac function and rhythm. While holding the hand to measure the radial pulse, it is often appropriate to measure the capillary refill time (CRT).

Primary Survey

C – Circulation

Bleeding: The presence of deformity of the extremities or torso should alert one to the possibility of substantial bleeding.

If open bleeding is found, the wound site should be compressed manually (beware compressing arterial bleeds from the head as there may be an underlying cranial fracture).

If the HCP is alone, place a circular compression bandage over the wound site and continue the primary survey.

Severe arterial limb bleeding may require the application of a tourniquet to stop exsanguination.

Inspection: Is the skin in the following forms:

1. Pale?
2. Clammy?
3. Moist?
4. Dry?

Are there large swellings?

Palpation: Palpate the radial or carotid pulse to evaluate the following:

1. Pulse frequency
2. Pulse quality
3. Pulse regularity

If there is an obvious gross extremity deformity, palpate a pulse distal to a suspected fracture to exclude the possibility of fracture induced distal ischemia.

Measure the CRT.

Auscultation: Auscultate the heart for heart sounds. Muffled or distant heart sounds may indicate cardiac tamponade.

Blood pressure: Apply an appropriate size of BP cuff to the upper or lower limb and measure the BP.

Treatment:

1. Establish IV access
2. Administer boluses of IV fluid to maintain the systolic BP to a minimum of 90 mmHg
3. Check for rhythm abnormalities (see Chapter 5)

If a team of HCPs is present, there may be sufficient time to insert an IV cannula and measure BP. If not, these procedures may be delayed if the transport time to the fieldside is short (e.g., football, courts, etc.). If the transport time is long (e.g., cross country skiing, marathon, etc.), consider inserting an IV line and measuring BP before transport.

Pulse: In a healthy exercising athlete, there would be an increased heart rate due to increased sympathetic stimulation and an increased systolic BP up to 220 mmHg (diastolic should remain relatively unchanged). The heart rate may increase more quickly if the athlete has a fever, is in pain, or is distressed. Normal pulse rate (pulse) for adults is between 45 and 95 beats per minute.

Pulse oximetry: Pulse oximeters offer quick, noninvasive, and relatively reliable readings of oxygen saturation (oxygen diffusion from the alveoli to the pulmonary capillaries and the subsequent binding to hemoglobin in the red blood cells). The percentage of oxygen bound to hemoglobin (SpO_2) can be determined using pulse oximetry. However, SpO_2 values within the normal range do not necessarily imply normal ventilation. In severe anemia (which may be associated with chronic renal failure), there will be low levels of hemoglobin but the hemoglobin may be 100% saturated, even though the body tissues are in a state of relative hypoxia.

In the otherwise healthy athlete population, low SpO_2 values usually indicate insufficient oxygen transfer to the pulmonary blood stream from the lungs (a compromised airway, pneumothorax, or hemothorax). Lung illness (high-altitude sickness, pneumonia, pulmonary edema, pulmonary embolism, chronic obstructive pulmonary disease (COPD), asthma, etc.) will also affect SpO_2 values but be aware of the potential for normal readings despite blood loss.

Finger pulse oximetry: Attach a pulse oximeter to a fingertip and measure SpO_2.

False readings: Most pulse oximeters are attached to fingertips and readings can be affected if the fingers are very cold, if the nail is varnished, if the probe is poorly attached, or if substances other than oxygen (carbon monoxide) are bound to hemoglobin.

Normal values: Normal SpO_2 values without supplemental oxygen are 94% or higher. Levels between 90% and 94% are potentially pathological and levels of 89% or lower would imply serious pathology. Falls in SpO_2 values are indicative of a failure of breathing or circulation. It is now recommended to titrate the inspired oxygen levels to achieve a SpO_2 of between 94% and 98% – high oxygen levels can cause cell damage and inhibit recovery.

The capillary refill time (CRT): Peripheral perfusion can be evaluated by measuring the CRT.

1. Lift the patient's finger higher than the level of the heart
2. Compress the athlete's fingertip pad with your own thumb and index finger until the skin becomes white (blanching)
3. Release the fingertip pressure
4. Note the time needed for normal skin color to return
5. Less than 2 seconds for the return of skin color indicates adequate perfusion

Poor peripheral perfusion may be an indication of hemorrhage-induced hypovolemia. The usefulness of CRT values in the prehospital setting is debatable as many factors, such as sex, age, gender, and ambient temperature may influence values. Some studies go so far as to call it an invalidated and unhelpful test. Larger studies on severely wounded military patients have shown that an abnormal CRT (i.e., >2 seconds) may be an indicator for the need for potential life-saving intervention. However, it cannot be regarded as an isolated predicator of life-threatening injury or illness.

If no serious findings major are discovered, continue to the primary survey of Disability (D).

Disability evaluation (D) As a detailed neurological examination can take 30 min or more to perform, the ED must have some form of abbreviated examination system that quickly but accurately reflects the patient's neurological status. Therefore, the neurological examination in the primary survey should take no longer than 1 min. No abbreviated examination will substitute a detailed neurological examination but the necessities of the primary survey demand a rapid evaluation before moving on to (E) exposure or environmental conditions. The time factor is particularly important if only one doctor is present and especially if there are several casualties that need evaluation. Similarly, if there are concerns about a patient's ABC, a shortened neurological evaluation can be performed before returning to do a more detailed examination in the secondary survey.

Many doctors use the AVPU evaluation system, others choose the more internationally accepted, but slightly more time-consuming Glasgow Coma Score. The Team Leader should perform the AVPU evaluation.

AVPU System

When time is of the essence, the AVPU system allows for a rapid but limited evaluation of the patient's responsiveness – this is a mnemonic for the following:

1. *A*lert: The patient is alert, conscious with open eyes, and is cooperative
2. *V*oice: Responds to a voice command, but is not otherwise alert

3. *P*ain: The patient only responds to a painful stimulus
4. *U*nresponsive: The patient is unresponsive to both verbal and painful stimuli

The advantage of this evaluation is that it takes no more than a few seconds to conduct. The AVPU scale is used by many as a "light" version of the GCS, which can be conducted during the secondary survey.

It is important to repeat the neurological evaluation at regular intervals and record results in order to detect and record any deterioration in responsiveness.

Glasgow Coma Score (GCS)

The GCS may be used in the primary survey but is more commonly conducted during the secondary survey. This useful system is used to assess the level of consciousness for both trauma and nontrauma patients after a head injury or cerebrovascular episode. The score evaluates eye movement, verbal response, and motor response, giving each an individual score. The maximum total score is 15 (totally awake and conscious) with a minimum score of 3 (totally unresponsive). Although a single GCS score will provide useful clinical information, it is important to repeat the assessment regularly as scores may change rapidly if a patient's condition deteriorates (see Chapter 10).

If no serious findings are discovered, continue to the Exposure (E) aspect of the primary survey.

Exposure (E) "E" is used to denote exposure, a reminder to the examiner to expose the patient in order to examine for otherwise unseen serious wounds, fracture deformities, or even petechia.

In some countries, "E" is used to denote an **environmental evaluation** concept to remind the examiner to do the following:

1. Expose the casualty
2. Exclude hypothermia as a cause of cardiac arrest
3. To consider hypoglycemia as the cause of coma or convulsions

This is dependent on local practice and having an appropriate number of HCPs in the team. In some systems, these investigations are part of the secondary survey.

If the trauma patient is in a critical condition, then undress the patient to see if there are fractures, wounds, deformities, or hemorrhages that are potentially life threatening and correct these if possible.

Once the "E" evaluation has been completed, initiate patient immobilization and transfer from the FoP.

Always consider patient privacy – If the event has spectators in close proximity or is being televised, the ED must balance the need for collecting further important clinical information with the athlete's need for privacy and possible cultural issues in certain countries. If the patient is unconscious and there are no clinical findings to explain the loss of consciousness, then it may be appropriate to expose the patient on the FoP to detect treatable life-threatening conditions. If this decision is made, then the ED should take all possible precautions to maintain the athlete's dignity using privacy screens, the careful use of blankets, or even outward facing FoP officials until the examination and treatment has been completed.

Transferring the Athlete from the FOP to the Fieldside

Perform any necessary life-saving treatment on the FoP. If the patient is stable, then secure and immobilize the patient before transporting to the fieldside, athlete medical room, or ambulance for further assessment or treatment. If a spinal injury is suspected, then extra attention must be given to spinal immobilization (see Chapter 19).

In serious injuries, rapid transfer to an appropriate treatment facility must be instigated. If the patient is unconscious, ask the coach, trainer, teammates, or bystanders if they have any relevant information before leaving the FoP.

If the patient can stand and walk unassisted, it is often wise to remove the athlete from the FoP to make a fieldside evaluation (including SCAT card evaluation – see Chapter 11, Figure 11.1) before allowing the athlete to return to play. Wherever possible, remove to the fieldside or another sheltered area before conducting detailed examinations or more complex treatments.

Do not, under any circumstances, be pressurized by officials into moving a seriously injured patient if you believe that movement would compromise life or limb; however, it may be necessary on some FoPs to make a rapid extrication to a safe area as the FoP arena is inherently dangerous to the athlete and the medical team.

If an athlete is unable to walk from the FoP, then assistance should be offered or the athlete should be carried from the FoP. Athletes will usually decide themselves if they are incapable of walking from the FoP unassisted, but should be encouraged to lie down and await stretchering if there is the potential for serious injury or lower extremity fracture. Consider carrying all athletes with head, chest, or pelvic injuries from the FoP.

Carrying a casualty from the FoP may seem simple but it does need training and repeated practice if it is to be carried out without injury to the athlete or the carrying team. Ensure that the equipment to be used is adequate for the size and weight of the athlete to be evacuated and that the team carrying the athlete is physically capable of lifting and carrying the casualty. The FoP medical Team Leader must coordinate and supervise the evacuation. Plan the evacuation route to be as direct as possible and to include stops to allow the carrying team rests or changes of position as necessary. Have a good understanding within the team that any team member can call for a stop at any time if they are unable to continue.

Fieldside Assessment

If the athlete is seriously injured but has been stabilized and immobilized, transfer the injured athlete directly to the ambulance and do not delay further by bringing the athlete to the athlete medical room before secondary evacuation.

It is important not to make prolonged examinations or undertake complex treatments on the FoP – in most cases, these are very exposed environments in a public arena and do not provide the patient due privacy or respect. Wherever possible remove to the fieldside or another sheltered area before conducting detailed examinations or more complex treatments.

If the athlete does not need immediate evacuation from the venue by ambulance or helicopter, then the athlete should be reevaluated at the fieldside or in the athlete medical room.

This evaluation includes the following:

1. Repeat the primary survey
2. Establish basic monitoring and record vital signs
3. Conduct a secondary survey (this should take no longer than 2–3 min)
4. Having confirmed that there is no life-threatening injury, take a focused history and conduct a focused examination

Prepare a management plan and initiate local treatment if possible.

Monitoring

It is important to monitor vital signs in order to detect deterioration or improvement. It is normal practice to monitor the following:

1. *Respiratory rate*: <8 or >30 rpm are considered to be indicative of serious pathology
2. *O_2 saturation (SpO_2)*: Maintain between 94% and 98% with supplemental oxygen
3. *Pulse*: Rate and volume – normal pulse rates for adults is between 45 and 95 beats per minute
4. *BP*: Endeavor to maintain a minimum systolic pressure of 90 mmHg
5. AVPU or GCS assessment
6. Pupil size, equality, and response – (see the subsequent text)
7. Blood glucose – (see the subsequent text)

While waiting for ambulance transportation, turn the patient into the recovery position (lateral recumbent position) in order to minimize the risk of aspiration should the patient vomit. It is particularly important to ensure that the neck, spine, pelvis, and lower extremities are adequately immobilized before turning the patient.

Pupils – Pathological Findings

Neither the AVPU nor the Glasgow Coma Scale includes pupil examination in their evaluation systems. A dilated or constricted pupil or a pupil that does not respond to light may be the first sign of an impending cerebral catastrophe and may be detected before major deterioration in the GCS occurs.

Examining the pupils is an essential part of every neurological evaluation. In the normal healthy patient, both pupils have a similar diameter and react equally to light. Reportedly, some 20% of normal individuals have unequal pupils (essential anisocoria), though both eyes will react to the light reflex. If a patient has fixed pupils, be they dilated or constricted, then suspect serious pathology. Classically, fixed constricted pupils are seen with opioid intoxication. However, this kind of drug abuse is not commonly seen in competing athletes. Both fixed constricted pupils and fixed dilated pupils can be found in a severe head injury. In a trauma patient, the finding of one or two dilated pupils should cause one to suspect a head injury with an intracranial hemorrhage. If one pupil reacts slower than the other, this may also indicate an intracranial hemorrhage.

Blood Sugar

Glucose levels can be easily measured in the prehospital environment with a sample obtained from a simple fingertip prick. A portable blood sugar measuring apparatus should be readily available at a sports event, as detection of severely low or high sugar levels allows the doctor to rapidly correct potentially serious conditions. Though severe hypo or hyperglycemic episodes are not common, they should not be unexpected occurrences at endurance events, in particular. Though most hypoglycemic episodes are mild with recognizable symptoms, the doctor can occasionally be fooled by hypoglycemia findings masquerading as the following:

1. Myocardial infarction
2. Pulmonary embolism
3. Cerebrovascular episode
4. Head injury
5. Intoxication or seizures

Blood sugar measurements should be taken when one of these conditions is suspected (see Chapter 26). Severe hypoglycemia occurs when the athletes are unable to independently treat themselves and may occur if levels are at 2.5 mmol/L or lower (45 mg/DL). Mild hypoglycemic symptoms can be detected at levels under 3.9 mmol/L (70 mg/DL).

Blood Pressure

Raised BP may also be associated with head injury and raised intracranial pressure. Low BP may be found immediately after a syncopal episode but low or falling BP may also indicate a severe injury such as the following:

1. Lung parenchymal damage
2. Splenic bleeding
3. Severe head injury
4. Spinal cord injury

During exercise or competition, an athlete will usually have an elevated BP, so the finding of low pressure should cause concern, particularly if there is a raised pulse simultaneously.

After trauma, the BP may fall due to the loss of significant amounts blood; however, the body compensates by increasing the heart rate (reflex tachycardia) and pumping more blood into the arterial system. A similar reaction occurs if the patient is dehydrated. Thus, the presence of low BP and increased pulse is significant. The BP is seldom measured before the patient is in an ambulance or in the athlete medical room, but can be measured on the FoP or fieldside if necessary. Normal BP in adults is as follows:

1. Normal systolic BP is between 90 and 140 mmHg
2. Normal diastolic BP is between 60 and 90 mmHg

Secondary Survey (Head-to-Toe Examination)

A secondary survey should be conducted to identify other serious (but not immediately life-threatening) injuries. The secondary survey should take no more than 2–3 min. The patient may deteriorate if too much time is spent examining other noninjured body parts. If deterioration is noticed, then the HCP should return immediately to the primary survey to restabilize the patient and only return to the secondary survey when the patient is stable.

1. Look for and palpate for pain *or* tenderness *or* bruising *or* deformity/distension, starting with the head and face, then the neck and throat, followed by the chest, abdomen, and pelvis
2. Measure the patient's BP
3. If the AVPU system has been used in the primary survey, then the GCS can now be estimated as a part of the secondary survey
4. Examine the pupils for light reflexes and rapidly assess vision in the responsive patient (double vision may be present with facial or cranial fractures)
5. If diabetic ketoacidosis or hypoglycemia is suspected, then take a blood sugar reading
6. Examine the extremities and then finally the patient's back if this has not already been done

Once the secondary survey has been completed, repeat the primary survey once more to reassess and reconfirm the patient's condition.

Focused History and Examination

If the patient is not seriously ill or injured, and having completed the primary and secondary surveys, take an appropriate and focused history. Ask about the current incident and other recent illnesses and injuries. Ask about previous head injuries and relevant illnesses, for example, asthma, diabetes, epilepsy, and so on. It may now be appropriate to make a focused examination with the goal of making a differential diagnosis in athletes with lesser injuries. Complete the SCAT3 form if appropriate (see Chapter 11).

Management Plan

Having monitored the patient continuously and completed the secondary survey and focused examination, a medical management plan should be devised which will include one of the following:

1. *Further fieldside observation*: Observe the athlete for a period of time at the fieldside.
2. *Transfer to the athlete medical room* (ambulance or other secluded area) for further evaluation or treatment (e.g. suturing) that is not appropriate at the fieldside. There are many reasons for moving away from the fieldside – patient privacy, availability of equipment, ability to conduct a proper examination (concussion evaluation and fundoscopy) and hygiene. So, if treatment can wait until the patient is in the athlete medical room or ambulance, wait – if not, treat immediately.
3. *Transfer the athlete to a hospital or specialized unit for further investigation, treatment, or observation.* Remember that athletes may be continuing on to other parts of the world and proper follow-up may be difficult for them to arrange.
4. *Make a return to play decision.* If, after a fieldside evaluation, the ED decides it is safe to allow the athlete to return to play and this is allowed under IF rules, then the athlete may reenter the FoP having informed the event officials as sport regulations require. Continued fieldside observation of the athlete on the FoP is mandatory in such situations and any signs of deterioration should signal withdrawal of the athlete from that competition. If the ED decides that return to play is not recommended, then a note of this must be made on the medical record, the relevant officials and team medics should be informed and all necessary documentation completed (including IF documents).
5. *Discharge the patient after fieldside treatment.* Ensure that copies of all documentation (medical notes, health, and safety reports) and athlete medical cards are given to the athlete and that the athlete receives and understands recommendations regarding training restrictions, rest periods, reoccurrence or worsening of symptoms (as with a head injury) as well as advice on contacting a physician for further follow-up if necessary. If the athlete is under the care and supervision of a national event medical team, the decision to return the athlete to their care should be discussed and agreed.

In all the above-mentioned, complete the medical records to include the initial examination findings, any treatment or drugs administered, and a description and rational behind the medical plan. Finally complete any necessary Federation or IOC incident reports and submit them in the appropriate confidential manner.

Athlete Medical Room Treatment

On arrival to the athlete medical room, repeat the primary survey and reevaluate the AVPU/GCS. Decide if further investigations/treatment are required and if the patient needs transport to another definitive treatment facility. Ensure that the patient's condition is stable, then secure the patient (immobilize if necessary) and transport to an appropriate medical center. If in doubt, either observe the patient for as long as necessary or transfer for further investigations/treatment. Observation should be for a preagreed period of time with decisions made in advance as to what to do if the patient does not improve during an agreed time period. Prolonged periods of observation in an athlete medical room are not appropriate and the patient should be moved to a medical center for ongoing evaluation, observation, and treatment.

If transferring the patient to another unit ensure that complete documentation of the medical findings and of any treatment undertaken accompanies the patient.

Finally, remember that the athlete medical room is only a temporary holding area and it is often better to transfer to a hospital or a more permanent medical facility early rather than to wait and delay observation and treatment while holding at the sporting venue.

Transportation to Hospital

If referring for further investigation or to hospital, ensure that the patient's condition is stable before transport, then secure and immobilize the patient as necessary, and transport to an appropriate medical center, having informed that unit before commencement of the transfer.

Ensure that the HCPs who will accompany the patient are capable of managing the patient's condition without detriment and that they have adequate equipment, oxygen and drugs to continue care of the patient through the transfer.

It may be necessary to decide if the patient is to be transferred to hospital by road (car/ambulance) or air. Air transportation should only be undertaken if the patient is seriously injured or road transport times are long and would thereby compromise patient safety. Air transport should be considered for exceptional cases only as it can actually take longer than a simple road transfer when considering the transfer from the venue to the helicopter, the flight time, and then the secondary transfer from the helicopter landing site to the hospital. If air transport is to be considered, it should be done in consultation with the air ambulance service and the receiving hospital.

Discharge

1. Reappraise the athlete after the event before discharging
2. Complete the SCAT3 card if appropriate
3. Enquire about home transport and the availability of caring observers in the forthcoming hours
4. Provide relevant written information to the patient (e.g. Head Injury card)
5. Ensure that the patient has adequate analgesia if required
6. Offer advice on warning symptoms and follow-up care

Also provide a report to the sport organizers/officials in non-detailed terms and keep up-to-date with the patient's progress. Finally, report serious injuries to the sport-governing body (most keep a record of serious and especially deaths).

Teamwork

The S-ABCDE mnemonic should be repeatedly drilled so that the FoP team automatically follows the correct procedure in an emergency situation. If a team of four competent doctors, paramedics, or nurses are present, then three individuals can perform several tasks at the same time as the Team Leader evaluates the data presented and coordinates the HCPs to perform relevant interventions within their particular skill base.

If a patient is unresponsive and has abnormal breathing, then the following tasks may be delegated.

Team member 1 controls the airway and head:

1. Shouts to the patient "Are you awake?"
2. Performs a chin lift/jaw thrust
3. Inspects the face/lips – listens for breath sounds
4. Inspects the airway – request suction if oral vomitus is suspected
5. Inserts oropharyngeal airway
6. Supports the oxygen mask and ventilates the patient if necessary
7. Intubates the trachea if necessary

Team member 2 controls the chest:

1. Exposes the chest and abdomen
2. Inspects the chest for deformities, asymmetrical chest expansion, and wounds
3. Palpates, percusses, and auscultates the chest
4. Performs needle thoracostomy if appropriate
5. Initiates chest compressions if appropriate
6. Attaches ECG leads if appropriate
7. Defibrillates if appropriate

Team member 3 evaluates peripheral circulation, extremity fractures, and pelvis:

1. Compresses major hemorrhage sites
2. Attaches pulse oximeter
3. Measures pulse
4. Measures blood sugar if appropriate
5. Inspects and palpates extremities
6. Compresses peripheral bleeding if appropriate
7. Measures BP if appropriate
8. Establishes IV access

Team Leader

The Team Leader has the overall management responsibility, coordinates the team, and records the results. When all the assessments have been made, then the team, led by the Team Leader, makes a joint decision as to the evacuation and continuing management of the casualty. It is the Team Leader's responsibility to communicate the FoP team findings and deliberations to the FoP officials and event organizers (with due respect for patient confidentiality) and make the necessary arrangements for the evacuation of the casualty to the fieldside/athlete medical room/ambulance. It may be necessary to hand over the ongoing care of the casualty to another HCP to allow the Team Leader to return to the FoP to continue medical supervision of the competition.

It is essential that all the HCPs on the FoP and in the athlete medical room work together as a fully integrated team. This will result in efficient and effective athlete medical care.

Bibliography

Niles, S.E., Miller, C.C., Hinds, D., Duke, J.H. & Moore, F.A. (2005) Prehospital physiologic data and lifesaving interventions in trauma patients. *Military Medicine*, **170** (**1**), 7–13.

Capillary Refill Time in Adults. Emergency Medicine Journal, 25, 325–326. doi:10.1136/emj.2007.055244

4 Cardiopulmonary Resuscitation on the Field of Play

Ruth Löllgen,[1] Herbert Löllgen,[2] and David Zideman[3,4,5]

[1]*Emergency Medicine, Children's Hospital at Westmead, Sydney, Australia*
[2]*German Federation of Sports Medicine, Remscheid, Germany*
[3]*Anaesthesia, Imperial College Healthcare NHS Trust, London, UK*
[4]*London Ambulance Service NHS Trust, London, UK*
[5]*Emergency Medical Services, London Organising Committee of the Olympic and Paralympic Games, London 2012, London*

Sudden cardiac arrest (SCA) is the leading cause of death in athletes during exercise and competition on the Field of Play (FoP). Such events are a rare but tragic occurrence. The reported incidence of SCA varies from 1:65,000 to 1:200,000 in athletes. SCA is the sudden, unexpected cessation of cardiac output in a previously seemingly healthy individual.

Cardiac emergencies on the FoP, such as sudden collapse or SCA may be due to various cardiac and noncardiac causes, both congenital and acquired. Structural heart disease (abnormality of the heart muscle) seems to account for 65–95% of the causes of SCA. Hypertrophic cardiomyopathy, arrhythmogenic right ventricular dysplasia, and congenital coronary artery anomalies constitute the most frequent causes in the under 35-year-old group and coronary artery disease in the over 35-year-old group. Ventricular fibrillation (VF) is the underlying pathophysiologic rhythm in SCA in all of these pathologies.

Commotio cordis is thought to account for 20% of SCA in the under 21-year-old group but seldom occurs after 21 years of age. VF is induced during the vulnerable repolarization period of the myocardium after sustaining blunt chest trauma from either solid objects such as a baseball or from collision with another player. Current research has shown that the object must be traveling with a velocity of 49 km/h and strike the chest within the cardiac silhouette within a 20-ms window of the upstroke of the T-wave.

Ruptured aortic aneurysm, myocarditis, aortic valve stenosis, mitral valve prolapse, and dilated cardiomyopathy are further structural causes of cardiac emergencies, predominantly in the elderly. SCA secondary to electrical or rhythmic abnormalities is observed in the young athlete. Causes include drug-induced cardiac rhythm abnormalities and ion-channelopathies such as long and short QT syndrome (caused by sodium or potassium ion channel genetic mutations), Brugada syndrome (defective

The IOC Manual of Emergency Sports Medicine, First Edition. Edited by David McDonagh and David Zideman.
2015 International Olympic Committee. Published 2015 by John Wiley & Sons, Ltd.

sodium channel gene), and familial catecholaminergic polymorphic ventricular tachycardia (CPVT) (abnormal ryanodine receptor regulating calcium release) and result in malignant ventricular arrhythmias.

Noncardiac causes of SCA comprise asthma, heat stroke, cerebral artery rupture, and exertional rhabdomyolysis secondary to sickle cell trait.

It has been proposed that SCA in athletes could be prevented by identification of athletes at risk, a preparticipation medical examination of athletes of all age groups, a close review of their family history, and a resting electrocardiogram (ECG). However, precompetition assessment is not yet mandatory in all sports, preparticipation cardiovascular screening is limited and it is difficult to interpret some of the clinical and investigative findings, particularly those which are borderline.

It would be expected that all members of the designated FoP medical team for all sporting events are trained, certified, and practiced in Basic Life Support and Automated Defibrillation. In addition, it would be anticipated that the majority of the same FoP team have been trained, certified, and practiced in Advanced Life Support and its various essential skills. It is essential that the FoP team is supported by a fully equipped ambulance with appropriately trained staff to complement the FoP team and transfer the patient to hospital.

Sudden Cardiac Arrest on the Field of Play

Management of SCA involves prompt recognition, immediate cardiopulmonary resuscitation (CPR), and early defibrillation where appropriate, by the fieldside healthcare professional medical team. It is paramount that these simple steps are commenced within seconds after the event, in order to achieve high resuscitation success rates. Successful cardioversion rates of >90% may be obtained if defibrillation is initiated within 1–2 min of the onset of the collapse. Rapid defibrillation, drug therapy, and advanced airway management increase the likelihood of return of spontaneous circulation (ROSC). Medical providers must be well trained in the recognition of SCA, including distracting pathologic features, such as seizures and agonal breathing. The aim of this chapter is to recommend a practical and systematic approach to the immediate management of SCA on the FoP, based on current international guidelines, but subject to local recommended practice.

It is recognized that most users of this manual have been trained and certified in CPR. This text is a reminder of the basic steps in establishing CPR. For those who have not been trained, this text alone will not be sufficient and the authors recommend that all FoP team members are trained and certified in Basic and Advanced Life support procedures.

Recognition of Cardiac Arrest

In sport, it is not unusual for athletes or team players to fall on the FoP, mainly following contact with an opponent or coplayer, sports equipment, or FoP furniture. In the majority of these incidents, little therapeutic action from the FoP medical team is required. Sudden collapse with or without a preceding collision must be regarded as a cardiac event until proven otherwise. Medical assistance and a speedy response are mandatory.

Following the collapse, enter the FoP immediately and approach the athlete (see Chapter 3). There may be apparent signs of life such as brief seizure-like activity or myoclonic jerks, as these occur after the collapse in 50% of SCA. Myoclonic jerk-like activity is thought to be secondary to oxygen deprivation to the brain following a nonperfusing cardiac arrhythmia. This distracting symptom may delay the recognition of SCA and the prompt initiation of life-saving CPR.

On approach, determine whether the casualty is conscious by gently shaking the shoulders and shouting "Are you alright?" If the athlete responds, leave in the position found and continue to determine the cause of the collapse (Figure 4.1).

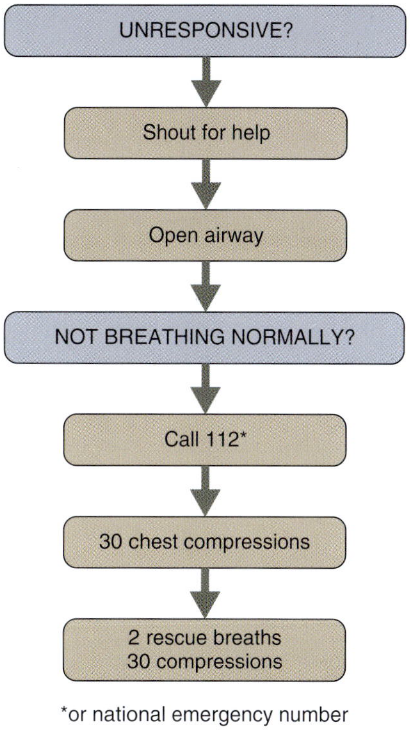

Figure 4.1 Adult basic life support (*Source:* Copyright European Resuscitation Council – www.erc.edu – 2014/012.)

If there is no response:

1. Call for help and for the automated external defibrillator (AED)
2. Turn the patient into the supine position
3. Open the airway by head tilt and chin lift
4. With the airway open – check for breathing (no more than 10 s)
   a. Look for chest movements
   b. Listen over the patient's mouth for breath sounds
   c. Feel over the patient's mouth for air movement
   d. Decide if any breathing efforts are normal and effective

If breathing is normal:

1. Turn the patient into the recovery position (see below)
2. Ensure that the airway is maintained using the head tilt/chin lift maneuver
3. Continue to monitor the patient
4. Remove the patient from the FoP for further observation and management

If there is no breathing:

1. Immediately commence chest compressions
2. Ensure that an AED is available

Combine chest compressions with rescue breathing:

1. After 30 chest compressions:
   a. Move to the head of the patient – if two or more FoP medical team members are present, then one should carry out chest compressions and the other deliver rescue breaths
   b. Open the airway using the head tilt/chin lift maneuver
   c. Give two rescue breaths (either as mouth-to-mouth or by bag-valve-mask)
   d. Immediately recommence chest compressions
   e. Alternate 30 compressions with two rescue breaths

On arrival of the defibrillator/AED:

1. Apply the defibrillator pads to the patient's exposed chest in the recommended positions
2. Analyze the rhythm
   a. For an AED:
      i. Follow the voice prompts
      ii. Defibrillate (shock) when instructed
      iii. Continue chest compressions and rescue breathing after each defibrillation attempt – the AED will analyze the rhythm following 2 min of post-shock compressions
      iv. If no shock is advised, continue CPR and reanalyze the cardiac rhythm every 2 min
   b. For a manual defibrillator
      i. Stop chest compressions
      ii. Analyze the ECG rhythm
      iii. If a shock is indicated, then continue chest compressions until the defibrillator is charged and briefly cease chest compressions (and stand clear) to deliver the shock
      iv. Immediately continue chest compressions post-shock
      v. Continue chest compressions for 2 min and then reanalyze the ECG rhythm
      vi. If no shock is required, continue CPR and reanalyze the cardiac rhythm every 2 min
3. Continue CPR until there is a ROSC
4. Arrange to transfer to the fieldside, medical room, or directly to an ambulance

The need for rapid assessment and the immediate commencement of CPR is the key to the success of resuscitation. Make an assessment of the athlete on approach, check for responsiveness, open the airway and check for breathing speedily, and commence chest compressions without delay. Do not interrupt the chest compressions apart from brief pauses for ECG analysis, defibrillation, and rescue breaths.

Field of Play Airway

Airway assessment begins as soon as the healthcare professional makes contact with the injured athlete. An alert, responsive athlete who is talking in a normal voice has a patent airway. Conducting an ongoing conversation with the athlete will not only provide information about any difficulties in breathing, but will also give the FoP doctor a continuous assessment of the athlete's conscious and mental state.

The unconscious athlete will not be able to maintain his/her own airway without intervention. Therefore, opening and maintaining a patent airway is of paramount importance and this must be secured before progressing to any other patient management procedures.

Airway management starts with the basic manual maneuvers and progresses to more complex interventions.

There are two simple airway maneuvers:

1. *Head tilt/chin lift maneuver*
   a. Approach the patient from behind the head
   b. Tilt the head by placing a hand on the victim's forehead and apply firm backward pressure
   c. Lift the chin with the other hand to bring the lower jaw upwards and forwards
   d. Do not press on the soft tissues in the floor of the mouth as this may cause obstruction by pushing the tongue into the airway

    e. Check for breath sounds over the mouth and nose. If there are no breath sounds, then reposition the head tilt and chin lift
2. *Jaw thrust*
    a. Approach the patient from behind the head
    b. Grasp the angles of the mandible between the index and middle fingers on each side
    c. Move the jaw forward and upward. This will lift the tongue from the back of the pharynx
    d. Maintain the head in the neutral anatomical position
    e. Check for breath sounds over the mouth and nose. If no breath sounds present, reposition the jaw thrust
    f. It will be necessary to maintain jaw thrust to provide an open airway

Jaw thrust is a painful maneuver and if the casualty does not react then they should be considered unconscious.

Jaw thrust is considered the procedure of choice if a spinal injury is suspected, as it can be achieved without having to move the head position; however, simple chin lift alone may be enough to open the airway.

Foreign Body Airway Obstruction (FBAO or Choking)

FBAO is a serious but treatable cause of airway obstruction.

If the patient is displaying signs of choking, this issue must be addressed immediately. Inspect the mouth and throat to see if the choking is due to a foreign body or damage to the airway. Remove any visible foreign bodies from the mouth if possible (if manual extraction does not work, a Magill forceps may be used). Choking is commonly caused by the tongue falling posteriorly into the hypopharynx (swallowing the tongue), which can usually be treated using a simple airway maneuver or, if necessary, following the choking algorithm (Figure 4.2).

If there is no visible foreign body to remove and the athlete is conscious and standing:

1. Bend the patient forward
2. Slap the patient in the center of the back up to five times

If this is unsuccessful, perform five abdominal thrusts: (artificial coughs)

1. Stand behind the patient
2. Place your arms around the patient's abdomen
3. Grasp your hands in front of the abdomen in a two-handed fist
4. Turn the fist inwards (thumbs toward the abdomen)
5. Pull inwards and upwards five times

Repeat alternate back slaps and abdominal thrusts until the foreign body is coughed up or the patient loses consciousness.

If the patient is lying on the ground, try to get the athlete to sit and then give up to five back slaps followed by five abdominal thrusts.

If the patient is unconscious, commence chest compressions to clear the foreign body from the airway.

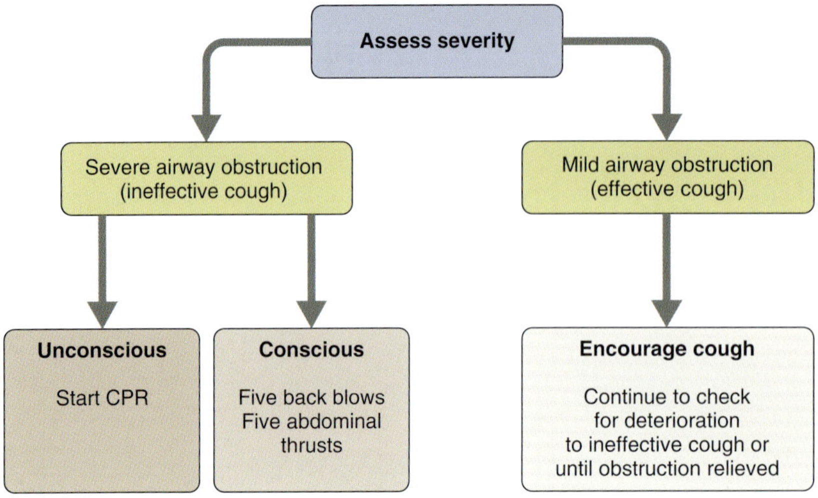

Figure 4.2 Adult foreign body airway obstruction treatment (*Source:* Copyright European Resuscitation Council – www.erc.edu – 2014/012.)

Field of Play Breathing

Having opened the airway, it is important to assess the efficacy of the patient's breathing. The simplest check is to look, listen, and feel for breathing. Apparent abnormal or agonal breathing patterns may be observed in cardiac arrest patients during the first few minutes of arrest while the brain has sufficient oxygen supply. However, these are not usually effective.

The patient who has spontaneous and effective breathing should be turned onto their side into the recovery position, as this will aid the drainage of fluids and foreign materials.

Recovery Position

1. Kneel beside the casualty, ensuring that both legs are straight
2. Place the nearest arm out at right angles to the body with the elbow bent and the hand palm uppermost
3. Bring the far arm across the chest and hold the back of the hand against the patient's cheek
4. Grasp the far leg just above the knee and pull it up to bend the knee, but keeping the foot on the ground
5. Keeping the hand pressed against the cheek, pull on the far bent leg to roll the patient onto their side
6. Adjust the upper leg so that both hip and knee are bent at right angles
7. Use head tilt or jaw thrust to make sure the airway remains open and adjust the hand under the cheek if necessary, to keep the head tilted and facing downwards to allow liquid material to drain from the mouth
8. Assess the patency of the airway by regularly checking for breathing

For the patient who is unresponsive and is not breathing, commence chest compressions immediately.

Field of Play Circulation

In cardiac arrest, the circulation is delivered by chest compressions. The delivery of high-quality CPR is dependent on performing efficient chest compressions with minimal interruptions.

Chest compressions must be delivered:

1. At an adequate rate (100/minute)
2. To a depth of one-third of the chest diameter or 5 cm
3. To the lower half of the sternum

It is important to allow for full chest recoil between individual chest compressions and to minimize interruption of chest compressions for any reason. Monitoring of the quality of chest compressions is encouraged. There are simple devices that can measure the depth and rate of chest compressions. If feasible, measure physiological parameters (ECG tracing, and the end-tidal CO_2 ($EtCO_2$)). The latter may correlate with cardiac output and coronary blood flow. During cardiac arrest, there is no delivery of CO_2 to the lungs and with the initiation of CPR, cardiac output is the major contributor to CO_2 delivery to the lungs. $EtCO_2$ will correlate well with cardiac output in *intubated* patients, using quantitative waveform capnography, if ventilation is constant. A persistently low $EtCO_2$ <10 mmHg may indicate that ROSC is unlikely.

In some arenas, the FoP team may be supplied with a mechanical chest compression device. Always start manual chest compressions immediately and transfer to the mechanical device, with minimal interruption, as soon as feasible. The advantage of mechanical CPR is that it maintains high-quality chest compressions even while the patient is being transferred from the FoP to the fieldside and also during the ambulance journey to hospital.

FoP: Combining Compressions and Ventilations

Combining ventilation with chest compressions completes the process of CPR. After 30 compressions, perform expired air ventilation until a bag-valve-mask becomes available.

Expired Air Ventilation

1. Open the airway using the head tilt/chin lift maneuver
2. Open the mouth maintaining the chin lift
3. Pinch the nares shut with the fingers of the other hand
4. Take a normal breath and seal your mouth over the patient's mouth
5. Blow into the patient for approximately 1 s and watch the chest rise
6. If the chest does not rise, then adjust the airway position
7. Perform two ventilations and return to performing chest compressions

When a bag-valve-mask becomes available, ventilate with this device:

Bag-Valve-Mask Ventilation (Two Rescuer Technique)

1. The first rescuer (airway)
   a. Open the airway using the head tilt/chin lift maneuver
   b. Place the facemask over the patient's face
   c. Seal the mask to the patient's face holding the mask onto the face with both hands
2. The second rescuer (compression and ventilations)
   a. Perform 30 compressions
   b. Ventilate the patient by squeezing the reinflating bag
   c. Perform two ventilations and return to performing chest compressions

It is critical to combine effective chest compressions and ventilation with 2-min cycles of defibrillation as described earlier and illustrated in the algorithm as follows.

The ability to adequately assess the presence or absence of a pulse has been deemphasized in CPR for both healthcare professionals and laypersons. The importance of commencing uninterrupted chest compressions as soon as possible is critical to success and should not be delayed for a pulse check. The pulse can be checked after 2 min of chest compressions post-defibrillation, if there is an ECG rhythm that would support a circulation.

Similarly, the "chest thump" has been removed from the CPR sequence. Not only was its efficacy in doubt, it resulted in a further delay in performing chest compressions while undertaking the post-thump pulse check.

FoP Removal

If the cardiac arrest occurs on the FoP, it is important to begin planning for removal of the patient from the FoP and away from spectators and the media as soon as possible. It should also be remembered that the team members and other athletes, coaches, and FoP officials might be distraught by the incident.

Removal can be accomplished as soon as there is ROSC. In this situation, the patient should be scooped and lifted in a basket stretcher or vacuum mattress and transferred directly into a designated ambulance for immediate transfer to hospital. The patient should continue to be monitored throughout this FoP removal and ventilation continued if required.

The difficulty arises when there has been no ROSC. It is recognized that chest compressions are not effective in a moving vehicle and will certainly have decreased efficacy, if they can be performed at all, during the removal from the FoP; unless an automated chest compression device has been used. Under these circumstances, it is still important to try and move the patient as soon as possible. CPR should not be continued for a prolonged period in this public arena nor should it be stopped, with the pronouncement of death, on the FoP. It is recommended that removal from the FoP should be planned and attempted after the third defibrillation, approximately 6 min into the resuscitation sequence, if there has been no ROSC. The efficacy of defibrillation diminishes after the third and subsequent shocks. Move the patient short distances, for example, FoP to fieldside, fieldside to medical room/ambulance, restarting chest compressions at every stop.

Rhythm Analysis

In addition to high-quality CPR, which delivers oxygen and metabolic substrates to the depleted myocardium and may reduce the right ventricular preload, defibrillation is the only rhythm-specific therapy for VF and pulseless VT that may improve survival to hospital discharge.

Cardiac arrest can be caused by four rhythms:

1. VF – disorganized electric activity
2. Pulseless ventricular tachycardia (VT) – organized electric activity of the ventricular myocardium but insufficient to generate a pulse.
3. Pulseless electric activity (PEA) – heterogenous group of organized electric rhythms with absent or insufficient mechanical ventricular activity to generate a pulse
4. Asystole – absence of mechanical ventricular activity with or without electric atrial activity

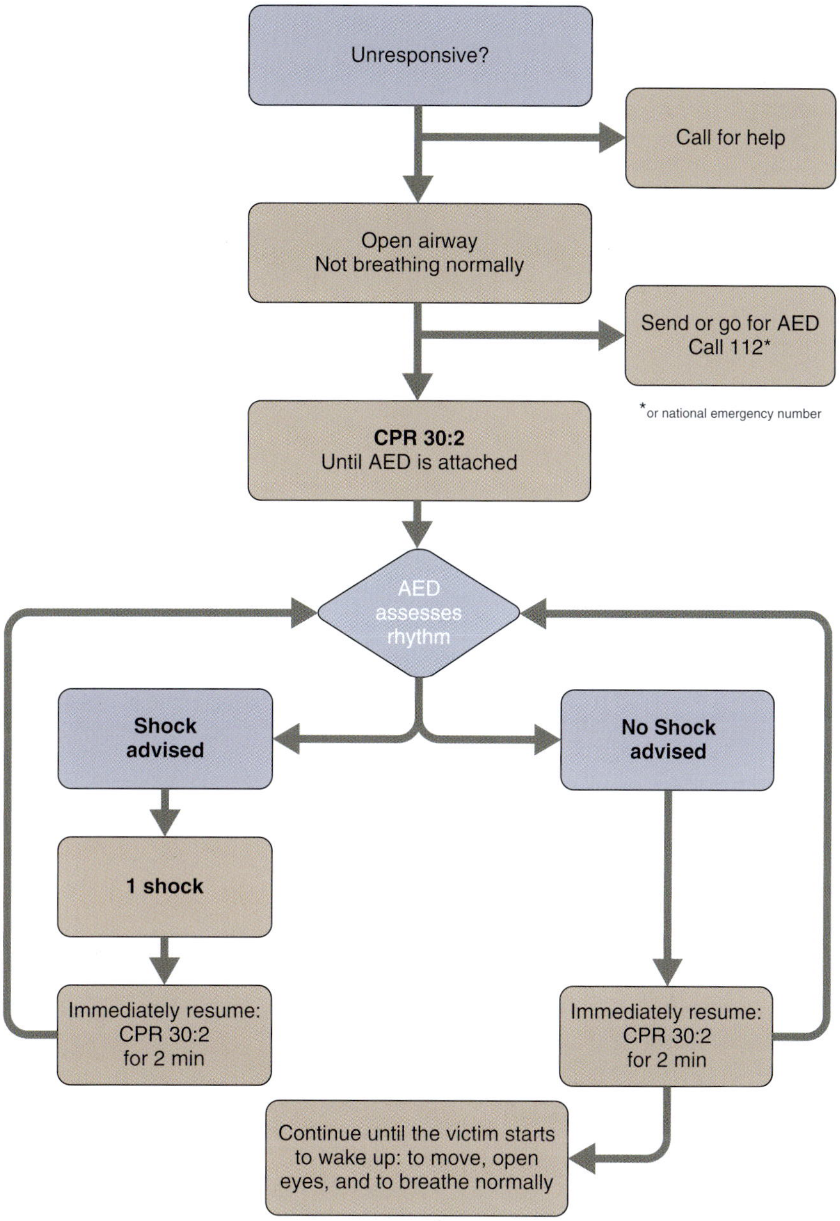

Figure 4.3 Automated external defibrillation algorithm (*Source:* Copyright European Resuscitation Council – www.erc.edu – 2014/012.)

VF and pulseless VT are shockable rhythms.

PEA and asystole are nonshockable rhythms.

AEDs are programmed to distinguish between shockable and nonshockable rhythms with a high degree of accuracy. It is recommended to follow the AED algorithm (Figure 4.3).

Shockable Rhythms

Defibrillation efficacy can be improved by the following:

1. Minimalizing the preshock pause by continuing chest compressions while the AED is charging. This technique does require good team leadership by the Team Leader and practice by the resuscitation team. Following charging of the AED,

the Team Leader calls "all clear" and visually checks that everyone is away from and no one is touching the patient. At this point, the Team Leader presses the defibrillation button and immediately commences chest compressions again. The preshock pause should not be longer than 5 s
2. The use of adhesive pads rather than paddles will also decrease the preshock pause as they are applied once, at the beginning of resuscitation and allow for ECG monitoring and deliver the defibrillation shock with no additional pause for positioning

It has been demonstrated that performing a fixed period of chest compression prior to the first defibrillation does not improve the likelihood of ROSC or improve long-term survival. However, the 2 min of CPR post-defibrillation and before a brief pause for rhythm analysis has been shown to improve rhythm stability and minimize post-shock myocardial stunning.

Defibrillation Energy Levels

The precise defibrillation energy levels have not been determined. Most modern defibrillators deliver a biphasic waveform. AEDs deliver a preprogrammed series of shocks, but manual defibrillators may have to have their energy level selected prior to charging. It is currently recommended to use:

First shock – an energy level of at least 150 J (some authorities use 120 J rectilinear biphasic waveform).

If the first shock is not successful and the defibrillator is capable of delivering a higher energy level, then it is recommended to raise the energy level for the second and subsequent shocks.

Nonshockable Rhythms

Pulseless electrical activity (PEA) and asystole cannot be treated with defibrillation and require continuous chest compressions and ventilation.

Reversible Causes (The 4H's and 4T's)

It is of paramount importance to diagnose and treat possible underlying or complicating causes for VF, VT, PEA, or asystole during each 2-min cycle of CPR. Consider the following reversible conditions to identify and treat appropriately:

H's	T's
Hypoxia	Toxins
Hypovolemia	Tamponade (cardiac)
Hypo–hyperkalemia/metabolic	Tension pneumothorax
Hypothermia	Thrombosis (pulmonary/coronary)

Advanced Life Support

Once basic life support has been established, then the procedures associated with Advanced Life Support can be considered (Figure 4.4). These procedures can be commenced on the FoP if the team has the appropriate skills, or it may be more appropriate to establish an advanced airway and venous access once removal from the FoP has been completed.

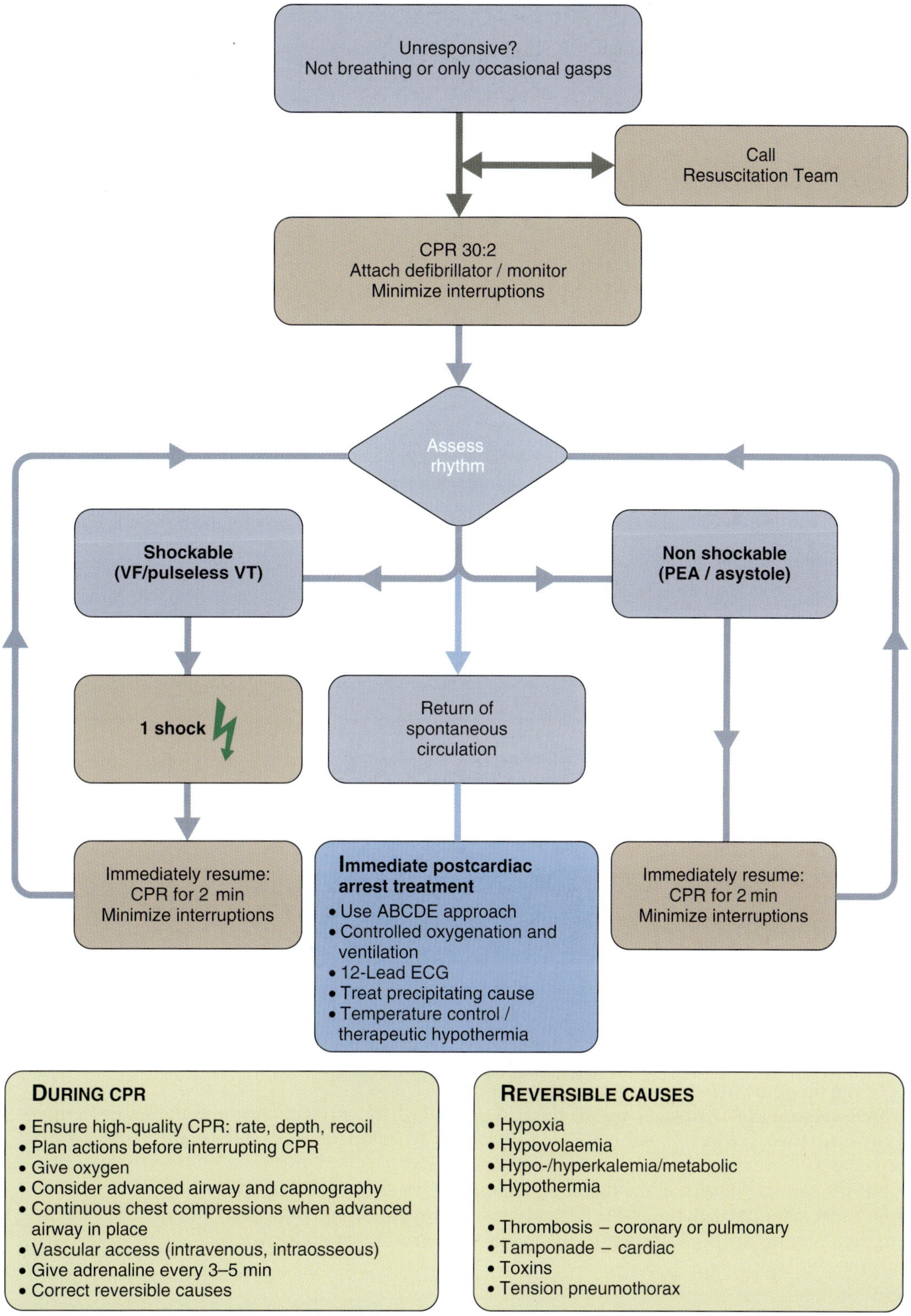

Figure 4.4 Advanced life support
(*Source:* Copyright European Resuscitation Council – www.erc.edu – 2014/012.)

Advanced Airway

Although endotracheal intubation is the optimal way of maintaining airway patency and adequate oxygenation during CPR, the incidence of complications of endotracheal intubation attempts by unskilled providers may be unacceptably high. Depending on the provider's experience and the victim's condition, adequate oxygenation may be more effectively delivered via bag mask ventilation rather than by unsuccessfully attempting repeated intubation attempts. It is recommended that advanced airway skills require frequent experience or retraining. If these advanced airway skills are not immediately available, focus on optimal bag mask ventilation with or without a simple airway adjunct, until more experienced/skilled support arrives.

Simple Airway Adjuncts

There are two simple airway adjuncts; the oropharyngeal airway (OPA) and the nasopharyngeal airway (NPA).

Inserting an Oropharyngeal Airway (OPA)

1. Select the OPA whose length matches the distance from the center of the incisor teeth and the angle of the mandible
2. Open the casualty's mouth using the cross-finger technique
3. Slowly insert the inverted OPA with the curve facing upwards and the tip pointing to the roof of the mouth
4. Gently rotate the OPA 180° to its correct orientation while advancing it forward until the flange rests at the front teeth. With the airway in place, reestablish chin lift or jaw thrust and reassess the patency of the airway
5. If the device does not assist airway positioning it should be removed

OPAs should never be forced into position. They cannot be used in patients with a clenched jaw or in conscious patients with a gag reflex.

Inserting a Nasopharyngeal Airway (NPA)

1. Select the NPA whose length matches the distance from the tip of the patient's nose to the tip of the earlobe
2. The diameter of the NPA should be such that it can fit inside the victim's nostril without blanching the skin of the nose. A rough guide is that a 6-mm diameter airway will fit a small face and a 7-mm diameter airway a larger face
3. Lubricate the outside of the NPA with a sterile, water-soluble lubricant
4. Gently insert the tip of the device into one nostril
5. Insert the NPA close to the midline, along the floor of the nostril and straight back into the nasopharynx
6. If there is any resistance, gently rotate the NPA a few degrees from side to side while guiding it forward
7. If resistance continues, remove the NPA and try the other nostril
8. When the NPA is correctly inserted, the flange should lie against the outside the nostril
9. Check for air movement through the NPA. If the casualty is breathing spontaneously but no air movement is felt, then remove the NPA and return to a chin lift or jaw thrust maneuver

The NPA performs a similar role to the OPA, but it can be used in a patient who has a functional gag reflex or even in those who are conscious.

The NPA must never be forced into the nasal cavity nor should it be inserted upwards into the nose; only insert backwards, parallel to the floor of the nose and the hard palate below.

Extreme caution must be used when attempting to insert an NPA with a suspected cribriform plate fracture or major facial injury as the NPA can unintentionally enter the skull and brain.

Advanced Airway Adjunct

Advanced airway management can be achieved using a supraglottic airways (SGA) or by traditional endotracheal intubation.

1. *SGA*
   The SGA airway has become the airway of choice for those without formal endotracheal intubation skills. It does not require direct visualization of the larynx with a laryngoscope, as the device is designed to be inserted directly into the upper supraglottic space. It sits above the glottic opening and does not pass into the larynx or the trachea. Two devices are commonly in use: the laryngeal mask airway (LMA) and the i-Gel airway.
   Other alternatives are the combitube and the laryngeal tube; both these devices are passed blindly into the trachea.
2. *Endotracheal intubation*
   Endotracheal intubation is the classic standard of airway management. Fortunately, it is rarely required on the FoP. It should only be attempted by those formally trained in the technique and, as it may require the administration of drugs, by those familiar and practiced in prehospital anesthesia management.
   The perceived problems with endotracheal intubation are the prolonged periods without chest compressions while intubation is attempted, the possibility of misplaced insertion of the tube into the esophagus rather than the trachea and the relatively high failure rate of tracheal intubation in the prehospital arena.

It is essential that $EtCO_2$ be monitored following the placement of an advanced airway device to confirm the devices correct placement in the airway.

The techniques for inserting these advanced airway adjuncts should be part of the intrinsic skills of the FoP team. These techniques require formal certified training and supervised clinical practice and are beyond the scope of this manual.

Venous Access

Establish peripheral venous access so that drugs can be administered following the initial defibrillation shocks. Endotracheal administration of drugs is no longer considered acceptable.

Venous access can be directly into a peripheral vein or, following two failed venous cannulations, via the intraosseous (IO) route.

Intraosseous Access

IO cannulation has been shown to be as efficacious as IV access. Drug and fluid administration into the IO space is slower but drugs reach the central circulation in a relatively short time. IO access can be established in the anterior tibia or the head of the humerus. New mechanized IO devices (EZ-IO or BIG) have made IO a safe and fast method of emergency venous access.

Drugs

The efficacy of drugs during resuscitation is currently being reevaluated and the FoP team should be fully up-to-date with the latest recommended local practice:

1. Adrenaline (epinephrine)
   Adrenaline (1 mg–10 mL of 1:10,000 solution or 1 mL of 1:1000 solution) is the first drug to be administered in cardiac arrest and is currently recommended to be administered every 3–5 min in the resuscitation sequence; in reality during alternate cycles. Adrenaline will improve both the chronotropic and inotropic cardiac response and, by its α-adrenergic action, raise peripheral vascular resistance and improve the end-diastolic pressure and coronary perfusion.
   There is currently no evidence to show that the administration of adrenaline improves the rate of neurological survival to hospital discharge.
2. Amiodarone
   Amiodarone, as an antiarrhythmic agent, has been shown to improve rates of survival from refractory VF to hospital admission. The initial dose of 300 mg IV is administered as a bolus injection after the first three defibrillation shocks, and a further dose of 150 mg can be given if the VF is still resistant to defibrillation.
3. Lidocaine
   Lidocaine is administered as an alternative antiarrhythmic agent in an IV dose of 1 mg/kg. It should not be given if amiodarone has already been administered.
4. Other drugs
   Atropine, magnesium, and bicarbonate have all been recommended in previous cardiac arrest guidelines. Current guidelines do not recommend the administration of these drugs.

Implantable Cardiac Defibrillators (ICDs)

Athletes who are at risk of spontaneous VT or VF are now fitted with an implantable cardiac defibrillator (ICD). In the event of a VT or VF rhythm developing, the ICD senses the pathological rhythm and automatically delivers a defibrillation shock of approximately 40 J though implanted leads directly to the heart. Visually it will appear that the athlete drops to the ground, has a very short whole body convulsion (the shock), then recovers, and will often sit up. The athlete should be removed from the FoP for further assessment. It would be hoped that any athletes with these devices would be confidentially identified to the medical team.

Occasionally, the ICD may need to deliver more than one shock to achieve conversion. On rare occasions, the ICD may fail. If the ICD fails, continue as for normal CPR and defibrillate as described, but placing the defibrillation pads away from the ICD.

Postresuscitation

If CPR is successful and there is ROSC, then the patient should be transferred directly to an appropriate hospital with full physiological monitoring and an experienced medical escort. There is a possibility that the patient may rearrest during transportation and will need further treatment. It may be necessary to maintain ventilation until effective spontaneous respiration returns.

There is discussion as to the effectiveness of prehospital therapeutic hypothermia following ROSC and local protocols should be followed.

If CPR is not successful, then it should be continued until the patient reaches hospital. The pronouncement of life extinct should not be made on the FoP or at the venue.

Bibliography

Nolan, J.P., Soar, J., Zideman, D.A. *et al.* (2010) European Resuscitation Council guidelines for Resuscitation 2010. Section 1. Executive summary. *Resuscitation*, **81** (**10**), 1219–1276.

American Heart Association (2010) American Heart Association guidelines for cardiopulmonary resuscitation and emergency cardiovascular care. *Circulation*, **122**, S640–S946.

Kramer, E., Dvorak, J. & Kloeck, W. (2010) Review of the management of sudden cardiac arrest on the football field. *British Journal of Sports Medicine*, **44**, 540–545.

5 Cardiac Emergencies on the Field of Play

Ruth Löllgen,[1] *Herbert Löllgen*[2] *and David Zideman*[3,4,5]

[1]*Emergency Medicine, Children's Hospital at Westmead, Sydney, Australia*
[2]*German Federation of Sports Medicine, Remscheid, Germany*
[3]*Anaesthesia, Imperial College Healthcare NHS Trust, London, UK*
[4]*London Ambulance Service NHS Trust, London, UK*
[5]*Emergency Medical Services, London Organising Committee of the Olympic and Paralympic Games, London 2012*

Cardiac emergencies in athletes on the Field of Play (FoP) are rare, but if present, may be life threatening. In this chapter, we discuss the several serious cardiovascular conditions.

1. Sudden cardiac arrest
2. Acute coronary syndrome (ACS)
3. Aortic aneurysm and aortic dissection
4. Myocarditis
5. Hypertensive crisis
6. Acute cardiac arrhythmias

Sudden Cardiac Death (SCD)

It is estimated that the incidence of SCD in adolescents and young adults under the age of 35 years is 1 in 100,000 per year. Despite all the benefits of a "healthy life style," statistics have demonstrated that young athletes may have a higher risk of sudden cardiac death (SCD) than their matched peer group. In Italy, the increased risk for young athletes (12–35 years) was estimated at 2.8 times that for nonathletes, compared with an increased risk of 1.7% for noncardiovascular causes. However, the risks vary geographically: Northern Italy has a quoted athlete FoP cardiac mortality of 2.3 per 100,000 rate compared to 0.5 per 100,000 in high school athletes in the United States. It is not surprising that there is also a difference in etiology between Italy and North America, with the primary diagnosis for Italy being arrhythmogenic right ventricular cardiomyopathy and hypertrophic cardiomyopathy for the United States.

SCD on the FoP or in the arena is mainly due to arrhythmias secondary to cardiac disease. However, structural changes of cardiac muscle (mainly cardiomyopathies) and structural electrophysiological diseases (such as ion channel–diseases–channelopathies) may also result in SCD. In reality, an undiagnosed underlying cardiac disease may first become manifest when the athlete collapses on the FoP.

The IOC Manual of Emergency Sports Medicine, First Edition. Edited by David McDonagh and David Zideman.

Acquired heart diseases that may cause SCD include the following:

1. Coronary artery disease
2. Arterial hypertension
3. Cardiac valve disease
4. Drug-induced long QT syndrome
5. Myocarditis
6. Commotio cordis

Structural abnormalities that can cause SCD are classified as being mechanical or electrical. Mechanical causes are almost always due to a cardiomyopathy which is caused by the following:

1. Hypertrophic, with or without outflow obstruction
2. Arrhythmogenic right ventricular dysplasia (ARVD)
3. Marfan's syndrome

Electrical causes of SCD are often ion channel diseases (channelopathies) and include the following:

1. Long and short QT syndrome
2. Brugada syndrome
3. Sudden unexpected nocturnal death syndrome (SUNDS)
4. Pre-excitation syndrome (WPW, Wolff–Parkinson–White)
5. Atrial tachycadia
6. Intermittent atrial fibrillation
7. Catecholaminergic polymorphic ventricular tachycardia (CPVT)

Observation of the sudden collapse of an athlete on the FoP without any trauma or direct contact with other athletes should cause the ED to suspect SCD until proven otherwise. It is essential to gain rapid access to the collapsed athlete and determine whether or not this is a cardiac event. The management of SCD has been dealt within Chapter 4.

FoP Management Non-traumatic Sudden Collapse

On approach, determine whether the athlete is conscious by gently shaking his/her shoulders and shouting "Are you alright?" If the athlete responds, leave in the position found and continue to determine the cause of the collapse.

If there is no response:

1. Call for help and for the automated external defibrillator (AED)
2. Turn the patient into the supine position
3. Open the airway by head tilt and chin lift
4. With the airway open – check for breathing (no more than 10 s)
    a. Look for chest movements
    b. Listen over the patient's mouth for breath sounds
    c. Feel over the patient's mouth for air movement
    d. Decide if any breathing efforts are normal and effective

If breathing is normal:
1. Turn the patient into the recovery position
2. Ensure that the airway is maintained using the head tilt/chin lift maneuver

3. Continue to monitor the patient
4. Remove the patient from the FoP for further observation and management

If there is no breathing:

1. Immediately commence chest compressions
2. Ensure that an AED is available

If the athlete's breathing is normal and there is a palpable regular pulse:

1. Consider a noncardiac cause for the collapse
2. If the patient is conscious, then ask a series of short focused questions to determine the clinical symptoms These include questions regarding the following:
   a. Acute chest pain
   b. Acute dyspnoea
   c. Acute palpitations and arrhythmias
   d. Dizziness
   e. Previous unexplained loss of consciousness (syncope)
   f. Acute hypertension with or without crisis

It would be hoped that the team doctor would know their athlete's previous medical history and that any serious concerns would have been communicated (confidentially) to the FoP Team Leader.

If a cardiac etiology is confirmed or suspected, the FoP medical team should immediately remove the athlete from the FoP to the sideline for emergency stabilization and then rapidly to the designated ambulance for immediate transfer to an appropriate hospital for definitive treatment.

At an Olympic Games, it would be expected that the FoP team would be equipped with a defibrillator, but many of these devices do not have an electrocardiogram (ECG) display or if they do, only have a one-lead ECG display. The nondisplay defibrillator (AED) only determines if the patient needs a defibrillation shock using its internal VF or VT algorithms. Thus, the AED will not diagnose or be of use in treating most cardiac rhythms associated with a palpable pulse. The defibrillator with an ECG display may be of limited use and the FoP doctor may be able to see some gross diagnostic features such as ST elevation or depression or heart block. The FoP team and most athlete medical rooms will not be equipped with an ECG monitor; however, most front-line emergency ambulances will carry a defibrillator/ECG device capable of providing a 12-lead or multichannel ECG. It is recommended that the athlete with cardiac symptoms is monitored as soon as possible with this device.

Acute Coronary Syndrome (ACS)

ACS may occur in athletes with abnormalities of the coronary arteries not previously diagnosed or, more rarely, due to genetic mutations. It may also be seen in FoP officials who may or may not have a prior history of cardiac disease.

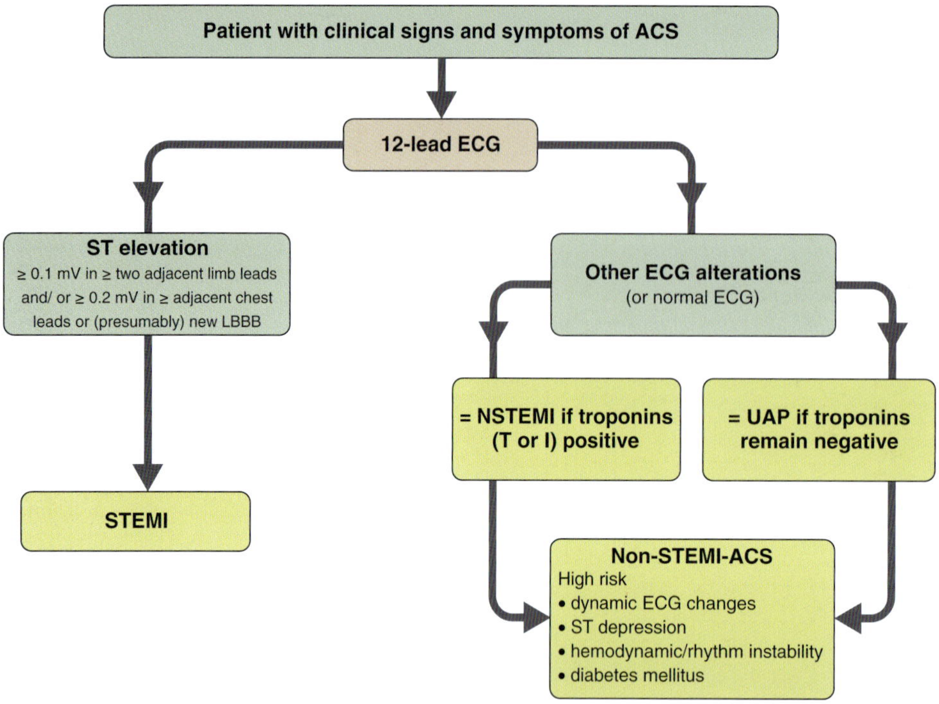

Figure 5.1 Diagnostic features of acute coronary syndrome (*Source:* Copyright European Resuscitation Council – www.erc.edu – 2014/012.)

Clinical Findings/Management ACS (Fig 5.1)

History: Typical history may feature exercise-induced pain within the last days or weeks. Precordial chest or left arm pain or discomfort is pathognomonic, sometimes radiating to the back, typically more to the left arm and left precordial chest wall. If the athlete is complaining of chest pain, conduct a primary survey on the FoP. If vital signs are normal, remove the patient from the FoP to the fieldside for further evaluation. Athletes may prefer to be sat up in a wheelchair or carry chair rather than laid flat on a stretcher. Repeat the primary survey at the fieldside, call for an ambulance, and take an ECG while preparing the athlete for transport to an appropriate hospital, preferably with a cardiac intervention facility if required. A doctor or experienced paramedic should accompany the athlete. Full physiological and ECG monitoring should be undertaken during transportation. It is essential to monitor oxygen saturation by pulse oximetry and only to administer supplemental oxygen therapy to patients who are hypoxic. High-flow oxygen has now been shown to be harmful to patients with uncomplicated myocardial infarction. Current recommendations are that treatment should be aimed at maintaining oxygen saturation between 94% and 98%.

Clinical examination: ACS may present with chest pain, pallor, and diaphoresis, representing reduced cardiac output and/or hypotension and cardiogenic shock. A parasternal or apical heave (precordial impulse) may be found on palpation as signs of right ventricular hypertrophy or severe left atrial enlargement. A third heart sound may be auscultated. Chest rales and crepitations and a systolic murmur may be present in severe mitral regurgitation, acute cardiac failure, and incipient pulmonary edema.

Diagnosis: Diagnosis is based on the history and typical ECG changes. A 12-lead ECG is mandatory if there is a suggestive history together with a positive clinical examination and the results could determine whether the patient is taken to a specific cardiac unit for active intervention. However, it should be remembered that in the early phase of an acute myocardial infarction (AMI), the ECG might not show typical changes and the diagnosis should be made on clinical grounds.Diagnosis of an acute ST elevation infarction (STEMI, ST segment elevation myocardial infarction) is a severe cardiac emergency requiring immediate transport to the hospital. Non-STEMI (NSTEMI) should be assumed until proven otherwise, and may develop into a STEMI subsequently. NSTEMI is a clearcut indication for hospital admission.

Treatment This should be in accordance with the latest guidelines and local protocols (See Fig 5.2)

1. Secure intravenous vascular access for the administration of IV drugs and analgesia
2. Administer 3–5 mg of morphine intravenously. Morphine can moderately decrease the preload

3. Administer the following:
   a. Nitroglycerine (if the systolic blood pressure >90 mmHg)
      i. Sublingual tablet (0.3–0.9 mg/dose)
      ii. Aerosol (0.4–0.8 mg/dose)
   b. Aspirin (160–325 mg) chewed
   c. Clopidogrel (75–600 mg) according to local protocol
   d. Consider an antithrombin according to local protocols
   e. Monitor pulse oximetry – oxygen should only be administered if the patient is hypoxic

Biomarkers, especially high-sensitive troponin and copeptin, in addition to CK-MB and C-reactive protein (CRP) are diagnostic of AMI but it is unlikely that these would be available in the venue. Fieldside blood collection or testing for troponin is not recommended.

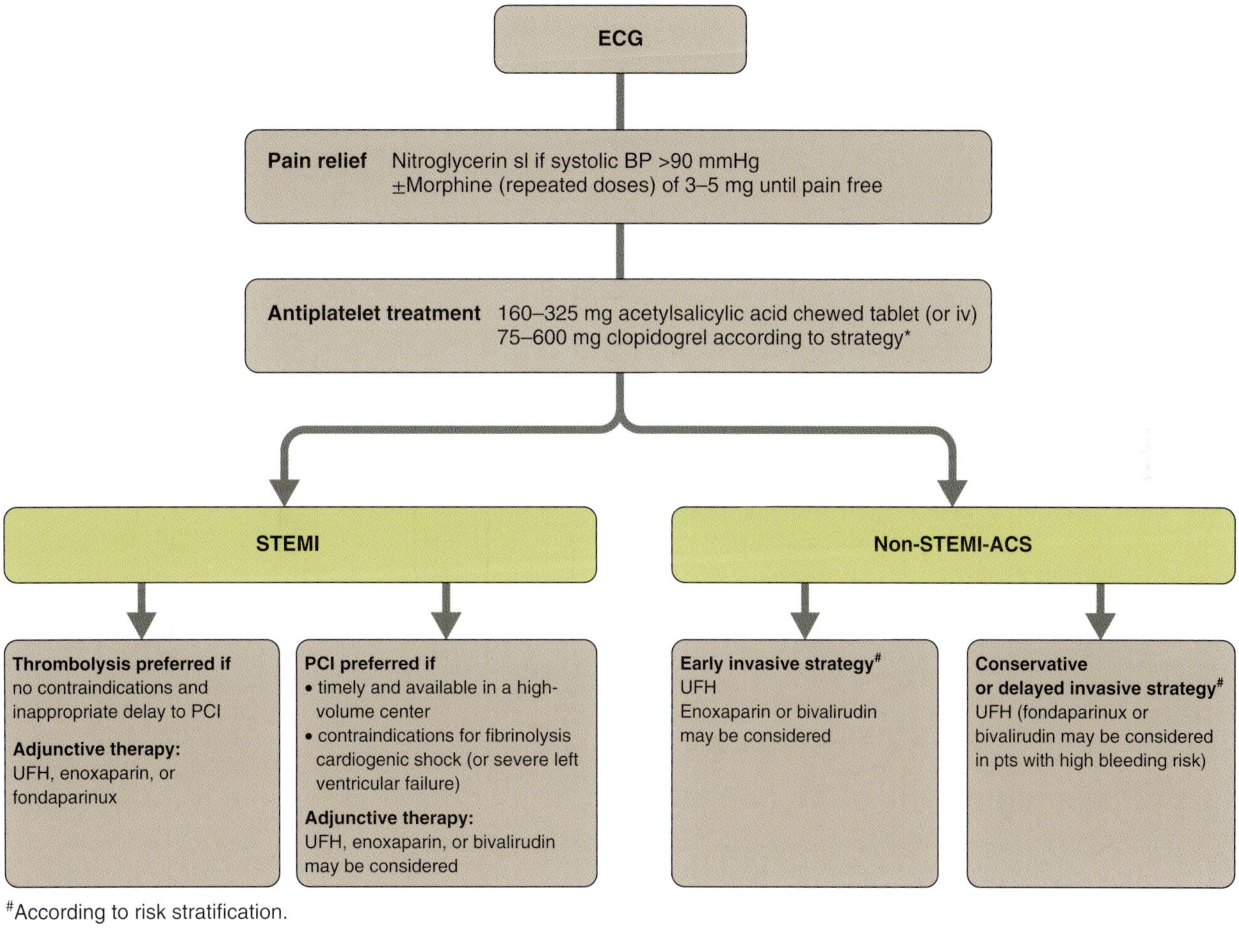

Figure 5.2 The ACS treatment algorithm
(*Source:* Copyright European Resuscitation Council – www.erc.edu – 2014/012.)

Aortic Aneurysm (AA) and Aortic Dissection (AD)

Acute out-of-hospital AA rupture cannot be prevented or treated in most cases and may lead to a catastrophic death. Aortic dissection is most often observed in tall athletes (body height ≥190 cm), for example, basketball, volleyball, or rowing athletes or patients with Marfan's syndrome. It can also be witnessed in cocaine abusers.

Clinical Findings/Management AA or AD

History: May occur spontaneously or after blunt or penetrating chest trauma.

Clinical examination: Pain associated with aortic dissection is characterized by its severity, sudden onset, and location to the back. The patient is often in circulatory failure or a precollapsed state.

Management:

1. Establish full physiological monitoring
2. Titrate high-flow supplemental oxygen to maintain oxygen saturation between 94% and 98%
3. Obtain IV access with two large bore cannula
4. Administer appropriate analgesia
5. Commence fluid resuscitation to maintain a systolic blood pressure at 90 mmHg
6. Arrange for immediate evacuation by stretcher from the FoP
7. If aortic dissection is suspected, transport immediately to a cardiothoracic surgical unit department with an appropriate skilled healthcare professional. Be aware that these patients may rapidly deteriorate, collapse, and arrest if the aneurysm ruptures or the dissection extends and perforates the external wall of the aorta

Pericardial Disease: Myocarditis

Viral myocarditis is often associated with a recent history of a febrile viral infection. The athlete will present with chest pain that will have to be differentiated from the symptoms of ACS. Classically the pain from myocarditis has a sudden onset and may last for hours or days before the athlete presents. ACS pain is typically a crushing pain that worsens with exercise and has a short-time course. It is estimated that myocarditis is a major cause of SCD associated with approximately 20% of deaths in adults less than 40 years old, including young athletes.

Athletes are strongly advised to take medical advice if they have a viral respiratory or gastrointestinal illness and wish to continue their training or before they actively participate in competition.

FoP Management of Myocarditis

History: There may be a history of recent viral infection. Sudden, sharp, stabbing, retrosternal, or left precordial area chest pain that is worse in the supine position or on inspiration pain: the pain may be accompanied by palpitations.

Clinical examination: Typically, a sharp friction rub during systole and diastole is heard on auscultation, which may change with the position of the patient. It can sometimes be intermittent, especially if there is an exudative component of pericarditis present. Heart sounds may be muffled, secondary to presence of a pericardial effusion. Cardiac tamponade may be impending and it is important to transfer these patients to hospital for urgent echocardiography. A pericardial friction rub may also occur during the late phase of a transmural myocardial infarction.

Managment:
1. Establish full physiological monitoring
2. Consider differential diagnosis of ACS
3. Titrate high-flow supplemental oxygen to maintain oxygen saturation between 94% and 98%
4. Obtain IV access
5. Administer appropriate analgesia
6. Remove from the FoP and transport to hospital with full monitoring

Hypertensive Crisis

Hypertensive crisis is defined as a systolic blood pressure of greater that 180 mmHg systolic or 120 mmHg diastolic, often associated with symptoms of severe headache, breathlessness, epistaxis, and severe anxiety. It is important to recognize and treat these crises as prolonged severe hypertension can give rise to stroke, heart attack, and renal failure. Approximately 1–2% of adults with hypertension will develop a hypertensive crisis.

Hypertensive crisis may be seen in paralympic athletes with spinal cord lesions above T6, known as autonomic dysreflexia. Athletes have been known to use this to "boost" the performance. The hypertension must be treated as an emergency as it can result in cerebral stroke. The simplest and usually most effective treatment is to manage the cause and empty the athletes' bladder or evacuate their bowels (see Chapter 23).

Clinical Findings/Management Hypertensive Crisis

History: The patient may complain of dizziness, nausea, headache, an altered level of consciousness (LOC), and may be associated with acute chest pain. Hypertension may cause the patient to collapse.

Examination: There may be a rapid pulse, with very high systolic and diastolic blood pressure measurements taken as part of the basic cardiovascular examination. There may be an altered AVPU (alert, voice, pain, unresponsive) or GCS (Glasgow Coma Scale) score.

Management:
1. Conduct a primary survey on the FoP
2. Remove the athlete from the FoP to the fieldside for further evaluation
3. If the systolic BP is >200 mmHg, the patient should be referred to hospital so that the blood pressure can be decreased cautiously, ideally in an intensive care unit setting, in order to avoid cerebral perfusion disturbances (cerebral stroke)
4. The goal of treatment is to lower the blood pressure by approximately 25% within 1–2 h *in a smooth and controlled manner*
   a. Consider administering antihypertensive drugs such as sublingual nitroglycerine (tablets or aerosol), sublingual nifedipine, or subingual captopril 12.5 mg
   b. Rapid and uncontrolled drops in blood pressure may result in cerebral, coronary, or renal ischemia or infarction
   c. Continue to monitor the blood pressure carefully
   d. In Paralympic athletes consider treating the primary cause (full bladder or rectum)

Acute Cardiac Arrhythmias

Cardiac arrhythmias are usually classified as a bradycardia or tachycardia. The simplest diagnosis on the FoP is by palpating the pulse and noting its rate and regularity. In addition, the athlete may describe irregular palpitations in the chest and a general feeling of being unwell. An ECG will provide more information and document the event.

Bradycardia

Sinus bradycardia with heart rates as low as 30 bpm at rest can often be observed in well-trained endurance athletes with the heart rate returning to normal levels during exercise. First-degree or second-degree heart block may be a physiological finding in well-trained athletes. Third-degree or complete heart block may be congenital or acquired with symptoms developing in patients aged more than 30 years and requiring the implantation of a pacemaker. Third-degree block in otherwise healthy elite athletes is extremely rare.

Clinical Findings/Management Bradycardia

History: Second-degree heart block may induce symptoms at rest such as dizziness, which will disappear during exercise. In outdoor sports, the physician should ask about a history of recent tick insect bites as these can induce bradycardia and will require antibiotic therapy (borreliosis).

Auscultation: A "canon sound" may be heard with third-degree block and alternating heart sound volume may be found in second-degree block.

Management: Follow the bradycardia algorithm (see Figure 5.3) or local protocols. Transfer to hospital for ongoing care early on the management sequence.

Assess using an ABCDE approach

1. Titrate high-flow supplemental oxygen to maintain oxygen saturation between 94% and 98%
2. Establish intravenous access
3. Establish physiological monitoring and record an ECG
4. Identify and treat reversible causes (see Chapter 4)
5. Assess the patient for adverse signs
   a. Cardiovascular shock
   b. Syncope
   c. Myocardial ischemia
   d. Heart failure
6. If there are no adverse signs, then observe and transfer to hospital for further management
7. If there are adverse signs consider the following:
   e. Administer atropine 0.5 mg intravenously
   f. Repeat the dose of atropine (maximum dose 3 mg)
   g. Consider the following:
      i. Isoprenaline infusion 5 mcg/min
      ii. Adrenaline infusion 2–10 mcg/min
      iii. Transcutaneous pacing
   h. Transfer to hospital for ongoing management

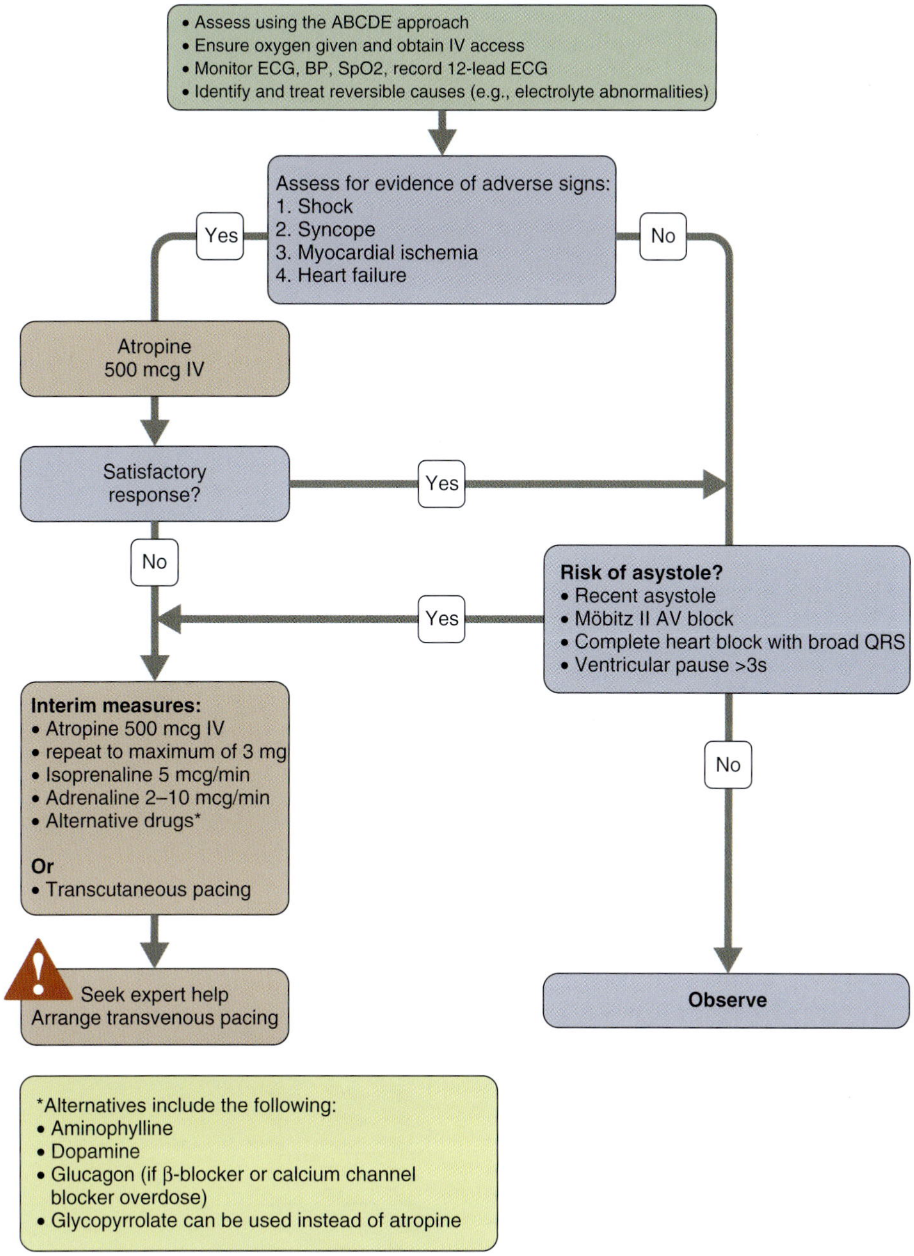

Figure 5.3 Bradycardia algorithm (*Source:* Copyright European Resuscitation Council – www.erc.edu – 2014/012.)

Tachycardia

Many tachycardias are simple and often self-limiting. However, their recognition and clinical management is critical to the overall general medical care, training schedule, and competitive ability of an athlete.

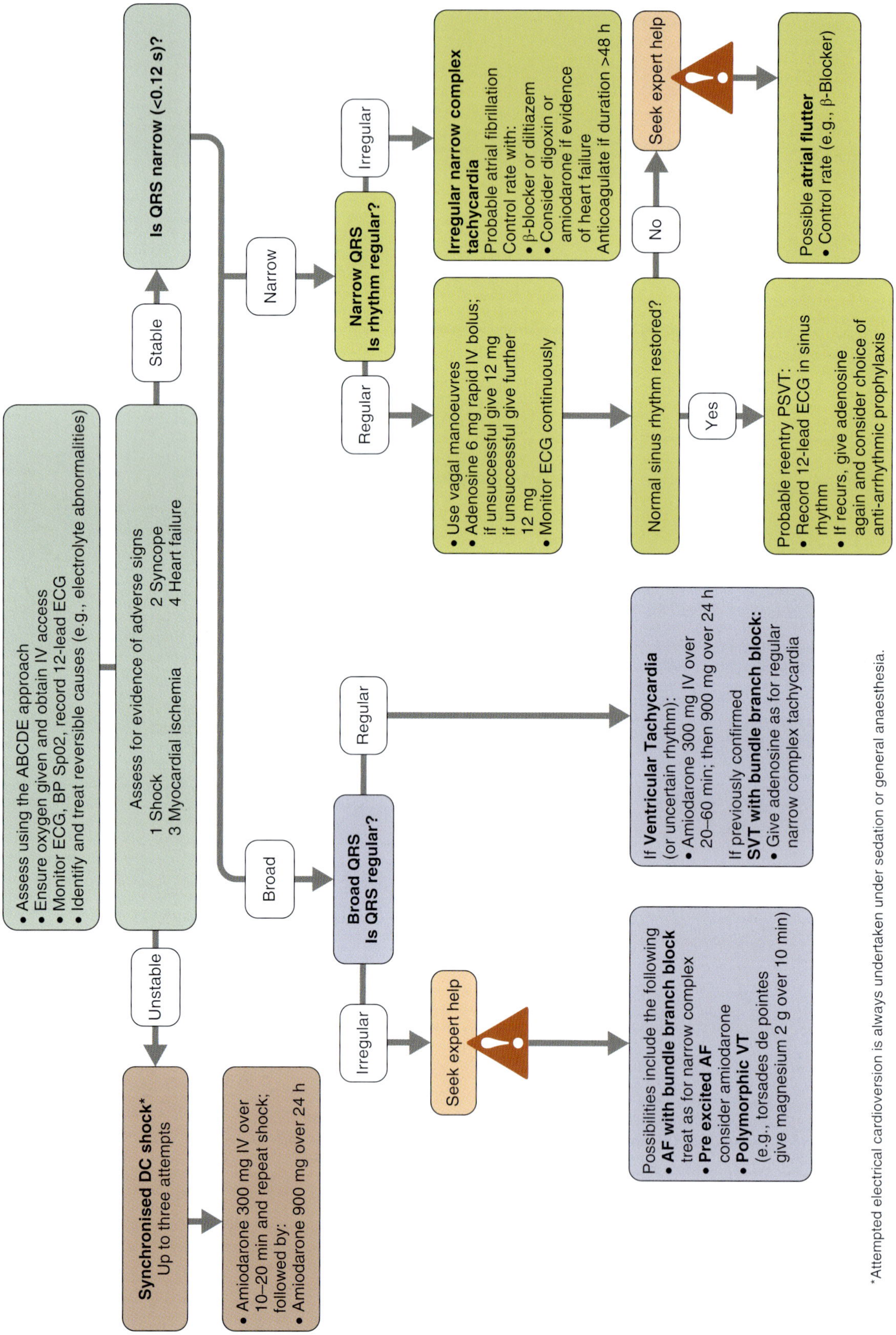

*Attempted electrical cardioversion is always undertaken under sedation or general anaesthesia.

Figure 5.4 Trachycardia algorithm
(*Source:* Copyright European Resuscitation Council – www.erc.edu – 2014/012.)

Clinical Findings/Management Tachycardia

History: Is this a first-time presentation or is there any prior clinical history and previous attempts at acute management. Symptoms include rapid heart beat, anxiety, dyspnea, dizziness, syncope, and even chest pain. The athlete should be removed from the FoP to the medical room for an ECG recording and monitored until the tachycardia has self-regulated or further treatment is required. The event should be carefully documented. In either case the athlete must be referred for a cardiology follow-up before undertaking further exercise.

Treatment: Follow the tachycardia algorithm (Figure 5.4) or local protocols. Transfer to hospital for ongoing care early on the management sequence.

1. Assess using an ABCDE approach
2. Titrate high-flow supplemental oxygen to maintain oxygen saturation between 94% and 98%
3. Establish intravenous access
4. Establish physiological monitoring and record an ECG
5. Identify and treat reversible causes (see Chapter 4)
6. Assess the patient for adverse signs
   a. Cardiovascular shock
   b. Syncope
   c. Myocardial ischemia
   d. Heart failure
7. *If cardiovascularly stable*: the treatment will depend on whether the QRS is narrow or wide. However, in most cases, these patients should be transported to an appropriate hospital for further medical care
   a. In a stable, narrow complex regular tachycardia consider the following:
      i. Vagal maneuvers
      ii. Intravenous bolus adenosine 6 mg, followed by two doses of 12 mg, if each successive dose is unsuccessful under full ECG monitoring. Beware that adenosine may induce short-duration A-V block or asystole and this should only be attempted by healthcare professionals with the required diagnostic and treatment skills
      iii. If treatment fails, transfer immediately to hospital as this may be atrial flutter
   b. In a stable, narrow complex irregular tachycardia consider the following:
      i. A diagnosis of atrial fibrillation
      ii. Controlling the rate with the following:
         - adrenergic blocker
         - Diltiazem
      iii. If there is evidence of heart failure, administer the following:
         - Digoxin
         - Amiodarone
         - *If cardiovascularly unstable*: Consider emergency DC cardioversion – this is an advanced procedure that may require sedation if the patient is conscious. It should only be undertaken by those with the required skill base and equipment
         - Do not attempt treatment unless the treating physician is trained and skilled in the management of tachycardia. In most cases it is simpler and safer to transfer to hospital immediately for definitive care.

Pulseless Ventricular Tachycardia and Ventricular Fibrillation

These life-threatening conditions require the immediate commencement of chest compressions and full cardiopulmonary resuscitation (see Chapter 4).

Bibliography

Nolan, J.P., Soar, J., Zideman, D.A. *et al.* (2010) ERC Guidelines Writing Group. European Resuscitation Council Guidelines for Resuscitation 2010 Section 1. Executive summary. *Resuscitation*, **81** (**10**), 1219–1276.

American Heart Association (2010) American Heart Association guidelines for cardiopulmonary resuscitation and emergency cardiovascular care. *Circulation*, **122**, S640–S946.

Pellis, T., Link, M., Antzelelvitch, C. & Kohl, P. (2007. Ch 63) Sudden death in athletes. In: Paradis, N., Halperin, H.R., Kern, K.B., Wenzel, V. & Chamberlain, D.A. (eds), *Cardiac Arrest*, 2nd edn. Cambridge University Press, pp. 1148–1200.

6 Control of Hemorrhage and Infusion Management

Kenneth Wing Cheung Wu and Hiu Fai Ho

Accident and Emergency Department, Queen Elizabeth Hospital, Hong Kong, China

Introduction

Major hemorrhagic incidents in sport are rare. When bleeding occurs, early intervention is important to prevent deterioration and circulatory collapse.

Fortunately, most of the bleeding wounds seen on the Field of Play (FoP) are minor and usually occur in collision with another athlete or competition apparatus. Many of these bleeding wounds can be managed immediately on the FoP or in the athlete medical room. In most sports, the athlete is allowed to return to play without being penalized for leaving the FoP for fieldside treatment (Rugby Union has the "blood bin" rule allowing athletes to return to play within 15 min after departing the FoP).

Crashes in high-speed sports such as downhill skiing, bobsleighing, cycling, motor racing, or equestrian sport may result in serious trauma. Serious injuries can also occur when a falling horse crushes the athlete and a major laceration or penetrating injury may be caused by sporting equipment, for example, the blade of a skateboot, the edge of a ski, a javelin, or a rifle bullet.

It is easy to make a diagnosis when the hemorrhage is visible. Depending on the size and the site of the wound, the bleeding can vary from minimal blood loss to exsanguination. Quick action is required to control the hemorrhage especially when dealing with an active arterial bleeding (see Chapter 3).

Sometimes bleeding is concealed and may be unnoticed in an internal organ injury. The injured athlete may appear well initially but later collapse with hypovolemic shock. Because recognizing the source of internal bleeding poses a diagnostic challenge in the acute setting of a sports event, a high index of suspicion is required when assessing athletes involved in a high-speed collision or blunt trauma. The mechanism of injury is a key indicator of potential injury. A systematic approach and detailed examination are required to ascertain whether or not the athlete has internal bleeding and if the athlete needs to be transferred to hospital for further

The IOC Manual of Emergency Sports Medicine, First Edition. Edited by David McDonagh and David Zideman.

investigation and treatment. While it is not required to make an exact diagnosis on the FoP, it is necessary to decide whether there is internal bleeding or not and if it is suspected, then to remove the athlete from the FoP and transfer to hospital as soon as possible.

When assessing bleeding wounds, underlying structures must also be assessed for injury, for example, bone, tendons, and nerves. Transfer the athlete to hospital for further treatment if underlying structural damage has occurred.

With the advances in digital technology, USG scanning techniques can be acquired and be applied at the fieldside to detect any concealed intraabdominal or intrathoracic bleeding. This does require training to expert level but it should be remembered that there might not be enough fluid in the cavity in the early stages to detect using USG scanning. The mechanism of injury, clinical signs and a high level of suspicion must remain of the primary diagnostic tools.

FoP Management

Apply the same FoP management principle as described in all FoP situations: SABCDE – safety, airway, breathing, circulation, disability, environment (or exposure). (See Chapter 3)

It is paramount to use Personal Protective Equipment to protect from blood-borne diseases when dealing with any body fluids, and universal precautions are mandatory. Vinyl or latex gloves are essential and wearing glasses or face visors may be necessary with profuse bleeding.

External Bleeding Wounds

Direct pressure on the bleeding site is the standard treatment for all bleeding wounds.

On the FoP, use clean (bottled) water to flush the wound of mud or debris. This cleansing method has been proven to be safe and efficient. Flush the wound with copious amounts of water if the wound is contaminated and use clean gauze to wipe the dirt and debris from the surface of the wound.

To stop the bleeding, put sterile gauze on the wound and apply direct pressure (caution should be exercised when compressing cranial fractures). Do not disturb any blood clot that has formed by exploring the open wound or removing the gauze to check if the bleeding has stopped. Apply a bandage to secure the gauze over the wound; the bandage should be tight enough to stop the bleeding but not so tight that it stops distal circulation if the bandage is around a limb. It is important to monitor the distal circulation intermittently after applying the bandage by checking the color of the limb, capillary refilling time (CRT), and distal pulses.

If the bleeding is profuse or there is an arterial bleed, pressure on the wound may need to be firmer and applied for a longer period of time. On some occasions, consider using an arterial tourniquet to stop the bleeding. A hemostatic suture may be necessary once the patient has been transferred to the athlete medical room.

If bleeding continues and is visible through the dressing and bandages, do not remove the dressings and bandages. If necessary, place more gauze over the established wound dressing to hold it in place or wrap the wound with additional bandages or cling film. Expedite removal of the athlete to hospital for definitive treatment.

Remember to remove all discarded contaminated swabs and dressings and dispose them in an appropriate waste container. In addition, ensure that any blood or body fluid is appropriately cleaned from the surface of the FoP or any FoP apparatus.

New Trends in Hemorrhage Control

New materials in combination with old hemorrhage control techniques introduced during the Gulf War are gaining popularity in prehospital settings. Although these methods are not commonly required in the FoP, they may be considered with severe hemorrhage.

Hemostatic Dressings (Clotting agents)

These come in powder or gel form and can be applied on the external bleeding wound directly or onto the gauze. Agents such as QuickClot absorb all the liquid in the blood, and leaving behind the clotting factors thus accelerating hemostasis. However their efficacy has been questioned. There is a risk of arterial thrombosis, so these clotting agents should be used with caution.

Celox gauze is a high-density gauze impregnated with hemostatic granules that has been proven to be effective in the prehospital arena. Apply the gauze to the wound and bandage securely in place. Do not remove until formal surgical intervention is available.

Tourniquet

Tourniquet techniques have been used to stop extremity bleeding in the battlefield and civilian settings. A tourniquet is applied proximal to the wound and tightened until the hemorrhage stops. The tourniquet should not be loosened or released until definitive surgical care and blood transfusion is available. It is recommended to use specifically designed equipment, for example, the combat application tourniquet (CAT) and that this should be applied by a healthcare professional. Occasionally, it may be necessary to apply a second tourniquet together with hemostatic dressings to establish full hemostasis.

While a tourniquet may be effective in stopping extremity bleeding, there is always the risk of distal ischemia and potential tissue infarction. Furthermore tourniquet may not stop arterial bleeding but conversely impair venous return, thus further decreasing the blood volume. This is usually only seen when the tourniquet has not been applied properly.

In a sports setting, a tourniquet should only be used if direct pressure on a wound cannot stop major bleeding. Having applied a tourniquet, record the time and expedite the athlete's transfer to the hospital. Maintain a written record of vital signs (respiratory rate (RR), pulse, oximetry, blood pressure, and GCS) during FoP extrication, treatment, and transfer.

Internal Bleeding

If internal bleeding is suspected, provide high-flow oxygen through a nonrebreathing facemask and titrate the inspired oxygen to a saturation level between 94 - 98%. Establish full cardiovascular monitoring and intravenous (IV) access. It is important to summon help, activate the emergency services, and initiate resuscitation, if required, as soon as possible. Immediate transfer to the nearest trauma hospital should be initiated.

Sources of internal bleeding include the liver, spleen, and kidney in the abdomen, or from pelvic or long bone fractures. Liters of blood can be lost into the body cavities resulting in the symptoms and signs of shock.

In the case of blunt trauma, the injury can look trivial; the athlete may appear to be relatively stable on initial assessment and may be allowed to continue to compete or even to be discharged from the venue. A high index of suspicion is required and repeated observation and reassessment is crucial to the athlete's continued wellbeing. Written or verbal instructions to the athlete and their coach/team must be given when the athlete is discharged from the venue.

In major pelvic fractures, the pelvis may appear to be both tender and unstable. The lower limb may appear shortened and rotated. Major hemorrhage can occur with venous and/or arterial bleeds. It is important to remember that once a pelvic fracture is suspected, no further examination of the pelvis should be conducted in order to avoid further damage and bleeding from the fracture sites. On the FoP, gently rotate both legs internally and then strap them together with a bandage to reduce the potential space inside the pelvis and thus pelvic volume. A commercially available pelvic splint, a triangular bandage, or a simple bed sheet can be used to wrap around the pelvis to bind and stabilize the unstable pelvis on the FoP (see Chapter 18).

If an injured athlete has been prescribed an anticoagulation medication or has clotting abnormalities, extra care is required and further observation and transfer to hospital is recommended.

Infusion Management

According to the 2014 WADA List, IV fluid infusion is permitted in emergency situations (see Chapter 31). However, it is essential that signs, symptoms, and the reasoning behind all treatments are carefully recorded.

It is difficult to assess the amount of blood lost with major injuries and attempts to do so have little value. Blood loss should be treated, not classified. In the sports setting, the heart rate will usually rise during the competition and recover after resting. In shock, the pulse rate gradually increases and pulse strength decreases. Be aware that in a well-trained and physically fit athlete, the cardiovascular system can compensate for blood loss and the regular signs and symptoms of hypovolemia may be delayed before a sudden and rapid circulatory deterioration occurs. Early intervention and continuous close physiological monitoring is therefore essential. Two large bore venous cannula should be inserted peripherally or alternatively intraosseous venous access obtained if peripheral vascular access cannot be obtained.

Permissive hypotensive resuscitation is now the mainstream of treatment in the trauma patient. The systolic blood pressure should be maintained at or around 90 mmHg with carefully measured and administered fluid boluses. The goal is to avoid the dilution of coagulation factors with large volumes of infused fluids and minimize the risk of dislodging blood clots at the wound site due to a sudden rise in local vascular pressures.

When assessing the circulation, blood pressure monitoring is essential. Place a noninvasive blood pressure cuff on an uninjured limb and take an early (manual) blood pressure. Where it is difficult to get a noninvasive blood pressure, use the peripheral pulses as an indicator of systolic pressure. An absent radial pulse indicates a systolic BP $\leq$ 90 mmHg. Administer boluses of 250 mL of crystalloid using the radial pulse as a guide to determine how much fluid is to be given.

For obvious reasons, the storage of blood products for blood transfusion is neither practical nor recommended on the FoP or medical room. However, some emergency services (especially helicopter emergency medical service (HEMS) services) are now carrying O Negative packed red blood cells and blood products. If there is an obvious need for blood, then the receiving hospital should be prealerted to prepare blood and blood products in anticipation of arrival of the patient in the emergency room.

As blood is usually not available, crystalloid fluid is the preferred choice for infusion. It is relatively cheap, has a long shelf life, and is easy to store. Among different crystalloid solutions, 0.9% saline or Ringer's lactate solution is the most commonly used. Where possible IV fluids should be warmed and general steps should be taken to ensure the maintenance of the injured athlete's core temperature.

Conclusion

The onfield management of hemorrhage requires event doctors to be vigilant and decisive. Although very serious injuries of this type are not common in sport, fast, accurate, diagnosis, and early intervention are essential in the proper management of hemorrhage.

Bibliography

AHA Journals (2000) *New guidelines*. AHA Journal Circulation online., retrieved November 20, 2013 at http://circ.ahajournals.org/content/102/suppl_1/I-77.full?sid=00a464f0-3e39-4e24-bb6a-e7fab0e65e85

Beam, J.W. (2006) Wound cleansing: water or saline? *Journal of Athletic Training*, **41** (2), 196–197.Retrieved on November 20, 2013 at http://www.ncbi.nlm.nih.gov/pmc/articles/PMC1472650/

Fernandez R, Griffiths R. Water for wound cleansing. Cochrane Database of Systematic Reviews 2012, Issue 2. Art. No.: CD003861. DOI: 10.1002/14651858.CD003861.pub3. The Cochrane Collaboration. Published by John Wiley & Sons, Ltd.

Max N (2003) *Blood clotter flopped in Iraq, sold at home.*, defensetech.org, June 11th, 2003. Retrieved November 20, 2013 at http://defensetech.org/2003/06/11/blood-clotter-flopped-in-iraq-sold-at-home/

Rall JM *et al.* (2012) *Comparison of novel hemostatic gauzes to Quikclot CombatGauze in a standardized swine model of uncontrolled hemorrhage.* Report #TR-2012-22. Naval Medical Research Unit, San Antonio.

Smith, A. *et al.* (2013) *Immediate Care in Sport Course Manual*, RFU.

Simpson E, Lin Y, Stanworth S, Birchall J, Doree C, Hyde C. Recombinant factor VIIa for the prevention and treatment of bleeding in patients without haemophilia. Cochrane Database of Systematic Reviews 2012, Issue 3. Art. No.: CD005011. DOI: 10.1002/14651858.CD005011.pub4.

The Cochrane Collaboration. Published by John Wiley & Sons, Ltd.

The American College of Surgeons, ACS/ATLS (2007) *American College of Surgeons/Advanced Trauma Life Support* [26] in Spahn D.R. *et al.*, *Critical Care*, 11:R17, retrieved on November 20, 2013 at http://ccforum.com/content/11/1/R17.

WADA, World Anti-Doping Program, (2011) *Medical information to support the decisions of TUECs*, : 1. Retrieved on November 20, 2013 at http://www.wada-ama.org/Documents/Science_Medicine/Medical_info_to_support_TUECs/WADA_Medical_info_IV_infusions_3.0_EN.pdf

7 Anaphylaxis

Andy Smith[1] and Jerry Nolan[2]

[1]Yorkshire Ambulance Services, Leeds Medical School, Leeds, UK
[2]Anaesthesia and Intensive Care Medicine, Royal United Hospital, Bath, UK

Introduction

The medical team should be fully aware of the allergies, medications, and past medical history within a known athletic population (athletes and management teams). Ideally, this information is readily available with the athlete's demographics and contact details and completed on a pre-prepared information sheet that will accompany the athlete to hospital if required. Use a structured approach to the history, such as the SAMPLE acronym:

1. S: Signs and symptoms
2. A: Allergies
3. M: Medications
4. P: Past medical history
5. L: Last meal and drink
6. E: Events and environment of the injury/illness

The general approach to an athlete with a medical emergency is the same as the approach to a patient with a traumatic injury: safe approach, Airway, Breathing, Circulation, Disability, Environment (or Exposure) (ABCDE). In the context of a medical emergency and collapse, cervical spine control is not usually indicated or required.

Anaphylaxis is a severe, life-threatening, generalized, or systematic hypersensitivity reaction. It is characterized by rapidly developing life-threatening airway and/or breathing and/or circulation problems usually associated with skin and mucosal changes.

Anaphylaxis is typically a Type I IgE-mediated (although many are non-IgE mediated) multisystem syndrome caused by the release of multiple inflammatory substances such as histamine in response to a known or unknown allergen. The release of these substances from mast cells and or basophils is responsible for the vasodilatation, edema, and increased capillary permeability.

Cases of anaphylaxis are increasing in some parts of the world, for example, the United Kingdom with approximately 20 anaphylaxis deaths reported each year. Anaphylaxis is triggered by a broad range of activators. Examples include the following:

1. Insect stings, for example, bee and wasp stings
2. Drugs: e.g., penicillin, nonsteroidal antiinflammatory drugs (NSAIDs), and aspirin

The IOC Manual of Emergency Sports Medicine, First Edition. Edited by David McDonagh and David Zideman.

3. Foods: e.g., nuts and seafood
4. Chlorhexidine
5. Latex: e.g., surgical gloves or equipment

In many cases of anaphylaxis, no cause is found and a significant number of anaphylactic cases are idiopathic, that is, non-IgE mediated. The severity of the anaphylactic attack is often more severe when the athlete has other medical conditions, especially asthma.

Signs and Symptoms

Severe anaphylaxis attacks often occur very soon after contact with the allergen. Reaction to medication can be severe within 5 min of intravenous (IV) delivery, within 10–15 min to insect stings, and within approximately 30–35 min to food, although with some foods, for example, seafood, it can be much shorter.

Using the ABCDE approach, the signs and symptoms include the following:

1. Airway – lip, tongue, pharyngeal, epiglottic swelling, causing the following:
   a. Airway occlusion resulting in difficulty breathing and swallowing and patients who describe "their throat closing up"
   b. Hoarse voice
   c. Stridor – a high-pitched inspiratory noise
2. Breathing – may develop bronchoconstriction from smooth muscle spasm and plugging, resulting in the following:
   a. Greater effort of breathing with increased respiratory rate (tachypnea)
   b. Expiratory wheeze due to the bronchospasm
   c. Cerebral hypoxia resulting in confusion
   d. Lethargy leading to exhaustion
   e. Respiratory failure with signs of cyanosis
   f. Respiratory arrest – if symptoms and signs are not recognized and treated promptly
3. Cardiovascular:
   a. Peripheral vasodilation with redness and feeling warm to touch
   b. Increased capillary permeability with loss of fluid from the circulation (edema)
   c. Increased heart rate (tachycardia)
   d. Profound hypotension resulting in collapse
   e. Possible myocardial ischemia and arrhythmias on electrocardiographs
   f. Cardiac arrest – if symptoms and signs are not recognized and treated promptly
4. Neurology:
   a. Confusion, agitation, and loss of consciousness due to the following:
      i. Hypoxia
      ii. Cerebral hypoperfusion
5. Skin:
   a. Pruritus – extensive itching
   b. Urticaria – hives, nettle rash, wheals, or welts
   c. Angioedema – swelling of deeper tissues (eyelids, lips, and oropharynx)
6. Gastrointestinal tract:
   a. Nausea and vomiting
   b. Abdominal cramps and diarrhea

Skin or mucosal changes *alone* are not a sign of an anaphylactic reaction.

Management of Anaphylaxis

Early recognition and aggressive management can prevent the progression of anaphylaxis.

The steps in anaphylaxis management are outlined in the anaphylaxis algorithm (Figure 7.1). Prompt recognition and early intramuscular (IM) adrenaline are the keys to successful treatment.

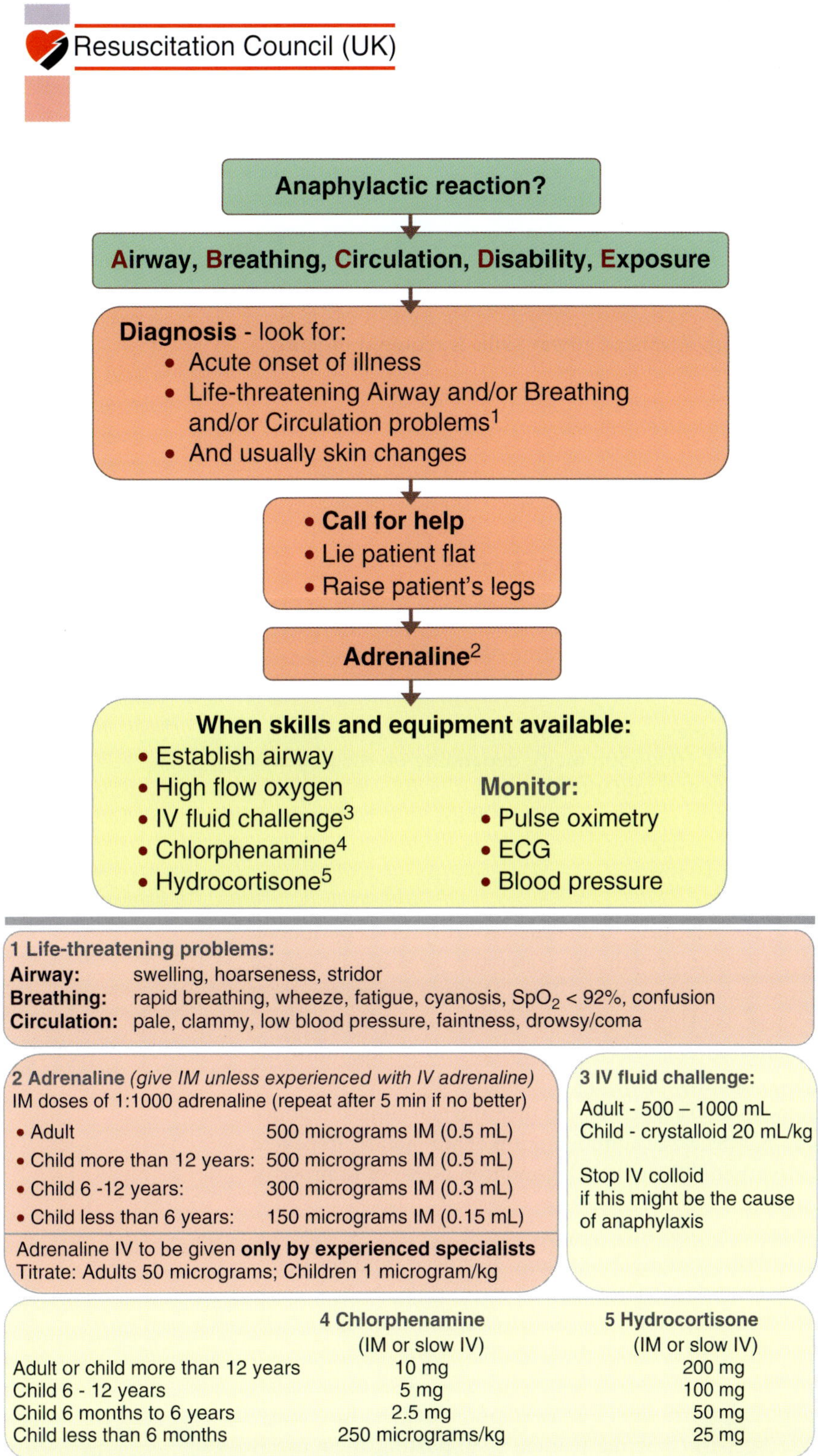

Figure 7.1 Anaphylaxis algorithm
(*Source:* Reproduced with the permission of the Resuscitation Council (UK).)

Use a systematic approach:

1. Check it is safe; ABCDE
2. Treat life-threatening problems as you find them
3. Remove from the Field of Play

4. Remove from any known or potential allergen
5. Get help early
6. Place the patient in a comfortable position; patients with respiratory compromise will often want to sit up to maximize their respiratory capacity. If the circulation is compromised, lying flat with the legs elevated will improve venous return, increase blood pressure, and increase cerebral perfusion. Unconscious patients who are breathing and have a pulse should be placed in the recovery position
7. Give high-flow oxygen via a nonrebreathing mask
8. Airway
   a. Protect the airway early
   b. If there are signs of airway swelling, give adrenaline 0.5 mg IM (as described under circulation below)
   c. Assessment by an individual with advanced airway skills is required urgently
9. Breathing
   a. Observe for the following:
      i. Wheeze
      ii. Tachypnea
      iii. Fatigue
      iv. Cyanosis (SaO_2 <92%)
      v. Confusion
   b. Wheeze will be improved with adrenaline IM (see below)
10. Circulation
   a. Observe for the following:
      i. Pallor
      ii. Clammy skin
      iii. Hypotension
      iv. Decreased level of consciousness
11. Administer IM adrenaline 0.5 mL 1:1000 (500 mcg); depending on the patient's response, further doses can be given at 5 min intervals
12. Obtain IV access and give fluids (large volumes – 500–1000 mL may be required)
   a. Administer IV hydrocortisone 200 mg
   b. Administer IV chlorphenamine 10 mg

Adrenaline is the essential drug in the treatment of anaphylaxis. It reverses peripheral vasodilatation, reduces edema, dilates the bronchi, increases the force of myocardial contraction, and suppresses the release of histamine. The IM route is best for most prehospital practice. Individuals who are known to be susceptible to anaphylaxis reactions may carry and self-administer adrenaline by an autoinjector syringe into the anterolateral aspect of the thigh (Epipen, Anapen). IV adrenaline should be used only by practitioners experienced in the use of vasopressors in their normal clinical practice but establishing IV access should not delay the administration of adrenaline. Repeated doses of IM adrenaline may be required if the patient's condition does not improve or continues to deteriorate.

Give rapid IV fluid challenges of 500–1000 mL crystalloid. Balanced fluid resuscitation based on the radial pulse or systolic blood pressure of 90 mmHg does not apply in anaphylaxis patients.

Hydrocortisone may shorten protracted reactions and prevent reoccurrence (a biphasic reaction). Antihistamines (e.g., chlorphenamine) may help to block the histamine-mediated vasodilation and bronchospasm but the evidence supporting their use is minimal.

If the patient becomes wheezy (with signs and symptoms similar to asthma) and following initial management with adrenaline, consider treating with repeated doses of nebulized salbutamol (5 mg), titrated to effect. If the patient continues to deteriorate, consider salbutamol IV, nebulized ipratropium, and magnesium IV. The vasodilator properties of magnesium may worsen hypotension.

Patients with signs and symptoms of anaphylaxis must be monitored closely and their pulse, respiratory rate, blood pressure, and pulse oximetry recorded regularly. Reassess after giving drugs. At the earliest opportunity, transport the patient urgently to the nearest hospital by emergency ambulance with a healthcare professional escort. Do not "stay and play" if it is possible to "scoop and run."

Airway compromise may occur rapidly in severe anaphylaxis, and advanced airway management may be required early if there are signs of pending airway obstruction, in particular, angioedema with swelling of the lips and tongue, hoarseness, and oropharyngeal swelling. In appropriately skilled hands, consider tracheal intubation early before the airway obstructs, making this procedure difficult. A surgical airway may be required if tracheal intubation is not possible.

When managing patients with severe anaphylaxis, the attending medical personnel should prepare for a possible cardiac arrest. Early involvement of skilled medical personnel is essential at scene or by emergency transfer to hospital.

Athletes who have had, or are suspected of having had an anaphylactic reaction need to be observed by appropriately trained medical personnel for at least 8 h in an appropriate medical facility that is capable of managing cardiac arrest. It is recommended that these patients are not kept by the Field of Play or in the athlete medical room. Symptoms may reoccur ("biphasic" reaction), and depending on the allergen, the risk may last for 24–36 h. In the presence of any of the following features, consider observing the athlete for longer before returning home or to the athlete village/accommodation:

1. Slow onset reaction
2. Those who have asthma or have had a severe asthmatic-type element to their reaction
3. Where there is a possibility of continuing absorption of allergen, for example, oral medication
4. Previous history of biphasic reactions
5. Where access to emergency care is limited
6. Limited ability to respond to deterioration

If there is any doubt as to how the reaction is progressing, the athlete should be transferred to an hospital for continued observation and management.

The postcare plan includes contact with the athlete's team doctor, education of the athlete and their medical team, and referral to a specialist allergy service consisting of healthcare professionals with the skills and competencies necessary to accurately investigate, diagnose, monitor, and provide ongoing management of suspected anaphylaxis. Consider prescribing an adrenaline autoinjector (plus instruction on its use) as an interim measure before the specialist allergy service appointment. Consider a medical alert bracelet or chain.

Bibliography

National Institute for Health and Clinical Excellence (NICE) Clinical Guideline 134 (2011) *Anaphylaxis: Assessment to Confirm an Anaphylactic Episode and the Decision to Refer after Emergency Treatment for a Suspected Anaphylactic Episode*. NICE, London. http://guidance.nice.org.uk/CG134.

Working Group of the Resuscitation Council (UK) (2008) *Emergency Treatment of Anaphylactic Reactions. Guidelines for Healthcare Providers*. Resuscitation Council (UK), London. www.resus.org.uk.

8 Asthma and Respiratory Emergencies

Joseph Cummiskey

Faculty of Sports and Exercise Medicine, Royal College of Surgeons and Royal College of Physicians of Ireland, Dublin, Ireland

This chapter focuses on the emergency diagnosis and treatment of severe thoracic medical problems in the prehospital sporting environment. On the Field of Play (FoP), it is important to be able to diagnose and treat the following conditions, some of which may be potentially life-threatening:

1. Acute asthma
2. Exercise-induced bronchospasm
3. Pulmonary embolism
4. Acute respiratory difficulty due to air pollution

Observation – From Outside the FoP and While Approaching the Patient

During the competition, the doctor should follow the event at all times if possible.

This allows the doctor to observe if the athlete has had a gradual or a sudden onset of symptoms and thus gather important information. Establish if the athlete is injured or has collapsed as a result of trauma. If no trauma has been involved, then one must suspect a medical cause. Especially relevant to this chapter is the question, is there known to be air pollution issues in the event area?

FoP Management of a Suspected Chest Medical Event

Initiate the primary survey following the ABCDE mnemonic (see Chapter 3). Exclude chest injuries, tracheal deviation, wounds in the throat, chest, abdomen and back, chest wall deformities, or asymmetric chest wall movements.

Primary Survey

Inspection: If conscious take a focused history. "Are you in pain," "Where is the pain," "Can you breath properly," and "What happened." Inspect the patient noting if they are or are not conscious (drowsiness may be a sign of brain hypoxemia), able to speak, in severe pain, cyanotic, or dyspneic. It is vital to hear the patient speaking as aspiration may block the upper airway. The patient may just point to their throat. Stridor from a throat pathology may be heard over the larynx as well as over the lungs, sometimes even without a stethoscope. On observation, note if the patient is cyanotic, the respiratory rate, the ratio of inspiration to

The IOC Manual of Emergency Sports Medicine, First Edition. Edited by David McDonagh and David Zideman.

exhalation, the presence of wheeze, and the presence of cough. A barrel-shaped chest is a sign of chronic air trapping.

Place the athlete in the most comfortable breathing position.

Palpation: Palpate the throat and chest for tenderness or deformity. There is usually an increased rate with moderate-to-severe lung disease though this may be due to the level of activity before the event or may be maintained due to pain. Cardiac conditions or hemorrhage may result in a raised pulse rate. A slower than normal rate may be found with cardiac arrhythmias, cardiac tamponade (both reduced rate and reduced pulse volume), and in deteriorating severely injured (often bleeding) patients.

Pulse oximetry has modified the management of airway-related conditions. Place the pulse oximeter on a peripheral digit and monitor the readings. Administer oxygen at a rate of 2–4 L/min if the athlete is dyspneic or the oximeter suggests oxygen is needed. Oxygen should be titrated at a level to keep oxygen saturation (SpO_2) between 94% and 98%. Consider the need for a reservoir bag on the oxygen mask if you have difficulty elevating the SpO_2.

Auscultation: Auscultate the chest to reveal abnormal chest sounds of wheeze or rhonchi often present in airflow obstruction. A silent chest or decreased chest sounds may be a sign of pneumothorax, hemothorax, atelectasis, lung contusion (if several hours have passed), pleural effusion, or severe asthma, possibly accompanied by cyanosis, variable consciousness, or cardiac arrhythmia. Prolonged exhalation, inspiratory, or expiratory rhonchi are typical of airflow obstruction with or without airway infections

Subtle auscultatory changes are often difficult to detect on the FoP and may only be detectable away from the FoP – evacuation of the athlete to the athlete medical room is usually recommended.

Management: Ensure that the patient is fit to move and remove them from the FoP or any polluted environment. Examine the patient in a quiet, well-lit, and secure location. Position the athlete with the chest at a 45° angle to the examination couch to assist diaphragm movement. Loosen clothing to assist air entry. Assess the severity of the condition. If the patient is standing and appears to be fully alert, then a pulmonary/cardiac examination may be made and a decision about return to play made. If the athlete is standing but obviously obtunded, lie them down before you begin your evaluation. Ensure that there is no adverse environmental condition that may have been responsible for triggering an acute asthmatic attack.

Fieldside Management of Chest Medical Conditions

Conduct a secondary survey by reexaming the patient after a few minutes to ensure that no progression or new signs have appeared in the time it takes to move them into a position where treatment is to be administered. If the patient cannot speak and is dyspneic, consider the management of an obstructed upper airway (see Chapter 4).

The presence of crackles or crepitation may be a sign of cardiac failure and pulmonary edema. This can occur from a primary cardiac condition or secondarily from a head injury. The mechanism of head injury causing pulmonary edema is the head impact that gives rise to an elevated systemic BP which then rapidly returns to normal but the after-load increase on the left ventricle causes pulmonary edema that takes longer to clear and may need therapy. Blood pressure may be slightly elevated due to a high activity level at the time of trauma. This can still be the case initially even in the presence of severe internal bleeding. A low blood pressure may be present if the cause is syncopal or if the patient is about to go into shock.

If a patient has had a severe respiratory event with no signs to suggest a diagnosis, a pulmonary embolus (PE), or an exercise-induced anaphylaxis should be considered. A pneumothorax may still be present despite the absence of external trauma signs.

Referred sounds are usually quieter than those generated by an underlying pathology. Bowel sounds can be auscultated in the thorax and their presence may indicate a diaphragmatic injury with parts of the stomach or intestines being trapped in the thoracic cavity. Bowel sounds may also be heard over a large pneumothorax due to the lack of lung tissue. Try to differentiate between referred sounds and sounds from the underlying tissue.

Attach electrocardiogram (ECG) electrodes if there is a suspicion of cardiac involvement. Be prepared to transfer the patient to get a chest radiograph as soon as possible.

1. Anaphylaxis (see Chapter 7)
   Administer 0.5 mg of adrenaline by intramuscular injection urgently and continue to monitor while transferring the patient to hospital. It may be necessary to administer a second dose to ameliorate symptoms.
2. Asthma
   Administer inhaled β-2 sympathominetics until there is improvement or side effects occur. Use either the athlete's own salbutamol- or albuterol-metered inhaler (two puffs of 100 μg per puff every 20 min) or nebulize 5 mg of salbutamol in an oxygen-powered nebulizer (repeat every 20–30 min). It is rare to have to administer intravenous salbutamol and this should be reserved for those where the inhaled nebulized administration is not considered reliable. If the reaction to salbutamol is poor, consider the administration of 500 μg nebulized ipratroprium bromide.

Systemic glucocorticosteroids (prednisolone 40–50 mg by mouth or hydrocortisone 100 mg intravenously) may be indicted for both anaphylaxis and asthma but they should not be used as an initial treatment of the incident. The onset of action of glucocorticosteroids on the vasculature of the lung airways is approximately 1 h.

All patients with anaphylaxis and those with resistant asthma must be referred to hospital for continued observation and management. These patients should be transferred by emergency ambulance with an appropriate healthcare professional escort.

It will be necessary to complete the appropriate WADA paperwork for all patients who receive treatment for anaphylaxis or asthma.

Pulmonary Embolism

This has been called the great mimicker. It can present spontaneously without history or physical signs as a potentially deadly disease. It is said to be the cause of 10% of all hospital deaths. At most it may only present with dyspnea, unilateral wheeze, or pleuritic chest pain without an obvious cause of these symptoms. Classically, the chest radiograph is clear; occasionally a small pleural effusion or classically a wedge-shaped lesion in the parenchyma may be present in large emboli.

A history of air travel for more than 5 h, prolonged rest over days or weeks as with an injury, bed rest due to a medical condition, or recent surgery are predisposing factors. A past history of a deep venous thrombosis (DVT) or PE is also an increased risk factor.

The source of the blood clot embolus is usually from the veins of the legs or pelvis. Physical examination of the legs may only be positive in 12% of patients. Other signs of a large DVT are unilateral leg edema and pain in the calf muscle.

Positive signs of the presence of a large PE are hypotension, severe dyspnea, hypoxemia manifested by blue lips, and expectorating blood with no other obvious cause of these symptoms. In these situations, the patient should be treated nonspecifically. Remove the athlete from the FoP, lie the patient down, give oxygen by facemask, attach full patient monitoring, and refer to hospital as an emergency.

Bronchial Asthma and Exercise-Induced Bronchospasm (EIB)

Asthma is the biggest medical problem in sport. Asthma affects from 3% to 50% of competing athletes. Asthma has no etiological agent. Exercise-induced bronchospasm

(EIB) is manifested by airflow obstruction on exercise only. This form of airflow limitation has a lymphocyte infiltration in the airways, responds differently to challenge tests, and has a lower exhaled nitric oxide as a manifestation of airway inflammation. Clinically patients only have symptoms when they exercise and respond poorly to corticosteroids by inhalation (ICS, inhaled corticosteroids). EIB may occur with atopic asthma.

Athletes with atopic asthma when screened may be positive for the following:

1. Conjunctivitis
2. Allergic rhinitis

There is a 33% chance of a family history of atopic asthma.

Clinical Manifestations of Asthma

Asthma is manifested by episodic symptoms of airflow obstruction often with dyspnea, cough, and wheeze (wheeze can occur with pneumothorax alone). Sputum may be of a thick, tenacious nature. Haemoptyis is a sign of severity, bronchial pathology, or trauma.

Respiratory symptoms such as recurrent breathlessness, cough, wheezing, chest tightness, and excessive mucous production are common in athletes and may be suggestive of asthma. A previous medical history and records of asthmatic attacks may assist in making a diagnosis.

As symptoms alone cannot be relied upon for making a diagnosis of asthma and clinical examination may be normal, objective physiological tests of bronchospasm are required to confirm the diagnosis.

Diagnosis depends on tests that include spirometry (forced expiratory volume in 1 s or FEV_1). Athletes may have an FEV_1 within or above the normal range but this does not exclude variable airway obstruction. If spirometry is normal, supernormal or airway obstruction is present, spirometry should be repeated after inhalation of a bronchodilator to test for reversibility. In the absence of airflow limitation, a bronchial provocation test, to establish the presence of bronchial hyperresponsiveness, is needed. If the results of these tests are negative, the following disorders should be considered in the differential diagnosis of bronchospasm (see Table 8.1).

• Other lung obstructive diseases
• Chronic bronchitis, emphysema, bronchiectasis, and bronchiolitis
• Interstitial lung disease
• Swimming-induced pulmonary edema
• Exercise-induced hypoxemia
• Vascular lung disease
• Hyperventilation with exercise
• Upper airway disease
• Vocal cord dysfunction – paradoxical movement
• Laryngeal prolapse
• Laryngomalacia with inspiratory stridor
• Gastroesophageal reflux

Table 8.1 Differential diagnosis of asthma

Medications in the Treatment of Asthma

It is always wise to check to see if the medication chosen is in the current WADA Prohibited List. (See Chapter 31)

Salbutamol

1. Two puffs (100 µg per puff) from a hand-held inhaler, starting inhalation at the end of forced exhalation, on inhalation hold breath for 5 s
2. A spacer will improve the delivery of the drug as will a nebulizer
3. Two puffs every 20 min until effective or side effects appear
4. Side effects
5. Peripheral muscle tremor especially in hands
6. Tachycardia (see Chapter 31)

The rationale for use of other beta-2 agonists are currently not obvious. The other allowed drugs in 2014 are salmeterol and formoterol. Terbutaline is currently a banned drug. The logical approach would be to allow β-2 agonists that have the least amount of β-3 activity and therefore exclude potentially anabolic agents in high doses.

Glucocorticosteroids

1. If the diagnosis and severity warrant it, administer systemic intravenous use of solumedrone 120 mg IV push stat followed by 120 mg every 6 h or by infusion 120 mg over 6 h.
2. There is an acute effect from IV steroids that can be seen in less than 1 h. This is felt to be an effect on the lung vasculature probably preventing the leakage of serum.

Delivery system for inhaled drugs

1. Hand-held cannisters with fluorocarbons and newer CFC-free canisters
2. Salbutamol, terbutaline, salmeterol, and formoterol
3. Controlled release cannisters
4. Turbohaler for steroid and terbutaline
5. Respiror for spiriva
6. Discus for dry powder salmeterol and flixotide
7. Nebulizers
   a. Steroids, anticholinergics, and β-2 sympathomimetics

Other therapies

1. Inhaled selective β-2s
2. Inhaled steroids
3. Antileukotrienes
4. Cromones
5. Xanthines
6. Anticholinergics
7. Calcium channel blockers
8. Inhaled local anesthetic
9. Inhaled frusamide
10. Anti-IgE antibodies

Drugs that work in various types of asthma

11. With eosinophilic asthma or allergic asthma
    a. Inhaled corticosteroids
    b. Antileukotrienes
12. With lymphocytic asthma or
    c. Airway damage bronchoconstriction due to challenge test
       i. β-2 sympathomimetic

The Effect of Environmental Conditions and Pollutants in Sport Activity

As the Summer Olympic Games are usually held in large cities, it is important for the FoP doctors to have an understanding of some of the outdoor environmental factors that can induce acute respiratory changes either indoors or outdoors (see Table 8.2).

Primary pollutants	
	CO, CO_2, SO_2, NO_2, metals, coal, graphite, and lead
Secondary pollutants	
	Ozone (O_3), HN_3, H_2SO_4, nitrate peroxyacetyl, and other inorganics

Table 8.2 Air pollutants

Several environmental factors are able to influence performances in different sports. Training schedules for top athletes may cause an important stress on the airways. They can increase the respiratory frequency with a 10- to 15-fold rise above the normal resting frequency and increase ventilation up to 100 L/min. At this high minute ventilation, the lungs are exposed to high ambient levels of pollutants, which enhance inflammation of airways. This reaction to allergens in humans is measured as decreased pulmonary function. Hyperventilation itself could be a trigger for exercise-induced asthma (EIA). The increased uptake of pollutants and their displacement to the smaller airways may worsen respiratory symptoms in professional athletes. Although the role of substances such as nitrogen dioxide (NO_2), sulfur dioxide (SO_2), particulate matter (PM), chlorine derivatives, and smoke has yet to be completely clarified, other factors such as allergens and climatic factors (temperature, humidity, and wind speed) have a well-defined influence in inducing respiratory symptoms in the general population as well as in athletes. The proven influence of these factors on the respiratory function of athletes highlights the need for special attention to be paid to the environments in which indoor and outdoor sports are performed. The local Organizing Committee should provide an air analysis derived from historic data and be able to predict abnormal levels of allergens and air pollutants based on predicted weather conditions.

Sports environments may be polluted by exterior pollutants or may be sources themselves of substances able to increase the airway's hyperreactivity. There is evidence that urbanization, with its high levels of vehicle emissions and a westernized lifestyle, is linked directly to the rising frequency of respiratory symptoms in the general population as well as in athletes. An estimated mean increase of 3% in prevalence of lower airway respiratory symptoms and 0.7% increase in upper respiratory tract symptoms every 10 m^3 of airborne PM has been calculated. Furthermore, as concentrations of airborne allergens and air pollutants are frequently increased at the same time, the enhanced airway's inflammation, together with an enhanced IgE-mediated response, can worsen respiratory symptoms in allergic subjects.

The pollutants, mainly derived from combustion engines, power generation, and industry, are subdivided into two main categories: primary (those that do not undergo chemical changes after their origin from a certain source) and secondary (those that are produced through a chemical reaction from natural precursors or emitted from artificial sources (Table 8.2)).

These pollutants cause bronchoconstriction in asthmatics and patients with bronchial hyperresponsiveness secondary to methacholine. They can increase the morbidity and mortality in patients with underlying chronic bronchitis, asthma, and cardiac disease. However, studies from Germany have shown no increase in the prevalence of atopy, hay fever, or asthma in children and adults. SO_2 is dissolved in the surface fluid layer of the airway epithelium and undergoes a variety of chemical reactions to yield sulfuric acid, sulfites, bisulfites, and sulfates. The final common pathway for damage is the release of inflammatory mediators.

Chlorine

Chlorine is a gas commonly used over the years as a sterilization agent for swimming pools and water supplies in general. It is considered as a strong irritating agent for all human mucous membranes, eyes, and skin. Exposure to this gas may cause pulmonary irritation. It should always be considered as a "chemical risk" in all competitive and training aquatic venues.

Ozone $(O)_3$

O_3 is mainly generated from hydrocarbons and NO_2 in the presence of ultraviolet radiation ("LA smog"). Concentrations of 20–40 ppm may occur in the morning, rising to 100 ppm in the afternoon in polluted environments. Ozone may cause respiratory symptoms and increase the annual rate of decline of FEV_1 at levels as low as 80 ppm when exposure occurs over 6 h per day. Ozone causes transient increases in airway responsiveness. EIA is not exaggerated by ozone but allergen responses are and can occur within 1 h in asthmatics exposed to 120 ppm.

Nasal allergen responses, via concentration of eosinophil and eosinophil cationic protein, are increased after exposure to ozone. The cellular and biochemical effects of O_3 are to increase neutrophils and prostanoids, such as prostaglandins E_2 and F_2 alpha and thromboxane B_2. Treatment or prevention is through the use of bronchodilators, antiinflammatory agents, and possibly antioxidants.

Nitrogen Dioxide (NO_2)

NO_2 is a combustion-generated oxidant gas. It is widely present in indoor and outdoor environments. In outdoors it is generated mainly by oil combustion and it is a precursor to particles and ozone. In indoors it is generated by kerosene or gas cooking and heating. Its damage on the airways derives from the oxidation of the cell membranes and consequent inflammatory response. It has an important role both in the modulation of the degree and the duration of the inflammatory response itself. Normal subjects do not have any consistent effects after exposure to NO_2. Subjects with pathologies associated with airway hyperresponsiveness (such as EIB) experience worsening symptoms and enhanced airway responsiveness to methacholine. NO_2 also enhances the airway's response to the hyperventilation of cold air.

Sulfur Dioxide (SO_2) and Particulate Matter (PM)

SO_2 and PM are also combustion-generated particles. They can be considered as the most important components of urban smog. Several epidemiologic studies have demonstrated the association of short-term exposure to these components with transient declines in pulmonary function, especially in children. Particulate matter of less than 10 μm (PM10) is deposited in the lower respiratory tract. They are associated with both SO_2 and ozone smog. They act as vectors to carry the acidity in the particles to the lower respiratory tract. This gives an increase in respiratory symptom exacerbations and deterioration in lung function. PM may also act by an oxidative effect.

These oxidative effects, such as the catalytic actions of transition metals, may alter the viscosity of blood and increase the cardiovascular (CV) risks in patients with previous CV disease. SO_2 is dissolved in the surface fluid layer of the airway epithelium and undergoes a variety of chemical reactions to yield sulfuric acid, sulfites, bisulfites, and sulfates. The final common pathway for damage is the release of inflammatory mediators.

High levels of SO_2 and PM air pollutants may induce bronchitis, giving rise to wheeze, chest tightness, cough, and sputum. They cause bronchoconstriction in asthmatics and patients with bronchial hyperresponsiveness secondary to methacholine. They can increase the morbidity and mortality in patients with underlying chronic bronchitis, asthma, and cardiac disease. Studies from Germany have shown that these high levels do not increase the prevalence of atopy, hay fever, or asthma in children and adults.

Pollens and Other Allergens

Twenty percent of the general population in industrialized countries experience allergies. This suggests that at least 2 out of 10 athletes are at high risk of developing allergic symptoms while competing. Indoor and outdoor allergens can influence sport performances in the form of allergic asthma, rhinitis, or conjunctivitis.

Epidemiologic data indicate that asthma and allergic rhinitis frequently coexist. At least 80–90% of asthma patients reported rhinitis symptoms, and 19–38% of rhinitic patients reported asthma symptoms. The severities of allergic asthma and rhinitis are correlated. Hay fever or pollinosis is frequently used to study the links between air pollution and respiratory allergy. Pollinosis is frequently used to study the links between air pollution and respiratory allergy.

Climatic influences can affect both biologic and chemical components of this interaction. Pollutants, attaching to the surface of pollen grains or of plant derived particles of paucicromic size, are able to modify the morphology and the allergenic potential of these molecules. Airway inflammation is induced by the pollutants. An increased permeability of the mucosal barrier, at bronchial and nasal level, favors the overcoming of these molecules and a consequent allergic response.

Extreme climatic conditions during pollen seasons, such as thunderstorms, can induce severe allergic reactions in pollinosis patients. The rupture of pollen grains induced by a thunderstorm may release their cytoplasmic content, enhancing the number of inhalable, allergen-carrying microparticles.

Positive skin-prick tests were found in 41% of a group of Australian athletes from Olympic sports and in 28% of 118 athletes from the Italian Olympic team. It may therefore be difficult for elite athletes who find themselves participating in competitions which are not determined on the basis of the pollen season.

Therefore, special consideration should be given to aerobiologic and climatic conditions, especially during pollen seasons. The most frequently implicated pollens vary from one country to another. During the 2004 Athens Olympics, an aerobiologic network (www.aeroallergen.gr) was set up to provide information to athletes, trainers, and medical staff regarding the most frequently implicated pollens. In that region, cypress, hazel, wall pellitory, plane, olive, grasses, goosefoot, mugwort, and fungi spores (*Alternaria* spp. and *Cladosporium* spp.) were most common. This kind of data should be made available at least 1 year before major competitions in order to help allergic athletes to achieve the best performances under the correct prophylactic measures.

In indoor sports, athletes should be aware of other kinds of allergens, such as house dust mite (*Dermatophagoides pteronyssinus* and *Dermatophagoides farinae*) and molds in high-humidity environments (changing rooms of swimming pools and other facilities).

Recently, new potential hazards for allergic subjects have been described. Compressed air diving has been shown to increase airway hyperresponsiveness. This can be enhanced by pollens trapped in the scuba tank, which can also induce very dangerous asthma attacks underwater.

In general, the choice of athletes' accommodation without moquette or carpets can reduce symptoms in sports persons sensitized to house dust mites.

Ice Skating Rinks

The use of propane- or gasoline-powered ice resurfacers and edgers raised a concern regarding the indoor air quality in ice rinks. In studies performed in different ice rinks, the ones with propane-fueled machines had a daily mean indoor concentration of 206 ppb, compared to 132 ppb for rinks with gasoline-fueled resurfacers and only 37 ppb for rinks served by an electric-powered resurfacer. Other studies (332 rinks studied worldwide) show a mean for NO_2 level of 228 ppb. World Health Organization (WHO) recommendations indicate a 1-h guideline value of 213 ppb. NO_2 for an indoor arena. Athletes exposed to this contaminated environment show a mixed eosinophilic and neutrophilic inflammation, as well as a high prevalence of EIB and a positive methacholine test. Electric ice resurfacers, increased ventilation, and emission control systems are therefore recommended to avoid the risk of airway hyperresponsiveness-related symptoms in athletes and workers operating in ice rinks. The presence of CO (also derived from ice resurfacers) in ice rinks is also a problem. CO may be adsorbed by athletes, thus raising their carboxyhemoglobin (COHb) up to 1%. An average environment concentration of 20 ppm for the duration of a hockey game (90 min) should be the warning level for indoor skating rinks to avoid dangerous enhancements of the COHb in athletes' blood.

Cross-Country Skiing

It is well documented that dry and cold air exposure, for longer than 5–8 min, is a trigger for EIB. These are the typical conditions for cross-country ski sports (cross-country and biathlon). The bronchial inflammation shows a different pattern in comparison with the classic asthmatic process. The inflammation shows a prevalence of lymphocytes and mastocytes in bronchoalveolar lavage of these athletes. A high prevalence of asthma in winter sports athletes is also shown from various studies.

Bibliography

Katelaris, C.H., Carrozzi, F.M., Burke, T.V. & Byth, K. (2006) Patterns of allergic reactivity and disease in Olympic athletes. Clinical Journal of Sports Medicine, **16**, 401–405.

9 Seizures and Epileptic Emergencies

Geraint Fuller

Department of Neurology, Gloucester Royal Hospital
Gloucester, UK

Epilepsy is a relatively common disorder with a prevalence of active epilepsy of 5–10 per 1000 population. Epilepsy is a collection of diseases but can be broadly classified as being either generalized epilepsy or focal onset (also called localization related) epilepsy. Generalized epilepsies typically start before the age of 21, and patients will typically have tonic-clonic, myoclonic, or absence seizures. Focal onset epilepsies can start at any age and patients can have simple partial seizures, complex partial seizures, or seizures with secondary generalization whose exact nature will depend on the part of the brain involved.

Most patients with epilepsy gain good control of their seizures on anticonvulsants. A minority will have ongoing seizures of varying frequency. Having active epilepsy may prevent or limit participation in some sports, particularly water sports or climbing, depending on the type of seizure and frequency and safety rules of the sport.

Preparation

There are several strategies to consider for patients who have epilepsy prior to competition:

1. Optimize their treatment before competition in conjunction with their treating neurologist
2. Avoid recognized triggers for seizures, particularly sleep deprivation or missed medication
3. Have a treatment strategy for the patient's typical seizures (which may involve some of the treatments outlined in the following)
4. Have an appropriate treatment strategy for each sport

Fieldside Observation

In sport if an athlete falls to the ground after a head injury, then loses consciousness immediately and starts to convulse, this is most likely to be a concussive convulsion. If the collapse and seizure after a head injury is delayed, the seizure may still be defined as a concussive convulsion, but the likelihood of a more serious traumatic brain injury needs to be considered which may require management itself.

The IOC Manual of Emergency Sports Medicine, First Edition. Edited by David McDonagh and David Zideman.

Seizures can be triggered by hypoglycemia. This is only likely to occur in athletes with diabetes. Symptoms and signs of hypoglycemia usually develop over some time and an athlete's performance will usually deteriorate before collapsing and convulsing. However, symptoms and signs may be masked in hardened athletes, particularly those with insulin-dependent diabetes, who for competition purposes, may have reduced their sugar intake, miscalculated their insulin dose, or are carrying an infection. This deterioration may not have been observed by the medical staff, particularly if the event being conducted is an outdoor long-distance sport such as cross-country skiing or a marathon event. Similarly in weight class sports, such athletes may be both hypoglycemic and dehydrated in order to make weigh-ins. Fieldside doctors need to be aware of any athlete who is on insulin and oral hypoglycemic agents.

Observations on Approaching the Athlete

If a seizure occurs during an aquatic event and the patient is in water, then drowning must be avoided by holding the head above the water level even during the tonic-clonic phase. Move the patient to shallow water if possible and then onto dry land once the seizure is over. The likely possibility of aspiration must be addressed when the rescue has been completed.

When approaching an athlete in a nonaquatic sport, the healthcare professional should observe the movement characteristics of the seizure. Classically, seizures can be described according to the different patterns, though in practice the major differential will lie between tonic-clonic seizures and convulsive syncope (see Table 9.1).

	Features	Comments
Tonic-clonic seizure	Tonic phase: the patient goes rigid, with arms flexed or extended. Frequently associated with a groan as air is expelled from lungs. May become cyanosed Clonic phase: limbs jerk. Goes on for a 1–2 min. Usually self-limiting Followed by sleep and confusion	Occur without warning in patients with generalized epilepsy or can be preceded by complex partial seizure in patients with focal onset epilepsy – for example, head turning to one side or one arm extending while flexing the other
Concussive convulsions	Occur immediately after head injury. Often involves tonic contraction of upper arms, with shoulder abduction and elbow flexion – "bear-hug" position. Lasts 2–10 s. May be followed by rhythmic jerking up to 3 min. Self-limiting	These events do not lead to a higher risk of seizures subsequently
Syncope	Usually has prodromal, typically of visual loss. Falls either flaccidly or rigidly. A total of 80% have arrhythmic multifocal or generalized myoclonic jerks that last for less than 30 s. Pale. Pulse is lost in the initial phase	More profound or prolonged hypotension, for example, if the patient is propped up, can trigger a convulsion
Nonepileptic attack or functional seizure	Highly variable. Frequently involves hyperextension of the back (opisthotonus). Normal color. May actively resist those around them. Variable duration, often prolonged. Cardiovascular markers, pulse, and blood pressure, are normal during the episode (a tachycardia will be commensurate with the level of physical exertion)	Initially may be difficult to distinguish from epileptic seizure. Important for those in secondary care to consider

Table 9.1 Classical clinical presentation of convulsive seizure types

Clinical Findings/Management Convulsing Athlete

Local inspection: Look for signs of injury such as bleeding, deformity, foreign bodies, and proximity of potential contact objects such as goalposts and fencing. If the athlete is convulsing, delay the initial primary survey with ABCDE evaluation and initially protect the patient by supporting or cushioning the head during the seizure. Remove any objects from around the athlete that might cause injury.

1. Do not try to put the patient in the recovery position until after the tonic-clonic phase of the seizure has finished
2. Do not try to finger sweep the mouth and do not insert an oropharyngeal tube but remove easily removable mouth guards
3. During the convulsive, inspect the patient and the surroundings for any obvious details of trauma and take a history from those around the incident: was there a blow to the head, is the patient known to have epilepsy, diabetes, or other disorders?

Palpation: Open the throat/neck straps if the patient is wearing a sports helmet (boxing, taekwondo, and rugby) though removal of motorcycle helmets and bobsleigh helmets is not recommended until after the convulsion has finished. Inspection of the head and throat regions is usually difficult and may give little information.

Management: If the tonic-clonic phase lasts longer than 5 min or if there are repeated seizures, then medication should be administered by IV, IM rectl, or buccal routes. Inserting an IV cannula in a convulsing patient may be difficult (see Chapter 10) but if successful administer either:

1. IV – 5 mg diazepam bolus, repeat with 2.5–5 mg increments if required
   or
2. IV – 0.1 mg/kg lorazepam IV bolus, repeat after 10–20 min if required
   If IV access is not accessible, administer:
3. Rectal – diazepam 10–20 mg, and if necessary, repeat after 15 min
   or
4. Buccal midazolam 10 mg, dripping the liquid into the buccal pouch (the recess between the gums and the cheek). The midazolam should not be swallowed but absorbed via the oromucosal route
   or
5. IM midazolam usual dose 10 mg, repeating dose once after 10 min if needed

Both rectal and oral absorption of benzodiazepines requires some time and 3–4 min may pass before seizures start to diminish. If the patient is still convulsing after 10 min, repeat the procedure. By this stage a capillary blood sugar sample should have been taken by pricking a fingertip with a needle and tested using a glucose test strip. Consider administering IV glucose (50 mL of 20% solution) if there are glucose values lower than 2.5 mmol/L (approximately 45 mg/dL). If the patient is hyperglycemic, this is important information when managing a head injury.

Most seizures are self-limiting, but in the case of prolonged seizures or status epilepticus, rapid transfer to hospital is mandatory. IV phenytoin or fosphenytoin is usually effective and if not, the patient will require general anesthesia and ventilation.

Arrange for a direct transfer from the Field of Play (FoP) to hospital and that the healthcare professional escort has the appropriate skillbase.

The FoP doctor should take adequate precautions to safeguard the confidentiality and personal respect of the patient if there is a need to administer drugs by the rectal route.

If possible the athlete should be removed to a sheltered discreet position or if this is not possible, the patient should be screened from public view.

It is also important to remember that the athlete may become incontinent during the seizure and that facilities may need to be provided to allow the athlete to clean themself before returning to the FoP or into the public arena.

Referral or Discharge?

If the patient recovers completely and has no sequelæ after a period of observation, it is appropriate to ask the athlete and supporting team if the athlete is known to have active epilepsy. If the athlete has had one of their typical seizures and is with a supporting team who are confident in managing seizures, then they may elect not to be referred to hospital. However, patients who have had seizures, particularly where this is the first event, should be referred to hospital.

Patients who have had a seizure triggered by head injury will need to be formally evaluated in relation to their head injury.

Differential Diagnoses of Seizures

The most common situation a FoP healthcare professional will face is an athlete having a tonic-clonic seizure.

These need to be differentiated from other causes of loss of consciousness.

Concussive convulsions are an important differential diagnosis for loss of consciousness in sport. Indeed they were first characterized in sport (Australian Rules Football) and are easily recognized as they occur on head impact and are usually brief. The immediate management is as for seizures. It is important to know of their existence as they have a very good prognosis, do not predispose to epilepsy, and will not prevent the athlete from driving or other epilepsy-restricted activities.

Syncope can be difficult to distinguish from a seizure, especially if the patient is supported upright when they may develop a convulsive syncope (also referred to as a reflex axonic seizure). The importance in recognizing syncope is twofold. Recognition of syncope allows the initiation of appropriate investigations, particularly if the syncope occurred during exercise (which may be more sinister). Secondly, it will prevent an inappropriate investigation for seizures and all the associated lifestyle restrictions that this often entails e.g. driving.

Nonepileptic attacks (also referred to as pseudoseizures or dissociative seizures) are psychologically induced events that can be difficult to distinguish from epileptic seizures. Investigation during an attack shows no significant abnormalities with, for example, normal oxygen saturation as well as normal EEG. *A normal EEG does exclude epilepsy.* While it is important to be aware of this entity, this is a diagnosis that will probably be made by a neurologist.

Other Causes

Seizures can be triggered by hypoglycemia and in these patients, usually diabetic patients who are on insulin, correcting hypoglycemia is essential. There are other rare causes or episodes of collapse such as narcolepsy or kinesogenic dyskinesia that will not be considered further.

High-risk sports: risk to life if seizure occurs even with safety measures	
White water kayaking	Bobsleigh
Motor sports	Downhill skiing
Hang-gliding	Rock climbing
Scuba diving	Cycling
Long-distance swimming	
High-risk sports: risk to life if seizure occurs – risk that can be reduced by safety measures	
Slalom skiing	Mountain biking
Single sculling	Water skiing
Medium-risk sports: risk to life if seizure occurs – that can be markedly reduced by safety measures; some risk of injury	
Field hockey	Ice hockey
Ice skating	Football (soccer)
Rowing	Rugby football
Sailing (should not sail alone)	Swimming
Low-risk sports: no risk to life if seizure occurs; risks of injury equivalent to other daily activities	
Athletics	Baseball
Cricket	Golf
Running	Squash
Tennis	

Table 9.2 Classification of risks associated with seizures in some sports. Direct evidence to support this (or any other) classification is lacking

It should be remembered that certain classifications within paralympic sports do have a higher risk of spontaneous epileptic seizure (e.g., Bocca). In many of these, the seizure should be treated as per the routine seizure management (as above) unless there has been specific advice given to the athlete or their carer. In some sports, play will be suspended until the athlete's seizure has finished, allowing the athlete to continue to compete without penalty or disqualification.

Bibliography

NICE Guidance (2008) *The epilepsies: the diagnosis and management of the epilepsies in adults and children in primary and secondary care*. Accessed at http://www.nice.org.uk/Guidance/CG20 Aug 2008 – Excellent guidelines covering the management of all aspects of the epilepsies.

Lempert, T. (1996) Recognizing syncope: pitfalls and surprises. *Journal of the Royal Society of Medicine*, **89**, 372–375. Pivotal study that describes the wide range of changes that can occur during syncope.

McCrory, P.R. & Berkovic, S.F. (2000) Video analysis of acute motor and convulsive manifestations in sport related concussion. *Neurology*, **54**, 1488–1491.. One of a series from these authors that defines concussive convulsions in sport.

10 Head Injuries

David McDonagh [1,2,3] *and Mike Loosemore*[3,4]

[1]*Emeregency Deptartment, St. Olavs Hospital, Trondheim, Norway*
[2]*Faculty of Medicine, NTNU - National University of Science and Technology, Trondheim, Norway*
[3]*Medical Commission, AIBA - International Boxing Association, Lausanne, Switzerland.*
[4]*English Institute of Sport, The Institute of Sport, Exercise and Health, University College London, London, UK*

Head injuries are not uncommon in sports and data from the United States suggests an annual incidence of approximately 3.8 million sports-related episodes. The sports with the highest incidences are American football, ice hockey, rugby, soccer, and basketball. In 2013, the American Medical Society for Sports Medicine (AMSSM) stated that as many as 50% of concussions may go unreported. The vast majority of head injuries in sport can be classified as mild or minimal, according to the Head Injury Severity Scale (HISS) (see Table 10.1) A head injury may also include damage to the brain: traumatic brain injury (TBI) is a nonspecific term describing blunt, penetrating, or blast injuries to the brain. TBI can be classified as mild, moderate, or severe, typically based on the Glasgow Coma Scale (GCS) and/or neurobehavioral deficits after the injury. In mild TBI, patients have a GCS of 15 and no neurological deficits. The term "concussion" has been used interchangeably with mild TBI and minimal or minor head injury; a consensus has not been attained regarding the definition. Other systems are available for recommending when a CT head should be taken (New Orleans Criteria, Canadian CT Head Rule) – see below.

Until recently, our understanding of head injuries (minimal and mild injuries, in particular) has been limited by the relative inaccessibility of the brain within the cranium. Recent imaging development and concerted research is helping to change this. Though severe and most moderate head injuries are usually relatively easy to diagnose (and more challenging to treat) in the acute phase, it can be difficult to differentiate diagnostically between minimal and mild head injuries. It is also easy to score a patient incorrectly when using the GCS, as the interpretation of clinical findings is seldom clearcut. The terminology used has also been confusing with the term concussion,

The scale is based on the GCS but also includes other criteria. The scale has five categories:
Minimal head injury (GCS score 15, no LOC)
Mild head injury (GCS score 14–15 with amnesia or short level of consciousness (LOC) or impaired alertness/memory)
Moderate head injury (GCS score 9–13 with LOC for more than 5 min or with a focal neurological deficit)
Severe head injury (GCS score 5–8)
Critical head injury (GCS score 3–4)

Table 10.1 Head Injury Severity Scale (HISS)

The IOC Manual of Emergency Sports Medicine, First Edition. Edited by David McDonagh and David Zideman.

for many, being synonymous with a loss of consciousness (LOC). Similarly, the terms head injury and TBI are often used. Fortunately, definitions are now becoming more precise, particularly in relationship to concussion, which is now defined as being a subclass of mild traumatic brain injury (mTBI). Conversely, not all mTBIs are concussions. Most experts now agree that a concussion can present with one or several different symptoms and that these symptoms may last for days or even months, so-called persistent postconcussive symptoms (PPCS). Much research is now being focused on defining what concussion is and how it should be diagnosed and managed in the sporting environment (see Chapter 11).

This current and positive focus on concussion must not lure the healthcare professional into considering all head injuries as concussion and the Healthcare professional must remain diligent in diagnosing and managing more severe head injuries before initiating the concussion evaluation. This chapter focuses on the emergency management diagnosis of more severe head injuries.

Sideline Observation

Observing an incident can offer the Field of Play (FoP) healthcare professional clues as to the anatomical location and potential severity of an injury and this is definitely the case with head injuries. If an athlete collapses after a significant blow to the head, then it is reasonable to assume that the athlete collapsed due to the force of that blow and that a potential head injury is present. Even if an isolated head injury is witnessed, the authors still recommend that the FoP doctor conduct a primary survey, starting with ABC before moving on to D (See Chapter 3). The rationale for this is that treatment modalities performed during the ABC processes may result in the brain receiving greater amounts of properly oxygenated blood. Always assume that the athlete has a cervical injury if a head injury is suspected.

However, the primary survey process must be delayed if a patient is convulsing.

FoP Management of a Convulsing Athlete

The fieldside doctor must try to ascertain if the patient has been exposed to trauma. It is usually, but not always, relatively easy to discern if an athlete has suffered a "knockout" or LOC. However, there are many nontraumatic causes of seizure such as hypoglycemia, intracranial bleeding, epilepsy, and intracranial pathology. In the phase immediately after a blow to the head, the patient may be unconscious, frothing at the mouth, making strange snorting or snoring noises with the whole body shaking with convulsive movements. These findings are typical for posttraumatic convulsions and are usually self-limiting and easily recognizable. Such convulsions often involve tonic contractions of the upper arms, with shoulder abduction and elbow flexion, "bear-hug" position, lasting for 2–10 s before being followed by rhythmic jerking for up to 3 min. The prognosis after a single traumatic convulsion is usually very good and does not appear to predispose to epilepsy and thus should have no consequences for the athlete's long-term ability to drive a car, work at heights, and so on (See Chapter 9).

As most convulsive episodes end peacefully within 2–3 min, the FoP Medical Team should use these minutes to observe the patient, usually while kneeling beside the patient, until the episode has ceased. Intervention is usually not recommended while the patient is convulsing.

The FoP team member will often experience this convulsive period as being inordinately long particularly if the event is being shown live on television. If media are present, it is advisable to quickly arrange screening from the audience and cameras. Patient management must never be compromised for television coverage.

It is advisable that the Emergency Doctor (ED) conducts a rudimentary primary survey, primarily based on inspection findings, before initiating more active intervention after the convulsions have ceased. If the convulsion is prolonged (5 min or more), consider administering benzodiazepines such as diazepam or midazolam. The preferred route of administration is rectal and is easily achieved when the patient is in the recumbent position. However, such a procedure may pose obvious privacy challenges if on an open FoP such as a tennis court or in boxing ring. The athlete needs to be covered in some way and privacy respected. Buccal spray is also an option but not always easy to administer if the mouth is clenched. Inserting an intravenous cannula in a convulsing patient is advised, but may be difficult in inexperienced hands. Do not attempt to move the convulsing athlete away from the FoP until convulsions have ceased.

Primary Survey – Convulsing Patient

If the patient is convulsing, evaluation of the airway and breathing is difficult. In the unlikely event of the athlete convulsing in a sitting position, carefully place the athlete into the recovery position. As the patient is making noises and moving, assume that the patient has some form of breathing and circulation. If the patient has a loose mouthguard try to remove this but surrender quickly if the patient resists. Never attempt a mouth sweep, jaw thrust, or an oropharyngeal tube insertion until the convulsion has ended, as these actions may induce vomiting in the patient. The ED also risks being bitten on the fingers. Bite sticks are no longer recommended. If possible and if needed, simple superficial suction of secretions or blood may help to keep the airway clear and assist in breathing. During a convulsion it is difficult to evaluate both Circulation (C) and Disability (D). For Exposure (E), look for obvious signs of external injury. If there is hemorrhaging, manual compression may be attempted. Many experts recommend turning the patient, with cervical spine support, into the recovery position in order to prevent aspiration after vomiting (See Chapter 3). Delay application of a neck collar until seizures have ceased. Wait until the convulsion has ceased before initiating a formal primary survey.

Oxygen may be administered if deemed necessary or if the convulsion is becoming prolonged.

Once the convulsion ceases, the patient may suddenly regain consciousness, often with a startled "what happened?" expression. Remove mouthguards once the convulsion ceases. It is often wise to give patients some minutes to recover, as they are usually confused and easily irritated. Speak gently to the patient and offer supplemental oxygen. If an oxygen mask has been placed over the mouth, it is often wise to remove the mask as the athlete awakens, some athletes rip off these masks in their confusion. Advise the athlete to remain lying down and inform them that you intend to stretcher them from the FoP. Cover the pelvic region with a towel or blanket if there are visible signs of incontinence. Sometimes athletes refuse both a stretcher and physical assistance while being escorted to the sideline. It is not unusual for these athletes to fall over a second time or to be extremely unbalanced while leaving the FoP after a head injury. The ED should recommend stretcher transport or should at least lend an arm while escorting an athlete from the FoP. Always demand a sideline evaluation after a head injury. International Federations (IFs) have different rules and practices regarding sideline concussion evaluations and return to play issues.

On rare occasions, the patient may remain unconscious after the convulsion ceases. The primary survey must now be performed. An inability to be aroused may be due to the effect of benzodiazepines, if they have been administered, but is more likely to be due to the presence of a more serious brain injury. Prolonged LOC must always be interpreted as a very serious finding and is often associated with a critical injury or illness. Unconscious athletes have often snoring like noisy breathing, so it is essential that the mouth be inspected for foreign bodies and that these are removed. Once the convulsion ceases, Open the airway with a chin lift or jaw thrust maneuver, taking into consideration any possible cervical spine injury. Clear the airway of any obstruction and if the noisy breathing continues, reposition the airway maneuver, consider a foreign body or an airway injury. Similarly, under the (E) investigation, remember that hypoglycemia may induce convulsions.

FoP Management of a Nonconvulsing Athlete with a Head Injury

The ED has limited diagnostic resources available and hence the main task is to identify potentially serious ABC and cervical spine pathology, to initiate correct management and evacuate the patient to a neurosurgical unit as soon as possible.

Primary Survey on the FoP

ABC as described in Chapter 3.

Look for seizures and try to evaluate the movements.

An alert, verbal stimuli response, painful stimuli response, or unresponsive (AVPU) evaluation should be conducted, but a further more detailed neurological evaluation should be delayed until the patient has been evacuated to the sideline.

If a head or neck injury is suspected, apply inline cervical spine immobilization and a semirigid cervical collar.

The patient should be turned to the recovery position with spinal precautions.

Maintain airway, respiratory, or ventilation support while transferring the patient to the sideline.

FoP Management of Head Injury with a Low GCS

On rare occasions, the athlete may suffer a serious head injury and have a low GCS. Classically this is described as a GCS less than 7.

In these cases, it may be necessary to ensure a patent airway initially using an oral or nasopharyngeal airway (see Chapter 4) or, in exceptional circumstances, performing an advanced airway maneuver. The advanced airway procedure should only be attempted by those with an adequate skillbase to perform a rapid sequence induction (RSI) of anesthesia and tracheal intubation or insertion of a supraglottic airway (LMA, laryngeal mask airway), plus maintenance of anesthesia to definitive medical care. Further descriptions of RSI procedures are beyond the scope of this book and should be performed according to local protocols.

Management of Head Injury with a GCS 12–14 on the FoP

The management of an athlete with a GCS 12–14 is a complex matter. Many of these patients have suffered a severe blow to the head and are confused and often aggressive. Many of these reactions are indicators of hypoxic brain damage. It may be necessary to exert control before the athletes harm themselves or others. Some clinicians have advocated sedation. However, this does not deal with one of the major underlying problems, hypoxia. It is therefore recommended that a Rapid Sequence Intubation (RSI) is performed with the insertion of an advanced airway device, but this should only be attempted by healthcare professionals with the required skillbase for both RSI and maintenance of anesthesia. RSI procedures are beyond the scope of this manual and should be performed according to local protocols.

Fieldside Evaluation

Once at the sideline, the doctor should repeat the primary survey, initiate monitoring, and then immediately conduct a secondary survey. After a head injury, this survey should include the following:

1. Examining the pupils for size, equality, and light reflex
2. Glasgow Coma Scale
3. Examining for cranial fractures, deformities, binocular hematomas, Battles sign, and cerebrospinal fluid (CSF) leakage
4. Otoscopy for blood (or blood behind an intact eardrum may indicate a basal fracture)
5. Neck pain, neck tenderness, and cervical range of motion (ROM)
6. A focused medical history

Secondary Survey at the Fieldside

Inspection: Inspect the scalp, skull, and face, looking for cuts, bruises, and deformities. Look for CSF and/or blood leakage from the ears, mouth, and nose. A bleeding nose may indicate a nasal fracture but also a fracture at the base of the cranium. If bleeding from the ear is observed always, suspect a cranial basilar cranial fracture. Battle's sign or binocular hematomas may develop after a basilar fracture, though some time may elapse before these signs manifest themselves clinically. Large swellings may indicate a fracture. The incidence ofTBI is increased with cranial fracture.

Palpation: Palpate gently for indentations or depressed skull fractures. There is always a danger of pushing loose fracture fragments further into the brain if unnecessary pressure is applied.

Neurological evaluation: Conduct a rapid neurological evaluation. Most doctors use the Glasgow Coma Score and record the result and time of the evaluation.

Focused history: If conscious, enquire about the sports event and judge if the athlete has amnesia. Enquire about a sweet taste of sugar in the mouth or palate. This may be due to CSF leakage.

If relatively pain free, conduct a gentle test of cervical spine range of movement but stop if pain or resistance is noticed (see Chapter 19).

If alert, responsive, stabile, pain free, and able to stand and walk unassisted, conduct a sideline concussion evaluation. There are several systems available including the Sport Concussion Assessment Tool (SCAT) card. This examination should include a symptoms checklist, cognitive evaluation (including orientation, past and immediate memory, new learning, and concentration), balance tests, and further neurological physical examination (See Chapter 11).

The AMSSM also commented that while standardized sideline tests are useful, there is limited documentation regarding the sensitivity, specificity, validity, and reliability of these tests in different ages and cultural groups and it questions their usefulness in the absence of baseline tests.

Management of Patients with Head Injuries

The treatment goal is complete and rapid physiologic resuscitation, by ensuring a patent airway, optimal respiration, and circulation. Continuous high-flow oxygen is recommended if no pulse oximeter is available; otherwise titrate to 94–98% oxygen saturation. Once the patient's ABC have been stabilized, rapid transport to a designated neurotrauma center should be instigated if a serious head injury is suspected.

Hypoxia and/or hypotension dramatically increase the mortality in patients with severe head injury. It is therefore important to monitor the patient's breathing and blood pressure.

Establish intravenous access and strive to ensure normotension.

Stop scalp bleeding and cover cranial wounds. Always suspect a cervical injury in the head-injured athlete and apply a semirigid cervical collar. Use head blocks if normal practice and transport with spinal immobilization using a spinal board/scoop stretcher/vacuum mattress following local guidelines.

Do not remove penetrating intracranial foreign bodies; bleeding will most likely worsen if these are removed.

Elevation of the head and upper body during transport is still recommended, though data supporting this procedure is not definitive. Protect the cervical spine as best as possible.

Continuous monitoring of the AVPU or GCS and rapid evacuation to a neurotrauma unit is essential.

Control of Intracranial Pressure

Severe head injuries may result in rises in intracranial pressure (ICP). These rises can be detrimental and should be controlled if possible. Simple procedures such as minimizing pain, preventing straining or coughing, and ensuring a patent airway (thereby minimizing hypoxia or carbon dioxide retention) may result in the need for induction of anesthesia and RSI if the professional skillbase is adequate. If anesthesia is induced, then it is recommended controlling ventilation to an expired carbon dioxide of 30 mmHg or 4.0 kPa ($PaCO_2$ of 4.5 kPa) to optimize cerebral vascular tone.

In some medical services, the administration of intravenous mannitol or hypertonic saline (6 mL/kg) is recommended to those patients showing the following:

1. Unilateral or bilateral pupil dilation and a GCS < 8
2. Progressive hypertension and bradycardia with a GCS < 8

Note on Glucocorticosteroids

The USA National Guideline Clearinghouse states that glucocorticoids are not generally accepted to improve the outcome with TBI; they do not appear to decrease ICP and do not decrease mortality.

Pupil Examination

Examining the pupils is an essential part of every neurological evaluation. In most normal healthy patients, both pupils have a similar diameter and react equally to light. However, some 20% of normal individuals have unequal pupils (essential anisocoria), though both pupils will react to the light reflex relatively proportionally. If a patient has fixed pupils, be they dilated or constricted, then suspect serious pathology. Classically, fixed constricted pupils are seen with opioid intoxication (unlikely to be seen in competing athletes).

In a trauma patient, the finding of one or both dilated pupils (or a difference in reaction) should cause the healthcare professional to suspect an intracranial hemorrhage.

It may be difficult to assess the patient's light reflex in bright outdoor sunshine as the normal pupil will be constricted. This is also the case in the dark, if a torch has to be used to visualize the eye before using another light source. The healthcare professional should repeat these reflex tests on entering an area with an "acceptable" level of lighting.

Glasgow Coma Scale

The GCS is almost universally accepted as being a reliable, if not perfect, rapid emergency neurological evaluation system, though it has several widely criticized shortcomings, such as the following:

1. Periorbital/ocular trauma or edema may affect eye response evaluation
2. Mandibular/throat trauma or edema may affect verbal response
3. Spinal cord, plexus, or peripheral nerve injury may affect motor response
4. The noninclusion of brain stem and pupillary reflexes
5. The difficulty some healthcare responders have in correctly evaluating the motor response

Despite these critiques, many believe the score to be the best system available for rapidly evaluating consciousness in the prehospital environment.

On occasions, a conscious patient cannot open their eyes due to swelling after trauma or edema. The E score may thus be invalid, but such swelling would imply major trauma and the possibility of a basilar or facial fracture and thus the need for urgent stabilizing treatment and referral (or if edema, the possibility of anaphylaxis).

If impossible to test the E response due to injury, one should still continue to measure the V and M response.

Eye-Opening (E Score – Maximum Score of 4)

By evaluating the patient's eye movements, the healthcare professional can assess the patient's arousal level:

1. The eyes open spontaneously – Example – the patient may have closed eyes due to pain, but opens spontaneously on command – "Hello, are you awake? Open your eyes!"– the patient does so immediately – Score 4E
2. The eyes open on verbal command – Example – the patient has closed eyes, does not open them spontaneously, but opens them after *repeated* commands: "Hello – Open your eyes! Do you hear me, open your eyes!" – Score 3E
3. The eyes open after a painful stimulus – Example – the patient does not open the eyes despite repeated verbal commands, but does so in response to application of a painful stimulus such as trapezium squeeze (caution when applying all painful stimuli) – Score 2E
4. The eyes do not open to verbal or painful stimuli – Score 1E.

Verbal Response (V Score – Maximum Score of 5)

After testing the patient's arousal ability, the next phase is to measure the patient's awareness.

Start the process by asking relevant orientated questions: "What is your name?" "Where are we?" (Maddock's questions are excellent here)

1. *Orientated*: If the patient answers correctly, a Score of 5V is awarded
2. *Confused*: The patient can formulate sentences and words but the answers to the questions are obviously wrong, a score of 4V is awarded
3. *Inappropriate*: The patient cannot articulate sentences, just a few words that do not answer the question appropriately – Example – "What is the score in this match?" the patient answers incorrectly with words that have no relationship to the question, often just swear words – Score 3V
4. *Incomprehensible sounds*: The patient answers with grunts or groans – Score 2V
5. *No response*: Despite both verbal and physical stimuli – Score 1V

Motor Response (M Score – Maximum Score of 6)

The final assessment is of the patient's motor response to verbal and pain stimuli.

1. *Obeys commands*: The doctor makes two commands which the patient completes – Example – " Squeeze my finger" and repeat "Do it again" – a score of 6M is awarded
2. *Localizes to central pain*: The patient does not respond to a verbal stimulus but responds appropriately to a painful stimulus – Example – by pricking the abdominal wall with a needle, the patient purposely moves the arm to remove the needle away from the abdomen. This gives a score of 5M
3. *Withdraws from pain*: Example – by pricking the abdominal wall with a needle, the patient may shift a little or just move an arm toward the source of the pain but fails to locate the source of the pain. Score 4M
4. *Flexion to pain*: The patient flexes the elbow and internally rotates the shoulder, bringing the forearms to the chest, even clenching the fists. Score 3M
5. *Extension to pain*: The patient extends the elbow and may be associated with internal shoulder, wrist rotation, extending the head backwards, and extending the legs and toes. Score 2M
6. *No response to painful stimuli*: Score 1M

It takes practice to be proficient in correctly identifying a correct GCS score, in particular, with evaluating the motor (M) segment.

A score of *14–15 pts* indicates a mild head injury. The patient is awake, has partial or total orientation, with no or minimal neurological findings, though may have headache, nausea, and vomiting.
9–13 pts indicates a moderate head injury. The patient will have reduced consciousness, performs on command, can be conscious, but may have focal neurological findings. These patients may deteriorate and need urgent referral to an appropriate hospital after oxygen has been administered and the spinal column has been adequately immobilized.
A patient with a GCS score of *4–8 pts* has a severe head injury, has significantly reduced consciousness, is unable to follow command, and is a critically ill patient. These patients may need an advanced airway intervention.
When a patient has a score of *3 pts*, the patient is clinically unresponsive and is deeply unconscious or not alive. They all require advanced medical care and interventions but some patients with a GCS score of 3 pts can recover.

Table 10.2 GCS Scoring

When summarizing the score, include each response in your total (GCS 14 – E4, V4, M6). Some neurosurgeons place more value on the individual E, V, M response scores than on the total accumulative score. Be aware that being proficient in performing a correct GCS evaluation requires practice on a regular basis, particularly when evaluating the various forms of flexion in the M response. There is some discussion around what constitutes an adequate or correct painful stimulus and to which anatomical site it should apply. Some sources advocate pressing a pencil on a finger nail, others prick the skin with a needle, while others recommend applying pressure to the supraorbital ridge, pinching the trapezius muscle or pressing knuckles on the sternum, or combinations of these to differentiate between localization.

Be aware that the patient must understand the doctor's language and instructions otherwise scores may not be representative!

Follow locally accepted practice and guidelines, but as always use common sense and remember "Primum non nocere – do no harm!"

Binocular Hematomas - Raccoon Eyes

The presence of bilateral periorbital ecchymosis, also called binocular hematomas, usually indicates the presence of a frontal base of the cranium fracture.

The cornea is clear and white as opposed to the blood red coloration seen with subconjunctival hemorrhages (which are not usually associated with trauma, though they can occasionally be seen with craniofacial fractures due to venous seepage from meningeal tears). Periobital ecchymosis may take several days to develop and are not always immediately obvious on inspection. If present, they should alert suspicion. Similarly, the presence of a similar discoloration behind the ear (Battle's sign or periauricular ecchymosis - see below) should alert the healthcare professional to the possible presence of a basilar fracture. If found and if the patient is alert, the healthcare professional should advise the patient to refrain from vigorously coughing or blowing his/her nose, as these activities may further worsen the tearing of the meninges.

Battles Sign

Battle's sign – or mastoid ecchymosis, indicates a posterior cranial basilar fracture, but its absence does not exclude a fracture.

CSF Leakage

In certain fractures of the cranium where there is damage to the dura, CSF may leak from the nose or ear. It can be difficult to identify CSF, as there is often also concomitant bleeding from the nose or ears. If a urine dipstick is dipped into this fluid, a positive reading for glucose may indicate the presence of CSF in the fluid leakage, thus indicating a cranial fracture.

A Focused Medical History

A medical history should be taken from the conscious patient and information should also be requested from nearby trainers, spectators, or others either during the secondary survey or even after the patient has been sent to hospital, if time is of the essence. Important information can then be forwarded to the hospital. Relevant data includes the following:

1. Time of accident
2. Cause of accident and injury mechanism
3. LOC – description by patient and/or observers and time involved
4. Amnesia – before the incident, after the incident, and time involved
5. Observed seizures
6. Vomiting – how many episodes
7. Nausea, headache, parasthesia, and weakness
8. Visual defects
9. Symptoms indicative of injury to other organs
10. Previous injuries and illnesses
11. Allergies
12. Medications – such as warfarin and aspirin
13. Family history of stroke/subarachnoid bleeding/bleeding disorders
14. Alcohol/drugs, and so on

Transfer to the Hospital

If the patient is still lying on a spinal board/scoop/vacuum mattress, the head end of the stretcher bed may be elevated so that the head is higher than the heart.

The patient should preferably not lie on a wound or fracture site.

Continuous respiratory, circulatory monitoring, and neurological evaluation is essential; use a checklist and inform the neurotrauma unit of any deterioration in status.

Do not allow the patient to become hypotensive or hyperglycemic as this may compromise cerebral perfusion.

Ensure careful lifting and movement of the patient, maintaining correct cervical and spinal immobilization until spinal trauma can be safely excluded.

Contact with Hospital

Before initiating the transport, inform the neurotrauma unit of the patient's condition and expected time of arrival, so that the trauma team can be prepared.

When Should the ED Request a Cranial CT?

There are many varying recommendations around the world, not only from country to country, but even from specialty to specialty (radiology, neurology, or neurosurgery). It is therefore difficult to recommend one guideline when writing for an international audience. The best advice is to follow local guidelines.

Canadian CT Head Rule - High Risk of Hemorrhage

The "Canadian CT head rule" states that there is a high risk of finding hemorrhage on a cranial CT if there is following:

1. A witnessed LOC
2. A definite amnesia or witnessed disorientation in a patient with a GCS score of 13–15 with any one of the following:
   a. High risk (for neurological intervention)
   b. GCS score <15 at 2 h after injury
   c. Suspected open or depressed skull fracture
   d. Any sign of basilar skull fracture: hemotympanum, binocular ecchymosis, otorrhea or rhinorrhea, and Battle's sign (ecchymosis of the mastoids)
3. Two or more episodes of vomiting
4. Age 65 years or older

Canadian CT Head Rule - Medium Risk of Radiographic change

The "Canadian CT head rule" suggests that there is medium risk for finding radiographic changes on CT if there is following:

1. Amnesia >30 min before impact (retrograde amnesia)
2. A dangerous mechanism (pedestrian struck by motor vehicle, occupant ejected from motor vehicle, and fall from height of >3 ft or five stairs)

The New Orleans Criteria

The New Orleans Criteria is used to predict which concussed patients are likely to have an intracranial hemorrhage when a head CT has been taken. These criteria recommend that a CT be taken if the following criteria are present:

1. A LOC
2. A GCS of 15
3. Normal findings after a brief neurological examination
   And any one of the following:
4. Headache
5. Vomiting
6. Age >60 years
7. Drug or alcohol intoxication
8. Persistent anterograde amnesia (deficits in short-term memory)
9. Evidence of traumatic soft tissue or bone injury above clavicles or seizure (suspected or witnessed)

Scalp Lacerations and Bleeding

Scalp wounds may, on occasion, bleed profusely and this blood loss must be stopped. Simple suturing is usually adequate but may not be possible on the FoP or fieldside. Applying moderate digital compression adjacent to the wound edges can often stop venous bleeding. Bleeding that does not stop may be arterial in origin and may be secondary to a cranial fracture. Digital compression should therefore not be excessive as there is a risk of pressing fractured bone further into the cranium. If necessary, cover the wound and apply a turban bandage. Occasionally intravenous fluid is required if blood loss is significant, or if the patient is losing consciousness.

Smelling Salts

Smelling salts are a combination of ammonium carbonate salt and water. Increasing the respiratory rate alone certainly has no beneficial pathophysiological effect on the nature or underlying cause of concussive injury. Whether the salts increase alertness, improve reaction times, or have other positive cognitive benefits, remains to be proven scientifically. In modern sports medicine however, when used correctly, smelling salts are unlikely to have significant benefit or cause significant adverse effects in sport-related head injury.

Bibliography

Clinical practice guidelines for mild traumatic brain injury and persistent symptoms (The College of Family Physicians of Canada – 2012)

Concussion (mild traumatic brain injury) and the team physician: a consensus statement (American College of Sports Medicine (ACSM), American Academy of Family Physicians (AAFP), American Academy of Orthopaedic Surgeons (AAOS), American Medical Society for Sports Medicine (AMSSM), American Orthopedic Society for Sports Medicine (AOSSM), and the American Osteopathic Academy of Sports Medicine (AOASM) – 2011)

Concussion and mild TBI (Centers for Disease Control and Prevention – 2012)

Clinical policy: neuroimaging and decision making in adult mild traumatic brain injury in the acute setting (American College of Emergency Physicians – 2008)

Head injury: triage, assessment, investigation, and early management of head injury in infants, children, and adults (National Institute for Health and Clinical Excellence – NICE –2007)

Traumatic brain injury: diagnosis, acute management, and rehabilitation (New Zealand Guidelines Group – 2006)

Harmon, K.G., Drezner, J.A., Gammons, M. *et al.* (2013) American Medical Society for Sports Medicine position statement: concussion in sport. *British Journal of Sports Medicine*, **47**, 15–26. doi:10.1136/bjsports-2012-091941

McCrory, P. (2006) Smelling salts. *British Journal of Sports Medicine*, **40**, 659–660. doi:10.1136/bjsm.2006.029710

11 Concussion – Onfield and Sideline Evaluation

Paul McCrory[1] *and Michael Turner*[2]

[1]*The Florey Institute of Neuroscience, Melbourne Brain Centre – Austin Campus, University of Melbourne, Parkville, Australia*
[2]*British Horseracing Authority, London, United Kingdom*

Introduction

In sports medicine, clinicians must be able to recognize and manage a spectrum of brain injury. Fortunately, serious brain injury is rare in team sport and the majority of head injuries seen are mild. Nevertheless, all individuals involved in athletic care need to have a thorough understanding of the early management of the head-injured athlete, the risks of deterioration, and the potential sequelae of such injuries that may impact on the athlete's ability to return to sport or even in later life.

Epidemiology

The crude incidence for all traumatic brain injuries is estimated at approximately 300 per 100,000 population per year with the majority (80–90%) of those suffering a mild TBI. The US Center for Disease Control estimates that 1.6–3.8 million sports-related concussions are hospitalized each year in the United States. Other studies suggest that the number of unreported concussions may be 10-fold higher.

Definition of Concussion

The "Concussion in Sport Group" (CISG) definition has now become the accepted clinical operational definition of this condition. This definition states that:

"Concussion is a brain injury and is defined as a complex pathophysiological process affecting the brain, induced by biomechanical forces. Several common features that incorporate clinical, pathologic and biomechanical injury constructs that may be utilized in defining the nature of a concussive head injury include:

1. *Concussion may be caused either by a direct blow to the head, face, neck or elsewhere on the body with an "impulsive" force transmitted to the head.*

The IOC Manual of Emergency Sports Medicine, First Edition. Edited by David McDonagh and David Zideman.
2015 International Olympic Committee. Published 2015 by John Wiley & Sons, Ltd.

2. *Concussion typically results in the rapid onset of short-lived impairment of neurological function that resolves spontaneously. However, in some cases, symptoms and signs may evolve over a number of minutes to hours.*
3. *Concussion may result in neuro-pathological changes, but the acute clinical symptoms largely reflect a functional disturbance rather than a structural injury and, as such, no abnormality is seen on standard structural neuro-imaging studies.*
4. *Concussion results in a graded set of clinical symptoms that may or may not involve loss of consciousness. Resolution of the clinical and cognitive symptoms typically follows a sequential course. However, it is important to note that in some cases symptoms may be prolonged.*"

Symptoms and Signs of Acute Concussion

The diagnosis of acute concussion usually involves the assessment of a range of domains including clinical symptoms, physical signs, cognitive impairment, neurobehavioral features, and sleep disturbance. These are outlined on the SCAT3 and (Concussion Recognition Tool (CRT) forms (Figures 11.1 and 11.2).

The suspected diagnosis of concussion can include one or more of the following clinical domains:

1. Symptoms – somatic (e.g., headache), cognitive (e.g., feeling like in a fog), and/or emotional symptoms (e.g., lability)
2. Physical signs (e.g., loss of consciousness (LOC), amnesia)
3. Behavioral changes (e.g., irritability)
4. Cognitive impairment (e.g., slowed reaction times)
5. Sleep disturbance (e.g., insomnia)

If any one or more of these components are present, a concussion should be suspected and the appropriate management strategy instituted.

The common symptoms of concussion have been examined in prospective studies and include headache, dizziness, blurred vision, and nausea. These symptoms are not specific to concussion and in some cases may present in a delayed manner, which highlights a key issue that acute concussion is an evolving injury.

Fieldside Recognition of Concussion

Frequently, in episodes of mild concussion ("bell ringers"), the athlete will be dazed or stunned for a period of seconds only and continue playing. Alert medical and training staff should closely observe the actions of a player who has received a knock on the head for any signs of impaired performance. Visual clues to the presence of concussion are outlined on the CRT (Figure 11.2) and include loss of responsiveness or lying motionless on ground, slow to get up, unsteady on feet or falling over, grabbing or clutching head, dazed or blank look, and unaware of surrounding plays or events.

Concussion Injury Severity and Recovery

The classification of severity of concussive injury is a contentious area. The CISG recommended that no specific anecdotal scale be used and that all concussive injury management measure individual recovery to determine return to play (RTP) rather than an anecdotal grading systems and arbitrary exclusion periods.

SCAT3

FIFA® IIHF FEI

Sport Concussion Assessment Tool – 3rd Edition

For use by medical professionals only

Name

Date/Time of Injury:
Date of Assessment:

Examiner:

What is the SCAT3?[1]

The SCAT3 is a standardized tool for evaluating injured athletes for concussion and can be used in athletes aged from 13 years and older. It supersedes the original SCAT and the SCAT2 published in 2005 and 2009, respectively[2]. For younger persons, ages 12 and under, please use the Child SCAT3. The SCAT3 is designed for use by medical professionals. If you are not qualified, please use the Sport Concussion Recognition Tool[1]. Preseason baseline testing with the SCAT3 can be helpful for interpreting post-injury test scores.

Specific instructions for use of the SCAT3 are provided on page 3. If you are not familiar with the SCAT3, please read through these instructions carefully. This tool may be freely copied in its current form for distribution to individuals, teams, groups and organizations. Any revision or any reproduction in a digital form requires approval by the Concussion in Sport Group.

NOTE: The diagnosis of a concussion is a clinical judgment, ideally made by a medical professional. The SCAT3 should not be used solely to make, or exclude, the diagnosis of concussion in the absence of clinical judgement. An athlete may have a concussion even if their SCAT3 is "normal".

What is a concussion?

A concussion is a disturbance in brain function caused by a direct or indirect force to the head. It results in a variety of non-specific signs and/or symptoms (some examples listed below) and most often does not involve loss of consciousness. Concussion should be suspected in the presence of **any one or more** of the following:

- Symptoms (e.g., headache), or
- Physical signs (e.g., unsteadiness), or
- Impaired brain function (e.g. confusion) or
- Abnormal behaviour (e.g., change in personality).

SIDELINE ASSESSMENT

Indications for Emergency Management

NOTE: A hit to the head can sometimes be associated with a more serious brain injury. Any of the following warrants consideration of activating emergency procedures and urgent transportation to the nearest hospital:

- Glasgow Coma score less than 15
- Deteriorating mental status
- Potential spinal injury
- Progressive, worsening symptoms or new neurologic signs

Potential signs of concussion?

If any of the following signs are observed after a direct or indirect blow to the head, the athlete should stop participation, be evaluated by a medical professional and **should not be permitted to return to sport the same day** if a concussion is suspected.

Any loss of consciousness?	Y	N
"If so, how long?"		
Balance or motor incoordination **(stumbles, slow/laboured movements, etc.)**?	Y	N
Disorientation or confusion **(inability to respond appropriately to questions)**?	Y	N
Loss of memory:	Y	N
"If so, how long?"		
"Before or after the injury?"		
Blank or vacant look:	Y	N
Visible facial injury in combination with any of the above:	Y	N

1 Glasgow coma scale (GCS)

Best eye response (E)	
No eye opening	1
Eye opening in response to pain	2
Eye opening to speech	3
Eyes opening spontaneously	4
Best verbal response (V)	
No verbal response	1
Incomprehensible sounds	2
Inappropriate words	3
Confused	4
Oriented	5
Best motor response (M)	
No motor response	1
Extension to pain	2
Abnormal flexion to pain	3
Flexion/Withdrawal to pain	4
Localizes to pain	5
Obeys commands	6
Glasgow Coma score (E + V + M)	of 15

GCS should be recorded for all athletes in case of subsequent deterioration.

2 Maddocks Score[3]

"I am going to ask you a few questions, please listen carefully and give your best effort."

Modified Maddocks questions (1 point for each correct answer)

At what venue are we at today?	0	1
Which half is it now?	0	1
Who scored last in this match?	0	1
What team did you play last week/game?	0	1
Did your team win the last game?	0	1
Maddocks score		of 5

Maddocks score is validated for sideline diagnosis of concussion only and is not used for serial testing.

Notes: Mechanism of Injury (**"tell me what happened"**?):

Any athlete with a suspected concussion should be REMOVED FROM PLAY, medically assessed, monitored for deterioration (i.e., should not be left alone) and should not drive a motor vehicle until cleared to do so by a medical professional. No athlete diagnosed with concussion should be returned to sports participation on the day of Injury.

SCAT3 SPORT CONCUSSION ASSESMENT TOOL 3 | **PAGE 1**

Figure 11.1 SCAT3 assessment tool

(*Source:* Concussion in Sport Group © 2013 – SCAT3. *British Journal of Sports Medicine* 2013; 47(5): 259.)

BACKGROUND

Name: ______ Date: ______
Examiner: ______
Sport/team/school: ______ Date/time of injury: ______
Age: ______ Gender: M F
Years of education completed: ______
Dominant hand: right left neither
How many concussions do you think you have had in the past? ______
When was the most recent concussion? ______
How long was your recovery from the most recent concussion? ______
Have you ever been hospitalized or had medical imaging done for a head injury? Y N
Have you ever been diagnosed with headaches or migraines? Y N
Do you have a learning disability, dyslexia, ADD/ADHD? Y N
Have you ever been diagnosed with depression, anxiety or other psychiatric disorder? Y N
Has anyone in your family ever been diagnosed with any of these problems? Y N
Are you on any medications? If yes, please list: Y N

SCAT3 to be done in resting state. Best done 10 or more minutes post excercise.

SYMPTOM EVALUATION

3 How do you feel?

"You should score yourself on the following symptoms, based on how you feel now".

	none	mild		moderate		severe	
Headache	0	1	2	3	4	5	6
"Pressure in head"	0	1	2	3	4	5	6
Neck Pain	0	1	2	3	4	5	6
Nausea or vomiting	0	1	2	3	4	5	6
Dizziness	0	1	2	3	4	5	6
Blurred vision	0	1	2	3	4	5	6
Balance problems	0	1	2	3	4	5	6
Sensitivity to light	0	1	2	3	4	5	6
Sensitivity to noise	0	1	2	3	4	5	6
Feeling slowed down	0	1	2	3	4	5	6
Feeling like "in a fog"	0	1	2	3	4	5	6
"Don't feel right"	0	1	2	3	4	5	6
Difficulty concentrating	0	1	2	3	4	5	6
Difficulty remembering	0	1	2	3	4	5	6
Fatigue or low energy	0	1	2	3	4	5	6
Confusion	0	1	2	3	4	5	6
Drowsiness	0	1	2	3	4	5	6
Trouble falling asleep	0	1	2	3	4	5	6
More emotional	0	1	2	3	4	5	6
Irritability	0	1	2	3	4	5	6
Sadness	0	1	2	3	4	5	6
Nervous or Anxious	0	1	2	3	4	5	6

Total number of symptoms (Maximum possible 22)
Symptom severity score (Maximum possible 132)

Do the symptoms get worse with physical activity? Y N
Do the symptoms get worse with mental activity? Y N

self rated | self rated and clinician monitored
clinician interview | self rated with parent input

Overall rating: If you know the athlete well prior to the injury, how different is the athlete acting compared to his/her usual self?

Please circle one response:

no different | very different | unsure | N/A

Scoring on the SCAT3 should not be used as a stand-alone method to diagnose concussion, measure recovery or make decisions about an athlete's readiness to return to competition after concussion. Since signs and symptoms may evolve over time, it is important to consider repeat evaluation in the acute assessment of concussion.

COGNITIVE & PHYSICAL EVALUATION

4 Cognitive assessment

Standardized Assessment of Concussion (SAC)[4]

Orientation (1 point for each correct answer)

What month is it?	0	1
What is the date today?	0	1
What is the day of the week?	0	1
What year is it?	0	1
What time is it right now? (within 1 hour)	0	1
Orientation score		of 5

Immediate memory

List	Trial 1		Trial 2		Trial 3		Alternative word list		
elbow	0	1	0	1	0	1	candle	baby	finger
apple	0	1	0	1	0	1	paper	monkey	penny
carpet	0	1	0	1	0	1	sugar	perfume	blanket
saddle	0	1	0	1	0	1	sandwich	sunset	lemon
bubble	0	1	0	1	0	1	wagon	iron	insect
Total									

Immediate memory score total of 15

Concentration: Digits Backward

List	Trial 1		Alternative digit list		
4-9-3	0	1	6-2-9	5-2-6	4-1-5
3-8-1-4	0	1	3-2-7-9	1-7-9-5	4-9-6-8
6-2-9-7-1	0	1	1-5-2-8-6	3-8-5-2-7	6-1-8-4-3
7-1-8-4-6-2	0	1	5-3-9-1-4-8	8-3-1-9-6-4	7-2-4-8-5-6
Total of 4					

Concentration: Month in Reverse Order (1 pt. for entire sequence correct)

Dec-Nov-Oct-Sept-Aug-Jul-Jun-May-Apr-Mar-Feb-Jan 0 1

Concentration score of 5

5 Neck Examination:

Range of motion | Tenderness | Upper and lower limb sensation & strength

Findings:

6 Balance examination

Do one or both of the following tests.

Footwear (shoes, barefoot, braces, tape, etc.)

Modified Balance Error Scoring System (BESS) testing[5]

Which foot was tested (i.e. which is the non-dominant foot) Left Right

Testing surface (hard floor, field, etc.)

Condition

Double leg stance: Errors
Single leg stance (non-dominant foot): Errors
Tandem stance (non-dominant foot at back): Errors

And/Or

Tandem gait[6,7]

Time (best of 4 trials): ______ seconds

7 Coordination examination

Upper limb coordination

Which arm was tested: Left Right

Coordination score of 1

8 SAC Delayed Recall[4]

Delayed recall score of 5

SCAT3 SPORT CONCUSSION ASSESMENT TOOL 3 | **PAGE 2**

Figure 11.1 *(contd.)*

INSTRUCTIONS

Words in *Italics* throughout the SCAT3 are the instructions given to the athlete by the tester.

Symptom Scale

"You should score yourself on the following symptoms, based on how you feel now".

To be completed by the athlete. In situations where the symptom scale is being completed after exercise, it should still be done in a resting state, at least 10 minutes post exercise.

For total number of symptoms, maximum possible is 22.

For Symptom severity score, add all scores in table, maximum possible is 22 x 6 = 132.

SAC[4]

Immediate Memory

"I am going to test your memory. I will read you a list of words and when I am done, repeat back as many words as you can remember, in any order."

Trials 2 & 3:

"I am going to repeat the same list again. Repeat back as many words as you can remember in any order, even if you said the word before."

Complete all 3 trials regardless of score on trial 1 & 2. Read the words at a rate of one per second. **Score 1 pt. for each correct response.** Total score equals sum across all 3 trials. Do not inform the athlete that delayed recall will be tested.

Concentration

Digits backward

"I am going to read you a string of numbers and when I am done, you repeat them back to me backwards, in reverse order of how I read them to you. For example, if I say 7-1-9, you would say 9-1-7."

If correct, go to next string length. If incorrect, read trial 2. **One point possible for each string length.** Stop after incorrect on both trials. The digits should be read at the rate of one per second.

Months in reverse order

"Now tell me the months of the year in reverse order. Start with the last month and go backward. So you'll say December, November ... Go ahead"

1 pt. for entire sequence correct

Delayed Recall

The delayed recall should be performed after completion of the Balance and Coordination Examination.

"Do you remember that list of words I read a few times earlier? Tell me as many words from the list as you can remember in any order."

Score 1 pt. for each correct response

Balance Examination

Modified Balance Error Scoring System (BESS) testing[5]

This balance testing is based on a modified version of the Balance Error Scoring System (BESS)[5]. A stopwatch or watch with a second hand is required for this testing.

"I am now going to test your balance. Please take your shoes off, roll up your pant legs above ankle (if applicable), and remove any ankle taping (if applicable). This test will consist of three twenty second tests with different stances."

(a) Double leg stance:

"The first stance is standing with your feet together with your hands on your hips and with your eyes closed. You should try to maintain stability in that position for 20 seconds. I will be counting the number of times you move out of this position. I will start timing when you are set and have closed your eyes."

(b) Single leg stance:

"If you were to kick a ball, which foot would you use? [This will be the dominant foot] Now stand on your non-dominant foot. The dominant leg should be held in approximately 30 degrees of hip flexion and 45 degrees of knee flexion. Again, you should try to maintain stability for 20 seconds with your hands on your hips and your eyes closed. I will be counting the number of times you move out of this position. If you stumble out of this position, open your eyes and return to the start position and continue balancing. I will start timing when you are set and have closed your eyes."

(c) Tandem stance:

"Now stand heel-to-toe with your non-dominant foot in back. Your weight should be evenly distributed across both feet. Again, you should try to maintain stability for 20 seconds with your hands on your hips and your eyes closed. I will be counting the number of times you move out of this position. If you stumble out of this position, open your eyes and return to the start position and continue balancing. I will start timing when you are set and have closed your eyes."

Balance testing – types of errors

1. Hands lifted off iliac crest
2. Opening eyes
3. Step, stumble, or fall
4. Moving hip into > 30 degrees abduction
5. Lifting forefoot or heel
6. Remaining out of test position > 5 sec

Each of the 20-second trials is scored by counting the errors, or deviations from the proper stance, accumulated by the athlete. The examiner will begin counting errors only after the individual has assumed the proper start position. **The modified BESS is calculated by adding one error point for each error during the three 20-second tests. The maximum total number of errors for any single condition is 10.** If a athlete commits multiple errors simultaneously, only one error is recorded but the athlete should quickly return to the testing position, and counting should resume once subject is set. Subjects that are unable to maintain the testing procedure for a minimum of **five seconds** at the start are assigned the highest possible score, ten, for that testing condition.

OPTION: For further assessment, the same 3 stances can be performed on a surface of medium density foam (e.g., approximately 50 cm x 40 cm x 6 cm).

Tandem Gait[6,7]

Participants are instructed to stand with their feet together behind a starting line (the test is best done with footwear removed). Then, they walk in a forward direction as quickly and as accurately as possible along a 38mm wide (sports tape), 3 meter line with an alternate foot heel-to-toe gait ensuring that they approximate their heel and toe on each step. Once they cross the end of the 3m line, they turn 180 degrees and return to the starting point using the same gait. A total of 4 trials are done and the best time is retained. Athletes should complete the test in 14 seconds. Athletes fail the test if they step off the line, have a separation between their heel and toe, or if they touch or grab the examiner or an object. In this case, the time is not recorded and the trial repeated, if appropriate.

Coordination Examination

Upper limb coordination

Finger-to-nose (FTN) task:

"I am going to test your coordination now. Please sit comfortably on the chair with your eyes open and your arm (either right or left) outstretched (shoulder flexed to 90 degrees and elbow and fingers extended), pointing in front of you. When I give a start signal, I would like you to perform five successive finger to nose repetitions using your index finger to touch the tip of the nose, and then return to the starting position, as quickly and as accurately as possible."

Scoring: 5 correct repetitions in < 4 seconds = 1

Note for testers: Athletes fail the test if they do not touch their nose, do not fully extend their elbow or do not perform five repetitions. **Failure should be scored as 0.**

References & Footnotes

1. This tool has been developed by a group of international experts at the 4th International Consensus meeting on Concussion in Sport held in Zurich, Switzerland in November 2012. The full details of the conference outcomes and the authors of the tool are published in The BJSM Injury Prevention and Health Protection, 2013, Volume 47, Issue 5. The outcome paper will also be simultaneously co-published in other leading biomedical journals with the copyright held by the Concussion in Sport Group, to allow unrestricted distribution, providing no alterations are made.

2. McCrory P et al., Consensus Statement on Concussion in Sport – the 3rd International Conference on Concussion in Sport held in Zurich, November 2008. British Journal of Sports Medicine 2009; 43: i76-89.

3. Maddocks, DL; Dicker, GD; Saling, MM. The assessment of orientation following concussion in athletes. Clinical Journal of Sport Medicine. 1995; 5(1): 32–3.

4. McCrea M. Standardized mental status testing of acute concussion. Clinical Journal of Sport Medicine. 2001; 11: 176–181.

5. Guskiewicz KM. Assessment of postural stability following sport-related concussion. Current Sports Medicine Reports. 2003; 2: 24–30.

6. Schneiders, A.G., Sullivan, S.J., Gray, A., Hammond-Tooke, G. & McCrory, P. Normative values for 16-37 year old subjects for three clinical measures of motor performance used in the assessment of sports concussions. Journal of Science and Medicine in Sport. 2010; 13(2): 196–201.

7. Schneiders, A.G., Sullivan, S.J., Kvarnstrom. J.K., Olsson, M., Yden. T. & Marshall, S.W. The effect of footwear and sports-surface on dynamic neurological screening in sport-related concussion. Journal of Science and Medicine in Sport. 2010; 13(4): 382–386

Figure 11.1 *(contd.)*

ATHLETE INFORMATION

Any athlete suspected of having a concussion should be removed from play, and then seek medical evaluation.

Signs to watch for

Problems could arise over the first 24–48 hours. The athlete should not be left alone and must go to a hospital at once if they:

- Have a headache that gets worse
- Are very drowsy or can't be awakened
- Can't recognize people or places
- Have repeated vomiting
- Behave unusually or seem confused; are very irritable
- Have seizures (arms and legs jerk uncontrollably)
- Have weak or numb arms or legs
- Are unsteady on their feet; have slurred speech

Remember, it is better to be safe.
Consult your doctor after a suspected concussion.

Return to play

Athletes should not be returned to play the same day of injury.
When returning athletes to play, they should be **medically cleared and then follow a stepwise supervised program,** with stages of progression.

For example:

Rehabilitation stage	Functional exercise at each stage of rehabilitation	Objective of each stage
No activity	Physical and cognitive rest	Recovery
Light aerobic exercise	Walking, swimming or stationary cycling keeping intensity, 70 % maximum predicted heart rate. No resistance training	Increase heart rate
Sport-specific exercise	Skating drills in ice hockey, running drills in soccer. No head impact activities	Add movement
Non-contact training drills	Progression to more complex training drills, eg passing drills in football and ice hockey. May start progressive resistance training	Exercise, coordination, and cognitive load
Full contact practice	Following medical clearance participate in normal training activities	Restore confidence and assess functional skills by coaching staff
Return to play	Normal game play	

There should be at least 24 hours (or longer) for each stage and if symptoms recur the athlete should rest until they resolve once again and then resume the program at the previous asymptomatic stage. Resistance training should only be added in the later stages.

If the athlete is symptomatic for more than 10 days, then consultation by a medical practitioner who is expert in the management of concussion, is recommended.

Medical clearance should be given before return to play.

Scoring Summary:

Test Domain	Score		
	Date:	Date:	Date:
Number of Symptoms of 22			
Symptom Severity Score of 132			
Orientation of 5			
Immediate Memory of 15			
Concentration of 5			
Delayed Recall of 5			
SAC Total			
BESS (total errors)			
Tandem Gait (seconds)			
Coordination of 1			

Notes:

CONCUSSION INJURY ADVICE

(To be given to the **person monitoring** the concussed athlete)

This patient has received an injury to the head. A careful medical examination has been carried out and no sign of any serious complications has been found. Recovery time is variable across individuals and the patient will need monitoring for a further period by a responsible adult. Your treating physician will provide guidance as to this timeframe.

If you notice any change in behaviour, vomiting, dizziness, worsening headache, double vision or excessive drowsiness, please contact your doctor or the nearest hospital emergency department immediately.

Other important points:

- Rest (physically and mentally), including training or playing sports until symptoms resolve and you are medically cleared
- No alcohol
- No prescription or non-prescription drugs without medical supervision. Specifically:
  - No sleeping tablets
  - Do not use aspirin, anti-inflammatory medication or sedating pain killers
- Do not drive until medically cleared
- Do not train or play sport until medically cleared

Clinic phone number

Patient's name

Date/time of injury

Date/time of medical review

Treatingphysician

Contact details or stamp

Figure 11.1 *(contd.)*

Pocket CONCUSSION RECOGNITION TOOL

To help identify concussion in children, youth and adults

RECOGNIZE & REMOVE

Concussion should be suspected **if one or more** of the following visible clues, signs, symptoms or errors in memory questions are present.

1. Visible clues of suspected concussion

Any one or more of the following visual clues can indicate a possible concussion:

Loss of consciousness or responsiveness
Lying motionless on ground/Slow to get up
Unsteady on feet / Balance problems or falling over/Incoordination
Grabbing/Clutching of head
Dazed, blank or vacant look
Confused/Not aware of plays or events

2. Signs and symptoms of suspected concussion

Presence of any one or more of the following signs & symptoms may suggest a concussion:

- Loss of consciousness
- Seizure or convulsion
- Balance problems
- Nausea or vomiting
- Drowsiness
- More emotional
- Irritability
- Sadness
- Fatigue or low energy
- Nervous or anxious
- "Don't feel right"
- Difficulty remembering
- Headache
- Dizziness
- Confusion
- Feeling slowed down
- "Pressure in head"
- Blurred vision
- Sensitivity to light
- Amnesia
- Feeling like "in a fog"
- Neck Pain
- Sensitivity to noise
- Difficulty concentrating

3. Memory function

Failure to answer any of these questions correctly may suggest a concussion.

"At what venue are we at today?"
"Which half is it now?"
"Who scored last in this game?"
"What team did you play last week/game?"
"Did your team win the last game?"

Any athlete with a suspected concussion should be IMMEDIATELY REMOVED FROM PLAY, and should not be returned to activity until they are assessed medically. Athletes with a suspected concussion should not be left alone and should not drive a motor vehicle.

It is recommended that, in all cases of suspected concussion, the player is referred to a medical professional for diagnosis and guidance as well as return to play decisions, even if the symptoms resolve.

RED FLAGS

If ANY of the following are reported then the player should be safely and immediately removed from the field. If no qualified medical professional is available, consider transporting by ambulance for urgent medical assessment:

- Athlete complains of neck pain
- Increasing confusion or irritability
- Repeated vomiting
- Seizure or convulsion
- Weakness or tingling/burning in arms or legs
- Deteriorating conscious state
- Severe or increasing headache
- Unusual behaviour change
- Double vision

Remember:

- In all cases, the basic principles of first aid (danger, response, airway, breathing, circulation) should be followed.
- Do not attempt to move the player (other than required for airway support) unless trained to so do
- Do not remove helmet (if present) unless trained to do so.

from McCrory et. al, Consensus Statement on Concussion in Sport. Br J Sports Med 47 (5), 2013

Figure 11.2 Concussion Recognition Tool (CRT)
(*Source:* Concussion in Sport Group © 2013 – Concussion Recognition Tool. *British Journal of Sports Medicine* 2013; 47(5): 267.)

Concussion Management

The practical management of concussion can be divided into three broad areas where the issues and treatment priorities differ considerably. These areas are immediate/onfield, early, and late management.

Immediate or Onfield Management

The key objectives when assessing any athlete who has sustained an acute head or brain injury are the following:

1. Institute an appropriate triage on the FoP
2. Conduct a proper secondary survey in conjunction with a sideline assessment of the injured athlete
3. Manage the injury appropriately, minimizing the risk of any "secondary" injury, such as might be seen with coexistent hypoxia or hypotension
4. Safely remove the athlete from the Field of Play to an appropriate medical facility for further investigation and assessment
5. Determine subsequently when it is safe for the athlete to RTP

The major priorities at this early stage are the basic principles of first aid, for example, ensure a patent airway with adequate oxygenation, ventilation, and circulation. Once these basic aspects of first aid care have been achieved and the patient is stabilized, then consideration of removal of the patient from the FoP to an appropriate facility is necessary. It is essential that all EDs who have an onfield injury management role in their sport have formal training and certification both in first aid and trauma management.

At this time, careful assessment for the presence of a cervical spine or other injury is critical. If an alert patient complains of neck pain, has evidence of neck tenderness or deformity, or has neurological signs suggestive of a spinal injury, then cervical immobilization and transportation with suitable spinal immobilization equipment is required. If the patient is unconscious, then a cervical injury should be assumed until proven otherwise.

Concussive convulsions in collision sport are an uncommon but dramatic association of minor head injury. Clinicians need to follow the first aid principles above and wait for the convulsion to spontaneously resolve (see Chapter 11). Following the convulsion, the athlete should be managed as for a standard concussion.

Once this first aid process has been completed and the patient is stabilized, a full medical and neurological assessment examination should follow. Onsite doctors are in an ideal position to initiate the critical early steps in medical care to ensure optimal recovery from a head injury.

When examining a head-injured athlete, a structured and focused neurological examination is important. Because the major management priorities at this stage are to exclude a catastrophic intracranial injury, this part of the examination should focus on key clinical findings such as

1. the level of consciousness (measured using the Glasgow Coma Scale);
2. pupil response and conjugate eye movement;
3. motor function; and
4. thorough examination of the skull and scalp for evidence of trauma.

The importance of this initial neurologic examination is that it serves as a reference to which other repeated neurologic examinations may be compared.

Vital signs must be recorded following an injury. Hypotension is rarely due to brain injury, except as a terminal event, and alternate sources for the decrease in blood pressure should be aggressively sought and treated. This includes major scalp lacerations especially in young children or a cervical spinal cord injury. Restlessness is a frequent accompaniment of brain injury and can be an early indicator of increased intracranial pressure, intracranial bleeding, or hypoxia, all of which can aggravate any underlying brain injury. If the patient is unconscious but restless, attention should be given to the possibility of increasing cerebral hypoxia, a distended bladder, or painful injuries elsewhere. When time permits, a more thorough physical examination should be performed to exclude coexistent injuries elsewhere in the body.

Early Management

This refers to the situation where an athlete has been brought to the athlete medical room for assessment. Assessment of injury severity is best performed in a quiet medical room rather than in the middle of a football field in front of 100,000 screaming fans. This assessment should be performed by a medical practitioner. If no doctor is available for this assessment, then the athlete needs to be referred to hospital where this can be performed.

When assessing the acutely concussed athlete, various aspects of the history and examination are important. The SCAT3 tool (see Figure 11.1) outlines a complete structured medical assessment of the injured athlete.

When examining a concussed athlete, a full neurological examination is important. Because the major management priorities at this stage are to establish an accurate diagnosis and exclude a catastrophic intracranial injury, this part of the examination should be particularly thorough.

In recent times, the application of simple cognitive tests has created considerable interest as a means to objectively assess concussed athletes. The standard approach of asking the orientation items (e.g., day, date, year, time, date of birth, etc.) has been shown to be unreliable following concussive injury. This aspect of memory remains relatively intact in the face of concussive injury and should not be used. More useful, as demonstrated in prospective studies, are questions of recent memory. These are incorporated in the SCAT3 tool (Figure 11.1).

Although a trainer or nonmedical person may utilize the CRT to suspect the diagnosis of concussion, all concussed athletes should be referred for an urgent medical assessment. Most high-level amateur and professional teams will, in fact, have their own medical staff who make the diagnosis, however, where teams lack this facility, then concussed athletes need to be referred to hospital for a medical assessment.

Having determined the presence of a concussive injury, the patient needs to be serially monitored until full recovery ensues. If the concussed player is discharged home after an initial assessment, then they should be in the care of a responsible adult. It is the author's policy to give the patient and the attendant a head injury advice card upon discharge. This is incorporated in the SCAT3 tool (Figure 11.1).

Who should be referred to hospital? The treating clinician at a sporting event also must decide who should be referred to hospital or directly to a neurosurgical center. There are a number of urgent indications that are listed in Table 11.1. While it is acknowledged that a number of these indications are based on anecdotal rather than evidence-based information, these are widely accepted. The overall approach should be "when in doubt, refer." Where no physician is present and the initial management is in the hands of an athletic trainer, physical therapist, or paramedic, then an urgent medical referral should be considered mandatory in all cases of head injury.

Fractured skull	Confusion or impairment of consciousness >30 min
Penetrating skull trauma	Loss of consciousness >5 min
Deterioration in conscious state following injury	Persistent vomiting or increasing headache postinjury
Focal neurological signs	Any convulsive movements
More than one episode of concussive injury in a session	Where there is assessment difficulty (e.g., an intoxicated patient)
Children with head injuries	High-risk patients (e.g., hemophilia, anticoagulant use)
Inadequate postinjury supervision	High-risk injury mechanism (e.g., high-velocity impact)

Table 11.1 Indications for urgent hospital referral and/or neuroimaging

Who needs diagnostic investigations?

The indications for urgent neuroimaging in the initial evaluation of the head-injured patient are the same as those outlined in Table 11.1. The primary goal of imaging is to establish whether there is an intracranial hemorrhage. A depressed level of consciousness and, in particular, a GCS ≤8, are the strongest predictors of intracranial hemorrhage. Other signs that suggest surgical pathology include focal motor weakness and an asymmetrical pupil examination.

An important and more difficult question is who needs a head computed tomography (CT) scan when his/her level of consciousness is normal (i.e., GCS is 15)? Guidelines such as the Canadian Head CT Rules and the New Orleans Criteria suggest that factors such as age >60 years, headache, vomiting, intoxication, retrograde amnesia, confusion, LOC, seizures, visible trauma above the clavicles, and injury mechanism indicate a need for a head CT. However, a normal head CT scan does not always exclude a traumatic brain injury (TBI) or the need for neurosurgical consultation. About 20% of patients admitted to hospital after even mild TBI may develop posttraumatic abnormalities on subsequent imaging even after the initial head CT scan was normal.

Late Management and Return to Play

This refers to the situation where a player has sustained a concussive injury previously and is now presenting for advice or clearance prior to resuming sport. The main management priorities at this stage are the assessment of recovery and the application of the appropriate return to sport guidelines. Any clearance to return to sport is the province of a medical practitioner, ideally with experience of these sporting injuries, and should not be undertaken by nonmedical personnel.

RTP decisions remains difficult. Expert consensus guidelines recommend that players should not be returned to competition until they have recovered completely from their concussive injury. Currently, however there is no single gold standard measure of brain disturbance and recovery following concussion. Instead, clinicians must rely on a number of indirect measures to inform clinical judgment. In practical terms, this involves a multifaceted clinical approach, which includes assessment of symptoms, modifying factors, physical signs (such as balance), and neurocognitive function. Furthermore, individual International Federations may have specific recommendations for return to competition and/or the FoP and these need to be considered as part of the RTP paradigm.

It was unanimously agreed at the CISG meeting that no RTP on the day of concussive injury should occur. There is data demonstrating that at the collegiate and high school levels, athletes allowed to RTP on the same day may demonstrate neuropsychological deficits postinjury that may not be evident on the sidelines and are more likely to have delayed onset of symptoms. The principal concern of premature RTP of a concussed athlete is that due to the impaired cognitive function (e.g., slowed information processing and reduced attention), the athlete will sustain further injury (both concussive and other) when returning to a dangerous playing environment.

The guiding policy should be that until completely symptom free, concussed athletes should not resume any training or competition. Once the acute concussive symptoms resolve at rest and exercise, a graduated plan of return to low-level aerobic training, followed by non-contact drills and finally contact play will allow close monitoring of the development of any adverse symptoms. Persisting or newly developing symptoms necessitate further follow-up and detailed medical evaluation. An outline of a graduated RTP strategy is presented on the final page of the SCAT3 tool (Figure 11.1).

Most sports-related concussive injuries are uncomplicated and recover fully over 1–3 weeks. However, it is worth noting that detailed neuropsychological testing shows that 20% or more athletes will still have unrecognized cognitive deficits 10 days after concussion. For this reason, reliance on nonscientific nostrums ("miss a week") or symptoms alone to guide RTP is not recommended as best practice care. This fact highlights the important role of neuropsychological testing to inform clinical decision making and as one of the cornerstones of management. In postconcussive athletes with persistent symptoms or cognitive deficits (>14 days), consideration of referral to a multidisciplinary concussion program may be worthwhile. At the end of the day, good clinical judgment should prevail over written guidelines.

One of the key problems to consider in this setting are mental health issues (such as depression, anxiety, and suicide) that have been reported as consequence of TBI including sports concussion. All players with ongoing symptoms or a prolonged clinical course should be screened for depression using standard clinical tools, for example, Hospital Anxiety and Depression Scale, Beck Depression Inventory, and so on.

Concussion in Child and Adolescent Athletes

The CISG evaluation and management recommendations can be applied to children and adolescents down to the age of 13 years. Below that age, children report concussion symptoms differently from adults and require age-appropriate symptom checklists as a component of assessment. An additional consideration in assessing the child or adolescent athlete with a concussion is that the clinical evaluation by the healthcare professional may need to include both patient and parent input, and possibly teacher input when appropriate. A child SCAT3 has been developed to assess concussion for individuals aged 5–12 years.

Because of the different physiological response and longer recovery after concussion and specific risks (e.g., diffuse cerebral swelling) related to head impact during childhood and adolescence, a more conservative RTP approach is recommended. It is appropriate to extend the amount of time of asymptomatic rest and/or the length of the graded exertion in children and adolescents. It is never appropriate for a child or adolescent athlete with concussion to RTP on the same day as the injury, regardless of the level of athletic performance.

Prevention of Concussion

There are relatively few methods by which concussive brain injury may be minimized in sport. The brain is not an organ that can be conditioned to withstand injury. Thus, extrinsic mechanisms of injury prevention must be sought.

Helmets have been proposed as a means of protecting the head and theoretically reducing the risk of brain injury. In sports where high-speed collisions, missile injuries (e.g., baseball) or falls onto hard surfaces (e.g., gridiron, ice hockey), there is published evidence for the effectiveness of sport-specific helmets to be of benefit in reducing head injuries, particularly skull fractures. For other sports such as soccer and rugby, no sport-specific helmets have been shown to be of proven benefit in reducing rates of head injury. Some believe that the use of protective equipment may alter playing behavior deleteriously so that the athlete actually increases his or her risk of brain injury.

Although the use of correctly fitting mouth guards can reduce the rate of dental orofacial and mandibular injuries, the evidence that they reduce cerebral injuries is largely theoretical, and clinical evidence for a beneficial effect in reducing concussion rates has not yet been demonstrated scientifically.

Consideration of rule changes (i.e., no head checking in ice hockey) and rule enforcement to reduce the head injury rate may be appropriate where a clearcut mechanism is implicated in a particular sport. For most sports, however, head injuries are an accidental byproduct of normal play and hence rule changes or rule enforcement has little effect on head injury rates. Nevertheless, the promotion of fair play and respect for opponents are ethical values that should be encouraged in all sports and by sporting associations. Education of players, coaches, parents, and other staff play an important part in ensuring these values are implemented on the Field of Play.

Neck muscle conditioning may be of value in reducing impact forces transmitted to the brain. Biomechanical concepts dictate that the energy from an impacting object is dispersed over the greater mass of an athlete if the head is held rigidly. Although attractive from a theoretical standpoint, there is little scientific evidence to demonstrate the effectiveness of such measures.

As the ability to treat or reduce the effects of concussive injury after the event is minimal, education of athletes, colleagues, and those working with them as well as the general public is a mainstay of progress in this field. Athletes and their healthcare providers must be educated regarding the detection of concussion, its clinical features, assessment techniques, and principles of safe RTP. Methods to improve education including various web-based resources (e.g., www.concussionsafety.com), educational videos, outreach programs, concussion working groups, and the support and endorsement of enlightened sport groups must be pursued vigorously.

Other Specific Issues

Diffuse Cerebral Swelling and Second Impact Syndrome

Second impact syndrome is frequently mentioned in the concussion literature but, surprisingly, has little scientific evidence for its existence. It is a term used to describe the potential catastrophic consequences resulting from a second concussive blow to the head before an individual has fully recovered from the symptoms of a previous concussion. The second head injury is believed to result in the loss of cerebrovascular autoregulation, which in turn leads to brain swelling secondary to increased cerebral blood flow. There is a lack of evidence to support the claim that the second impact is a risk factor for diffuse cerebral swelling. However, there is evidence that acute (and delayed) brain swelling may occur following a single blow to the head, in association with a structural injury such as a subdural hematoma and also in disorders of calcium channels, suggesting a possible genetic basis for some of these cases. Such events are virtually only seen in children and adolescents. The diagnosis is usually made with an urgent CT brain scan or magnetic resonance imaging (MRI).

Clinical examination, for example, papilledema on fundoscopy, decerebrate posturing, may also provide a clue to the diagnosis. If cerebral swelling is suspected or noted on imaging studies, an urgent neurosurgical consultation is required. Mortality in this condition approaches 100%.

Chronic Traumatic Encephalopathy

Tremendous media attention surrounding sport-related concussion has been directed toward the potential for long-term problems in athletes with high exposure to head contact (i.e., both concussive and subconcussive impacts) during a career in contact sport. This attention has been fueled by the publication of autopsy case studies of retired professional athletes and research reporting increased mortality rate due to neurodegenerative diseases in former professional athletes. There is also evidence from retrospective surveys supporting an association between long-term cognitive, psychiatric, and neurobehavioral problems and participation in sport. In this setting, there is limited neurophysiological and radiological evidence to suggest persistent disturbance of brain function in the absence of overt pathological change that may occur following concussive injury. In recent years, chronic traumatic encephalopathy (CTE) has been redefined from the original condition resembling Alzheimer's disease in professional boxers to a new condition observed in athletes, military personnel, and other nonsporting individuals that shares many features with known psychiatric disorders and other forms of dementia. Although the clinical phenotype is not yet clarified, CTE is characterized by distinct neuropathological findings. The strongly presented causal assumptions in the literature relating to concussive and subconcussive brain impact exposure derived from the case studies are scientifically premature, especially given the absence of prospective, or longitudinal studies on the topic. In addition to the limitations associated with verifying clinicopathological correlation, further research is required in order to better delineate this disease process.

Conclusion

Management of head injury in sport is a critical aspect of sports medicine care. As the ability to treat or reduce the effects of brain injury after the event is minimal, education of athletes, colleagues, and the general public is a mainstay of progress in this field. Athletes, referees, administrators, parents, coaches, and healthcare providers must be educated regarding the detection of concussion, its clinical features, assessment techniques, and principles of safe RTP. Methods to improve education including web-based resources, educational videos, and international outreach programs are important in delivering the message. In addition, concussion working groups, plus the support and endorsement of enlightened sport groups such as FIFA, IOC, IRB, and IIHF have enormous value and must be pursued vigorously. Fair play and respect for opponents are ethical values that should be encouraged in all sports and sporting associations. Similarly, coaches, parents, and managers play an important part in ensuring that these values are implemented on the Field of Play.

Bibliography

Echemendia, R.J., Iverson, G.L., McCrea, M. *et al.* (2012) Role of neuropsychologists in the evaluation and management of sport-related concussion: an inter-organization position statement. *Archives of Clinical Neuropsychology*, **27** (**1**), 119–122.

Giza, C.C., Kutcher, J.S., Ashwal, S. *et al.* (2013) Summary of evidence-based guideline update: evaluation and management of concussion in sports: report of the Guideline Development Subcommittee of the American Academy of Neurology. *Neurology*, **80** (**24**), 2250–2257.

Harmon, K.G., Drezner, J.A., Gammons, M. *et al.* (2013) American Medical Society for Sports Medicine position statement: concussion in sport. *British Journal of Sports Medicine*, **47** (**1**), 15–26.

Herring, S., Bergfeld, J., Boland, A. *et al.* (2006) Concussion (mild traumatic brain injury) and the team physician: a consensus statement. *Medicine and Science in Sports and Exercise*, **38** (**2**), 395–399.

McCrea, M., Iverson, G.L., Echemendia, R.J., Makdissi, M. & Raftery, M. (2013) Day of injury assessment of sport-related concussion. *British Journal of Sports Medicine*, **47** (**5**), 272–284.

McCrory, P., Meeuwisse, W.H., Aubry, M. *et al.* (2013) Consensus statement on concussion in sport: the 4th International Conference on Concussion in Sport held in Zurich, November 2012. *British Journal of Sports Medicine*, **47** (**5**), 250–258.

12 Throat Injuries

Jonathan Hanson[1,2,3], *Padraig B. Sheeran*[4,5,6], *Brian Carlin*[7] *and David Zideman*[8,9,10]

[1]*Broadford Hospital, Skye, Scotland*
[2]*Department of Sport and Exercise Medicine, Musgrave Park Hospital, Belfast, UK*
[3]*Scottish Rugby Football Union*
[4]*Department of Paediatric Anaesthesia and Paediatric Critical Care, Our Lady's Children's*
[5]*Hospital Crumlin, Dublin, Ireland*
Connacht Rugby, Ireland
[6]*Sports & Exercise Medicine, Royal College of Surgeons in Ireland, Dublin, Ireland*
[7]*UCD Centre for Emergency Medical Science School of Medicine, University College, Dublin, Ireland*
[8]*Anaesthesia, Imperial College Healthcare NHS Trust, London, UK*
[9]*London Ambulance Service NHS Trust, London, UK*
[10]*Emergency Medical Services, London Organising Committee of the Olympic and Paralympic Games, London 2012, London*

General principles of trauma to the neck refer to blunt or penetrating injuries. Some sports do involve potential for penetrating trauma but a majority of sporting injuries to the anterior neck are due to moderate blunt trauma as may occur in a tackle, a grapple hold with traction or sustained pressure on the neck, or direct contact with a piece of equipment such as a stick, ball, or puck. Establishing the mechanism of injury will often be helpful in the overall management of the injury. The magnitude of force contributing to the injury varies considerably between sports.

With blunt trauma, the area injured may be larger than one specific zone. Injuries may present in variable time frames. In arterial dissection, the clinical presentation of the injury may occur either immediately or may be several days after the injury. As with all injuries presenting to the Field of Play (FoP) medical team, serious injuries may evolve (or wane) with time and there is considerable value in repeated schematic reassessment.

Penetrating trauma in sport is much more unusual but may occur as an unanticipated consequence of some sports such as, tree branches in downhill mountain biking or ice skate blades in ice hockey. An injury is not considered to have significantly penetrated the neck unless the injury pierces the platysma muscle layer. Injuries through the platysma and injuries crossing the midline usually cause a higher degree of damage to a greater number of critical anatomical structures. The angle of entry into the neck may mean that structures have been injured in other zones.

The IOC Manual of Emergency Sports Medicine, First Edition. Edited by David McDonagh and David Zideman.
2015 International Olympic Committee. Published 2015 by John Wiley & Sons, Ltd.

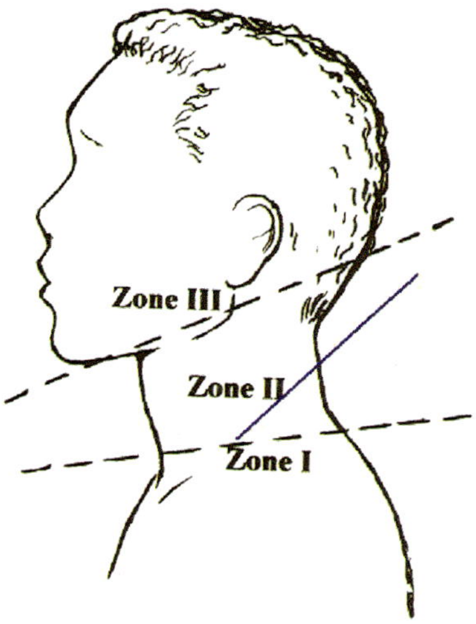

The anterior neck or throat is a complex anatomical structure divided into tight fascial compartments. The common carotid arteries transcends on either side of the neck across Zones I, II, and III (Fig 12.1) parallel to the trachea and is protected by deep connective tissue, muscles, and fascia (as are the internal jugular veins and the vagus nerve on the left). The carotid arteries do not lie against either the trachea or the cervical spinal column. Multiple vital structures are concentrated in the relatively unprotected anterolateral aspect of the neck. The organization of the fascial compartments in the neck can limit hemorrhage and contribute to the tamponade effect on a vascular injury. However, such tightly contained swelling risks additional pressure on the soft posterior trachea and other compressible structures in the neck.

Clinical examination may not be sensitive enough to detect such complex and involved injuries, hence the need for the FoP medical teams to have a high index of suspicion, perform a proper primary survey onfield, transfer the athlete to the fieldside for proper secondary evaluation, be prepared for life-saving intervention, and facilitating safe packaging and rapid transfer to definitive hospital care.

Trauma to the anterior lateral neck can generally be considered to potentially damage four main groups of structures:

1. Larynx and trachea – contusion and fracture
2. Tracheobronchial transection
3. Vascular structures
4. Esophagus and gastrointestinal tract

Other injuries such as cranial nerve injuries, thyroid injuries, or thoracic duct injuries can also all occur but are unlikely to be of direct consequence to the FoP medical team.

Penetrating Trauma

Penetrating injuries are very rare in sport but may occur in skating sports, skiing, or mountain biking. Penetrating injury to the trachea can have a high immediate mortality. In 30% of penetrating injuries to the anterolateral neck, multiple structures are involved (see Table 12.1). Vascular injury occurs in up to two-thirds of penetrating trauma. The angle and depth of a penetrating wound will vary and it is often impossible to predict which structures are injured. Hence, the rescuer may be dealing with both a significant airway injury and an expanding hematoma due to a vascular injury.

Zone	Landmarks	Contents
1	Clavicle to cricoid cartilage	Arteries – common carotid, vertebral, and subclavian trachea, esophagus, thoracic duct, thymus
2	Cricoid cartilage to angle of mandible	Arteries – internal and external carotid Veins – internal and external jugular Pharynx, larynx, esophagus, recurrent laryngeal nerve, spinal cord, trachea, thyroid, parathyroids
3	Angle of mandible to base of skull	Arteries – extracranial carotid and vertebral Veins – jugular

Table 12.1 A clinically relevant zonal system for detecting potentially injured neck structures

Clinical Findings/Management Penetrating Neck Wound

Inspection: Look for obvious foreign bodies and wounds. Is there a visible wound and track? Do not remove any deeply embedded foreign bodies.
Is there any obvious bleeding or swelling?

FoP management:
1. If severe, stem any bleeding. Preserve a patent airway by airway maneuvers or by inserting an airway adjunct. Ensure adequate breathing. Measure circulatory parameters. Assess disability.
2. If possible, sit the patient up and administer oxygen.

If both an airway and expanding vascular injury are present, it is essential that trained staff secure a definitive airway as soon as possible (see Chapter 4).

Significant vessel injury, particularly arterial injury, may result in external hemorrhage as well as rapid swelling resulting in a significant threat to airway. In the presence of major bleeding from a carotid arterial laceration, direct pressure must be applied, possibly with a hemostatic dressing (Celox gauze). Attempts to explore the wounds or occlude via Foley catheters are not recommended in the prehospital environment. High-flow oxygen should be administered and intravenous access with a wide bore cannula must be established. Intravenous crystalloid should be administered in 250 mL boluses until there is a palpable radial pulse, roughly equivalent to a systolic pressure of 90 mmHg. This permissive hypotension will encourage active clot formation at the site of injury. Transfer the patient directly to hospital immediately as an emergency, accompanied by an experienced medical team. It is essential to prewarn the receiving hospital.

Blunt Trauma

Any signs of injury such as abrasion, bruising, swelling, or wounds should alert the rescuer to the potential for injury to structures described in Table 12.1. Given the high concentration of critical structures in the anterior neck, symptoms (or lack of) may be misleading with regard to the sensitivity or specific location of injury. Symptoms can however be specific enough to allow localization.

Clinical Findings/Management Blunt Neck Trauma

Symptoms: Pain is often transient and a general symptom in the relatively small anatomical field of the anterior neck. There is always a possibility of a spinal cord injury with any neck injury. Blunt trauma may present with an athlete with a hoarse or weak voice, difficulty in breathing due to larngospasm or difficulty in swallowing due to a leak from a gas-containing structure with resultant surgical emphysema.
Inspection: there may be obvious bleeding, bruising, swelling, or deformity.
Palpation: Wounds that are not actively bleeding should not be probed or examined in any great detail on the FoP for fear of disrupting an established clot and precipitating further hemorrhage. There may be subcutaneous emphysema.
Auscultation: Auscultation for bruits may not be feasible in a noisy sports stadium.
Always conduct a full primary survey of the airway, cervical spine, breathing, circulation, and disability.
Management: On first approach, any athlete with an injury above the clavicle should be considered to have a significant cervical spine injury. Initial management priorities are to address airway patency, breathing, circulation, and disability, especially the maintenance of inline cervical spine immobilization. A history

of the mechanism and suspicious symptoms may raise the possibility of blunt vascular injury. Administer high-flow oxygen via a nonrebreathing mask. Package the athlete to protect the cervical spine and minimize the risk of movement of any injured vessel or of movement-assisted propagation of a vessel dissection. The packaging procedure will depend on local protocols but should include a semirigid collar (see later), cervical spine blocks, and straps and full-length spinal immobilization with an appropriate device.

If there is gross evidence of vascular injury such as swelling or hematoma, the management priorities may alter slightly due to the potential effect on the airway. The pressure exerted by a semirigid collar on a hematoma may compromise the trachea and larynx. The rapid loss of a patent airway is a significant risk, and securing a definitive airway using a cuffed endotracheal tube is a priority in the athlete with any degree of respiratory distress. In a conscious athlete, this would require a prehospital rapid sequence induction of anesthesia (RSI) and the use of paralytic drugs. Only a skilled and properly equipped doctor should undertake this procedure; when this skill is not available on the FoP, rapid emergency transport to the nearest hospital is the best and safest option.

Laryngeal Contusion

Laryngeal injury may vary from a mild contusion to a dramatic fracture, resulting in immediate respiratory compromise. Blunt anterior neck injuries are most common in zone 2 (cricoid cartilage to the angle of the mandible, including the larynx) due to the relative protection of the jaw and chest area over levels 1 and 3.

Sudden mild-to-moderate forceful contact with zone 2 of the neck and larynx can result in sudden spasm of the various intrinsic laryngeal muscles. This results in short-lived anxiety and difficulty in breathing in the athlete. The majority of cases recover onfield over a couple of minutes and can be managed with simple reassurance together with exclusion of other more significant injuries. If the magnitude of force is sufficient to cause an inflammatory response, the injury may persist with pain and hoarseness over a couple of days.

Clinical Findings/Management Laryngeal Contusion

Minor laryngeal contusions are usually self-limiting and recover rapidly onfield.
More significant contusions will be painful; the athlete becomes breathless, distressed, and hoarse.
FoP Management:
1. Sit athletes up to alleviate the sense of breathlessness and panic
2. Give high-flow oxygen at a rate of 15 L per minute
3. Protect the cervical spine if there has been a suspicion of spinal injury
4. Transfer to the fieldside for a secondary survey

If the athlete remains symptomatic or there are signs of deformity, refer to an Ear, Nose, and Throat specialist for further advice.

Laryngeal Fracture

Laryngeal fracture is a significant and life-threatening injury. Fracture of the thyroid cartilage results in immediate respiratory distress, the rapid development of surgical emphysema, and a palpable step in the laryngeal cartilage. In reality, the emphysema and distress may make it difficult to accurately establish the presence of a palpable step. Hemorrhage can occur that will give focal swelling around the step. Such swelling will also be intraluminal and progressively compromise the airway.

Clinical Findings/Management Laryngeal Fracture

General inspection: The athlete may be in respiratory distress and holding the throat as if choking.
Local inspection: There may be swelling due to bleeding in the anterior neck.
Palpation: A palpable step in the thyroid cartilage may be felt.
Auscultation: Over the larynx may reveal stridor.
Management: Although there may well be potential for cervical spine injury, optimal airway and breathing management is the priority at this stage. Athletes should be sat up and given high-flow oxygen, protecting the cervical spine as best possible. Simple airway maneuvers and adjuncts such as jaw thrust or oropharyngeal airways are unlikely to be of use as the injury is distal to the upper airway. If the athlete loses consciousness, due to initial concussive impact of the injury and the laryngeal trauma is in fact stable with a patent lumen, then simple airway maneuvers may be effective.

Some skilled physicians may feel comfortable to attempt rapid drug-assisted RSI, gently passing the endotracheal tube over a bougie past the laryngeal injury (there is a high risk of formation of a false passage) and this may be the only immediate and life-saving option. Others may feel more confident and experienced in performing surgical cricothyrotomy to gain airway control and to provide ventilation, but this is not a common or a necessarily appropriate skill among the majority of sport healthcare professionals. If a surgical airway is attempted, then the operator must be aware of the distorted anatomy due to surgical emphysema, hematoma, and athletic body habitus, all of which will make prehospital surgical dissection complex.

The safest option is to undertake a rapid emergency transfer to the nearest hospital capable of performing drug-induced RSI or a surgical cricothyrotomy. The unit should be given notice of the suspected pathology so that they can have experienced specialist staff ready for the patient's arrival.

Performing a Cricothyrotomy

This is a life-saving emergency procedure for patients with severe upper airway damage. The two techniques are needle and surgical cricothyrotomy. Unfortunately, needle cricothyrotomy is extremely precarious and it is not reliable enough for patient transfer. This method may allow the doctor to provide a *short* period of emergency oxygenation while awaiting more skilled assistance. The FoP team may feel that maintaining oxygenation is a more appropriate goal rather than attempting to provide a definitive airway and ventilation. Surgical cricothyrotomy is a procedure, which should be reserved for the peri-arrest athlete in whom *all other airway maneuvers have failed.*

Needle Cricothyrotomy

1. Choose a 14-gauge intravenous cannula
2. Insert the cannula, in the midline and angle it at 45° in a position superior to the cricothyroid membrane, and into the trachea through the cricothyroid membrane
3. Connect a 1 metre length of oxygen delivery tubing between the oxygen supply and the cannula
4. Cut a small side-hole in the tubing
5. Supply oxygen via the tubing at 15 L/min
6. Cover the hole in the tubing until the chest is seen to rise and then release it for a similar time to allow for passive expiration
7. It may be necessary to insert a second or third cannula to allow for sufficient expiration for further inspiration and oxygenation

Surgical Cricothyrotomy

1. Ensure effective wound suction available
2. Locate the cricothyroid membrane, superior to the cricoid cartilage in the anterior neck. It is a palpable dimple beneath the thyroid and cricoid cartilages
3. Consider injecting local anesthetic
4. Use a sharp scalpel to cut a 1.5 cm horizontal incision through the skin and the cricothyroid membrane in the midline
5. Insert a tracheal hook and lift the cartilage superiorly
6. Pass an appropriately sized endotracheal tube into the wound and the trachea and inflate the cuff
   It may be safer to pass a tracheal bougie through the hole in the cricothyroid membrane and into the trachea and then gently railroad an endotracheal tube over the bougie into the trachea
7. Listen to the chest to ensure bilateral ventilation and check for expired CO_2
8. If breath sounds are not heard and/or expired, CO_2 will not be detected; remove the tube immediately, reexplore the surgical wound and pass the endotracheal tube again. It is not uncommon to pass the tube anteriorly or laterally to the trachea

Tracheobronchial Injury

Blunt injury to the upper trachea is rare. Rupture is extremely difficult to manage effectively and has a high mortality at scene. Clinical features are usually evident with acute respiratory distress and concurrent surgical emphysema.

Attempting to perform endotracheal intubation in a tracheobronchial injury is a hazardous procedure with a high risk of failure and the formation of a false passage, but it may be the only immediate life-saving option.

Vascular Injury – Carotid Artery Dissection or Aneurysm

Blunt vascular injury in trauma patients is relatively rare; however, it is more common in school age athletes. Lateral flexion, hyperextension, and hyperflexion as may be seen in wrestling neck holds, football tackles or diving incidents, or direct blunt trauma can lead to shearing or tears to the intimal layer of the artery. The relatively high pressure in the carotid arteries can lead to dissection within the arterial wall with clotting of the trapped blood. Ultimately, the resulting clot will restrict the blood flow and may result in cerebral ischemia and stroke. More than 50% of people with a carotid artery dissection will develop a stroke over the first few days.

Dissection is a leading cause of stroke in young adults. When trauma causes a dissection, 58% of patients are eventually discharged from the hospital with some form of permanent neurological deficit. If damage to the vessel is more extensive, the injury may balloon outwards as an aneurysm with the direct risk of rupture of the vessel or compression of the trachea or larynx.

Signs of carotid dissection occur at two distinct times; immediately at the time of injury, or several hours to days later, when neurological symptoms caused by the dissection begin to develop. A detailed history about recent sporting activity may identify the traumatic trigger to the pathology.

VASCULAR INJURY - Clinical Findings Acute Vascular Neck Injury

Symptoms: The athlete may complain of sudden onset pain, described as throbbing or sharp, which may gradually worsen.
Inspection: May reveal swelling, abrasions, or bruising.
Palpation: Carotid pulsation may be unchanged on palpation.
Auscultation: An audible bruit may be present on the affected side. This assessment is best carried out in the medical room.
Conduct a rapid primary survey to exclude other life-threatening injuries.

Clinical Findings Delayed Presentation Vascular Neck Injury

Symptom presentation can be highly variable with a myriad of neurological symptom. These include the following:

1. Headache – classically ipsilateral
2. Facial pain/weakness
3. Ophthalmoplegia (weakness/paralysis of the eye muscles)
4. Hemiplegia (often incomplete)
5. Blurred vision
6. Blindness
7. Pulsatile tinnitus (ringing in the ears)
8. Loss of taste sensation or difficulty swallowing
9. Visual field disturbances
10. Anxiety

The differential diagnosis for such a presentation in the young athletic population would be an atypical migraine or cardiac anomaly such as a patent foramen ovale or ventricular septal defect.

Aerodigestive Tract

In the acute setting, injuries to the upper digestive tract in the neck are perhaps of lesser immediate significance than airway or vascular injuries. Nevertheless they are important injuries. The clinical signs may initially be confused with respiratory injuries and they most certainly do have a significant mortality and morbidity if they are missed. The close association of the pharynx and larynx and the posterior position of the digestive tract mean that isolated injury is unlikely. Pharyngeal hematomas have been described, which give painful swallowing or cause concurrent injuries to the laryngeal structures; they must be considered life-threatening in patients who are taking anticoagulants or have blood clotting abnormalities.

1. Rupture of the pharynx is unlikely due to its wide funnel shape and close communication with the nasopharynx
2. The proximal esophagus is slightly more at risk of rupture due to the cricopharyngeus muscle; however, rupture is more common distally
3. Rupture of the esophagus at any level will result in the release of gas into the mediastinum with resultant surgical emphysema, dysphonia, and dysphagia. A pneumomediastinum, while still important, is of lesser significance than other causes of surgical emphysema such as laryngeal, tracheobronchial, or lung injury
4. Esophageal rupture will present hours to days later usually with sepsis and mediastinitis

Management Aerodigestive Track Injury

Perform a primary survey on the FoP with cervical spine considerations, and treat any life-threatening injuries. Arrange for immediate transfer to hospital if major trauma is suspected.

Bibliography

Miller, M.D. (2013) Blunt trauma injuries in the athlete, Clinics in sports medicine **32** (**2**), 211–338.

Tator, C.H. (2008) *Catastrophic Injuries in Sports and Recreation. Causes and Prevention. A Canadian Study*. University of Toronto PressISBN: 0802089674.

13 Facial Injuries

David McDonagh[1,2,3] *and Mike Loosemore*[4,5]

[1]*Emeregency Deptartment, St. Olavs Hospital, Trondheim, Norway*
[2]*Faculty of Medicine, NTNU - National University of Science and Technology, Trondheim, Norway*
[3]*Medical Commission, AIBA - International Boxing Association, Lausanne, Switzerland.*
[4]*English Institute of Sport, University College London and International Boxing Association Medical Commission, London, UK*
[5]*Medical Committee International Bobsleigh and Skeleton Federation, Lausanne, Switzerland*

Injuries to the face are not uncommon in sport, with bruises and small cuts (the most common injury in boxing after the removal of the helmet) being predominant. Serious injuries are rare: at the London Olympic Games only one serious facial injury required Field of Play (FoP) removal. Facial injuries can be classified in several ways, either anatomically (eye, ear, nose, mouth, jaw, and bony structures) or sectional (upper face, midface and mandibular or upper, middle, and lower third).

The most immediate concern with a facial injury is that of airway damage. Fractures of the maxilla, palate, and mandible can affect the patency of the airway as can bleeding and swelling in the mid and lower face. As significant energy is required to fracture the maxilla, fractures of the midface (and mandible) are often associated with traumatic brain injury (TBI) and cervical spine injuries. Similarly, a temperomandibular joint (TMJ) dislocation may significantly affect the patient's ability to draw air into the larynx. Dislocated teeth, braces, or mouth guards can become foreign bodies and may obstruct the airway. Injury to carotid vessels at the angle of the jaw may lead to cerebral ischemia, aneurysm formation, or other potentially life-threatening conditions. As facial injuries lead to potential airway and circulation problems, as well as being associated with TBI and cervical spinal injuries, it is important that all athletes with facial injuries receive a thorough, precise, and rapid evaluation on the FoP, followed by a more detailed fieldside evaluation.

Facial fractures are usually caused by collisions, crashes, and blows from clubs, bats, or from other competitors. Traditionally, injuries have been classified as low-energy fractures (nasal, zygomatic, and dental) and high-energy fractures (mandible, maxilla, and orbit). Both types of fractures can occur in most sports. If there is a high-energy accident, as may occur in skiing, ice hockey, rugby, American football, diving, and boxing, then fractures to the orbit, mandible, and maxilla may be seen.

FoP Management Serious Facial Injuries

On approaching the patient, the doctor will observe if the patient is standing or lying down holding the face. The patient may be unconscious, convulsing, and have bleeding

The IOC Manual of Emergency Sports Medicine, First Edition. Edited by David McDonagh and David Zideman.

from facial wounds. The Emergency Doctor (ED) must always suspect a TBI or spinal injury with a facial injury particularly if the patient has an altered level of consciousness or other head/spinal injury findings.

Initiate the examination by conducting a primary survey.

Facial Injury - Clinical Findings/Management Serious Facial Injury

General inspection: Deformities of the face, mouth, and jaw may be immediately obvious. Similarly, swellings and deformities to the neck and throat must be recognized. The patient may be cyanotic and have breathing difficulties and altered breathing patterns.

Inspection of the airway: Is the patient breathing and is this breathing normal? Are there abnormal breathing sounds? In the obtunded patient, open the airway with a careful chin lift. This may not be possible with a fractured or dislocated jaw due to resistance and the patient may react with pain or spasm. If the jaw or parts of the jaw or palate are loose, then there may be great difficulty in achieving an open airway. If it is possible to open the mouth, do so using a chin lift and carefully inspect for and remove any foreign bodies. If it is not possible to open the mouth or perform a chin lift or jaw thrust, consider performing a head tilt but be aware that the patient may have a concomitant cervical spinal injury so follow manual inline stabilization (MiLS) principles. If this procedure does not adequately improve the patient's condition and/or should the patient deteriorate (become cyanotic, rapid rise or fall in respiratory rate (RR), heaving chest, and falling O_2 saturation), then advanced airway intervention is probably required. Intubation of such a patient will most likely require an anesthesiologist. Cricothyrotomy may be the only option for the nonanesthesiologist ED. This is, of course, a specialized skill and should probably not be performed by nonexperts.

Breathing: Expose the chest. Look for chest movement symmetry, deformities, and wounds. Count the RR. Owing to a potentially blocked airway, there may be dramatic changes in the chest. In the absence of noisy breathing, normal findings in the chest and RR in an alert patient would indicate that there is adequate airway patency and respiratory function. The patient should be turned to the recovery position.

Circulation: Bleeding from facial wounds are seldom life-threatening, unless there is hemorrhage in the mouth causing airway obstruction. This hemorrhage may be difficult to stop with digital compression, either due to the lack of accessibility in the mouth or due to the danger of displacing loose bony fragments or teeth. Airway drainage may be achieved by placing the patient in the recovery position and performing careful suction. Other facial wounds may bleed profusely particularly if the superficial temporal artery is involved. Significant digital compression may be required to stop bleeding, so the ED must be certain that there is no underlying temporal bone fracture/dislocation. Compression can be applied more proximally in the preauricular area over the zygoma if there is concern about compressing fractured temporal bone.

Swellings in the anterolateral aspect of the neck below the angle of the mandible should cause concern as these may represent significant bleeding from neck arteries (see Chapter 12).

Disability: An alert, voice, pain, unresponsive (AVPU) evaluation should be conducted immediately, but a further more detailed neurological evaluation should be delayed until the patient has been evacuated to the fieldside. The patient's condition may deteriorate, so regular neurological evaluations must be conducted until the patient has left the arena. If a head or neck injury is suspected, apply a semirigid cervical collar.

Management: The patient should be correctly immobilized and carefully transported to the sideline, maintaining airway, respiration, and ventilation support.

Fieldside Management Serious Facial Injury

Once at the fieldside, the ED should repeat the primary survey, initiate monitoring, and then immediately conduct a secondary survey. If the patient is alert but appears to have bleeding from the scalp or face, it may be better to transfer the patient to the athlete medical room where the scalp and facial wounds can be washed and cleaned carefully to decrease the risk for infection and improve visualization of wounds and injuries. The secondary survey starts with an examination of the head, neck, then scalp, and then face. This examination must also include the following:

1. Upper third
   a. Forehead evaluation – sensory and motor function
   b. Inspection and palpation of the area around the frontal sinuses
   c. Inspection of wounds to the forehead and scalp
2. Middle third
   a. Examining the pupils for size, equality and light reflex. Positional nystagmus may be seen with a temporal fracture
   b. Palpation of the bones of the midface, palate, and upper teeth
3. Lower third
   a. Examine for mandibular fractures, possibly with open or crossbite deformities
   b. Examine the ears – look for Battle's sign. Otoscopy may reveal blood in the canal or blood behind an intact eardrum (hemotympanum), indicative of a fracture of the base of the cranium (basilar fracture). Look for cerebrospinal fluid (CSF) leakage from the ears and nose - the "halo" sign (see below). A laceration in the canal or hemotympanum may represent a skull base fracture
   c. Neck tenderness, neck pain on movement, and cervical range of motion (ROM)

Clinical Findings/Management Serious Facial Injury

Inspection: Inspect the scalp, skull, face, and neck for cuts, bruises, and deformities. Look for CSF and/or blood leakage from the ears, mouth, and nose (see Chapter 10). A bleeding nose may indicate a nasal fracture but also a fracture of the base of the skull; with bleeding from the ear always suspect a fracture of the base of skull. Battle's sign or binocular hematomas may develop after a cranial base fracture – though some time may elapse before these signs manifest themselves clinically. Large swellings may indicate fracture. The incidence of TBI is increased with cranial and facial fractures. Inspect the eyes for abnormality. Inspect the open mouth.

Palpation: Palpate gently for indentations or depressed skull fractures and swellings, eye and orbit tenderness, bridge of the nose, the nose, frontal bones, jaw bone, and TMJ. Subcutaneous emphysema may be indicative of a maxillary fracture.

Neurological evaluation: Conduct a rapid neurological evaluation – most doctors use the Glasgow Coma Score.

Focused history: Take a focused history. Enquire about vision changes. Is there a sweet taste of sugar in the mouth or palate?

Range of Movement (ROM): If relatively pain free, conduct a gentle test of cervical spine ROM but stop if pain or resistance is noticed (see Chapter 19).

Management: If alert, responsive, stabile, pain free, and able to stand and walk unassisted, conduct a fieldside concussion evaluation (See Chapter 11).

It is important to be able to diagnose and manage the following conditions, some of which may be associated with potentially life-threatening complications:

1. Maxillary fractures
2. Mandible fractures
3. TMJ dislocation
4. Orbital fractures
5. Zygomatic fractures
6. Ear lacerations and contusions
7. Eye injuries (see Chapter 14)
8. Nasal fractures
9. Naso-ocular-ethmoidal fractures

10. Septal hematomas
11. Epistaxis
12. Oral/dental injuries (see Chapter 15)
13. Lacerations (see Chapter 27)

Maxillary Fractures

Maxillary fractures can be associated with life-threatening cranial and cerebral injuries. Fracture lines often follow the Le Fort classification:

1. Le Fort I is a transverse fracture crossing the maxilla below the nose and above the teeth
2. Lefort II is a pyramidal fracture that extends through the maxillae and across the bridge of nose
3. Lefort III is craniofacial disjunction fracture line that extends across the floor of the orbit and through the nasofrontal area. It may present with the classical "Dishface" appearance, with a flat elongated face

Clinical Findings/Management LeFort Fracture

Le Fort 1 fracture	Le Fort 2 fracture	Le Fort 3 fracture
Bruising of upper lip and lower half of midface	Periorbital bruising	Facial bruising
Mobility of whole of tooth-bearing segment of upper jaw	Infraorbital nerve damage – including hyperesthesia of the cheeks	Severe facial deformity –Deformity with palpable step in orbital rims, zygomatic arches, nose, and maxilla
Disturbed occlusion	May have bilateral subconjunctival hematomas and diplopia	May be unconscious and have breathing difficulties
Hematoma in palate	Symmetry/palpable step deformities of orbital rims, zygomatic arches, nose, and maxilla	Often infraorbital nerve damage including hyperesthesia
Palpable crepitation in upper buccal sulcus	Movement of dental arches and mobile maxilla	May have bilateral subconjunctival hematomas and diplopia
	Fractured/avulsed/mobile teeth	Often mobile palate/dental arches
		Palate hematoma
		Bloody nasal discharge – with CSF

Management: The first priority is to ensure adequate airway, respiration, and circulation. Look for and expect to find signs of cranial injury with Le Fort 3 and possibly with Le Fort 2 fractures. Continuous neurological evaluation is necessary. Rapid transportation to hospital is indicated with all Le Fort fractures but especially Grade 2 and 3 fractures. Continuous monitoring of the airway and respiration is obligatory.

Mandibular Fractures

Mandibular fractures are not infrequent and often occur after falls or high-energy blows to the chin. Fractures usually occur at the following sites: body (35%), angle (25%), condyle (15%), symphysis (10%), and ramus (5%). Double fractures can occur.

Clinical Findings/Management Mandibular Fracture

Inspection: Look for facial distortion, swelling, bruising, malocclusion of the teeth, gaps, or steps between the teeth which may be present with dislocation of a fractured segment.
Palpation: May be painful, examine for deformity along the mandible or at the TMJ.
Movement: Abnormal mobility of portions of the mandible or teeth. Inability to open the mouth or pain on doing so. Inability to close the mouth.
Management: Prehospital management is conservative. Ensure that the athlete has an adequate airway, normal ventilation. Suspect concomitant facial, cranial, cervical, and throat injuries. All patients with suspected mandibular fractures should be hospitalized. Analgesia may be required.

Traumatic Temperomandibular Joint (TMJ) Dislocations

TMJ dislocations may occur but are unusual. While a dislocation may occur after a blow (boxing), it may also occur after excessive opening of the jaw (tired, long distance runners). In most cases, the mandibular condyle luxates anteriorly so that the jaw appears to be prognatic and gaping. The surrounding muscles (masseter, temporalis, and internal pterygoid) often go into spasm, thus preventing autoreduction. The condition often occurs bilaterally but a direct blow may lead to a unilateral dislocation. Condyle fractures may occur, so radiological examination should be conducted before reduction is attempted. The clinical findings are usually very obvious after history taking and clinical examination. The patient will have difficulties in speaking and with swallowing; drinks and food should be avoided until the condition has been corrected.

Orbital Fractures

Trauma to the upper face may result in fractures of the orbit (see Chapter 14), which may vary from small defects in the orbital floor, to blowout fractures, to fractures involving all four orbital walls and more complex facial fractures. Isolated blow-in fractures have also been described, but are rare.

Blowout fractures usually occur after a direct blunt blow to the eye by a ball or bat. Forces may be transmitted downwards through the eye fracturing either the thin inferior orbital floor or medially into the ethmoid bones. The orbit sinks into the fracture recess and becomes entrapped. The infraorbital rim may be intact.

Fractures may also occur at the infraorbital rim and may extend into the inferior orbital floor. This type of injury is often caused by being hit by a golf ball, squash ball, and handle of an ice hockey stick. Not all orbital fractures are blowout fractures.

Clinical Findings/Management Orbital Fracture

Symptoms: Lid ecchymosis or edema, painful extraocular movements, diplopia (due to orbital muscle entrapment or globe malposition), decreased sensation of the lower eyelid, cheek, and upper lip.
Gross inspection: Proptosis (abnormal protrusion of the eye), enophthalmos (abnormal posterior displacement of the eye), or rotation of the eye may be present along with ecchymosis (swelling or black eye).
Pupil inspection: May be normal.
Pupillary reflex: May be normal.

Palpation: May reveal bony tenderness, subcutaneous emphysema, or numbness under the eye and on the cheek due to infraorbital nerve damage.
Gross visual acuity: May be double vision.
Eye movement: Classically, there may be restriction of ocular movement particularly during upward gaze, as a result of entrapment of the extraocular muscles.
Fundoscopy: May be normal.
Management: If a fracture is suspected, then the athlete must not return to play. Melting ice can be applied gently to the infraorbital area, but pressure must not be applied to the eye itself. Nose blowing should be avoided to prevent pressure displacement of sinus contents into the orbit.

Radiological referral is advised and the athlete should be evaluated by an eye specialist or facial surgeon.

Analgesia may be required. Patients with grossly displaced fractures or fractures with persistent double vision, ocular entrapment, or pain are usually candidates for surgical repair.

Zygomatic Fractures

Fractures may be isolated or associated with serious midface trauma. If there is an isolated uncomplicated fracture with no or minimal displacement of the zygoma, conservative management is recommended. The athlete should be sent for radiological evaluation. The athlete should avoid blowing his/her nose (to avoid subcutaneous and orbital emphysema). Displaced zygomatic fractures may require surgery. Some fractures are complicated with cranial, cerebral, orbital, ocular, facial, and cervical injuries, so the ED must remain alert and exclude these potential injuries. As always, it is essential to ascertain that the airway is not compromised.

Clinical Findings/Management Zygomatic Fracture

Inspection: Look for swelling and bruising around the eye, which is called the subconjunctival hemorrhage. Look for Malar flattening.
Palpation: There may be painful, palpable deformity (swelling or depressed fracture). Gently palpate the orbital walls. Impairment of sensation below the eye (infraorbital nerve) may indicate a maxilla fracture.
Eye: Inspect the eye, checking for damage to the globe, enophthalmos, and exophthalmos. Check visual acuity and visual fields. Check for diplopia and examine eye movements.
Jaw: Displacement of the fractured fragment may cause pain on chewing. Trismus can occur (spasm of the masseter muscle), making chewing difficult and painful. Examine TMJ movement.
Management: If a fracture is suspected, radiological referral is advised and the athlete should be evaluated by an Ear, Nose, and Throat (ENT) or facial surgeon. Analgesia may be required.

Ear – Lacerations, Avulsions, Contusions, Burst Eardrums, Discharges

Cuts to the ears are relatively rare but can occur and should be managed in the same manner as cuts elsewhere in the body; wounds must be cleaned and covered and the athlete removed from the FoP to the medical room for further wound cleansing, repair, and closure (See Chapter 27). Precise matching of structures is important for optimal cosmesis when suturing the ear.

If there is an open wound involving a small tear of the cartilage, it is often adequate for the doctor to suture the skin only, using the folds of the ear as alignment landmarks. Suturing cartilage can occasionally lead to cartilage destruction and resorption. The dressings play an important splinting role and should support the pinna on both sides; the dressings may also help prevent the formation of a hematoma.

For larger cartilage tears, the cartilage must be sutured. Wounds to the ear are commonly irregular, and if there is cartilage exposure due to skin loss, refer to a specialist.

Avulsed ear If the ear or parts of the ear are avulsed, it is important to locate and salvage the avulsed parts by placing them in a cold clean saline solution. Cover the injured ear with a saline bandage and support the bandage with a circular elasticized turban bandage around the head. Bleeding may be profuse and intravenous (IV) fluids may be necessary. The patient should be transported to hospital with the head elevated.

Repetitive bruising of the ear may lead to the development of an auricular hematoma, the so-called "cauliflower ear," which is particularly predominant in rugby and boxing. An acute hematoma should be managed with ice compression and possibly early needle aspiration in very large swellings as the hematoma may cause baronecrosis of the auricular cartilage (similar to the processes involved in a nasal septal hematoma).

Burst eardrum Tympanic membrane ruptures occur after falls or blows to the side of the head (boxing) but also after exposure to loud noises (acoustic trauma) or acute pressure (barotraumata). The condition is painful with varying degrees of hearing loss. Some patients experience tinnitus or vertigo. There may be bleeding or discharge from the ear. Otoscopic examination will usually reveal the extent of the condition.

Management involves rest and avoidance of new injury while the drum heals. Infection may delay this process. Elective surgery is sometimes indicated.

Barotrauma Barotrauma is mostly seen in water sports such as diving and water skiing. The patient may present with pain, reduced hearing, bleeding or discharge, tinnitus, nausea, and vertigo. Rest is recommended, antibiotics may be appropriate with infections, and nasal decongestants may help reduce pain and swelling. Initial symptoms usually disappear within 2–3 days. If not, consider specialist referral. A ruptured eardrum usually heals without surgical intervention.

Ear – fluid or blood discharge from the ear Discharge from the ear may occur when there is an underlying cranial fracture and may contain blood, CSF, or a mixture of both. CSF may be difficult to detect – place some tissue paper in the discharge, leave for a minute, and inspect the paper – there will be blood at the point of paper contact and possibly an orange/lighter colored ring outside the blood stain, the so-called "halo" sign. Eardrum and blood vessel ruptures can occur in the absence of fracture but their presence should raise concern. The most common cause of discharge is, of course, infection.

Nasal Fractures

When examining for nasal injuries, the ED considers the following:

1. Is the airway patent and is the athlete breathing adequately?
2. Is there epistaxis (see below)?
3. Are there any symptoms or signs of concussion and associated head injury?

4. Are there associated facial or cervical spine injuries?
5. Is there a nasal bone, nasal cartilage, or nasoethmoidal fracture?
6. Is there a septal hematoma?

Airway patency and breathing will be evaluated in the primary survey, as will the patient's responsiveness. Head injury must be excluded with all nasal injuries. The face will be examined in more detail during the secondary survey at the fieldside. Most nasal fractures in sport are the result of minor or moderate trauma after a punch or elbow to the face. The ED should examine all bony structures of the face, including the orbits, interorbital area, maxilla, zygomatic arches, mandible, teeth, and palate. Any swellings, cuts, bruises, and deformities of or around the nose should be noted and the eyes should be examined for ocular injury, diplopia, and blowout fractures.

Clinical Findings with a Nasal Fracture

Symptoms: Pain, inability to breath through the nose, bloody nose.

Inspection: There may be deformity and swelling of the nose, epistaxis, edema, and bruising of perinasal and periorbital structures. Blood may be visible in the pharynx behind the uvula. If epistaxis persists, there may be a fracture present despite limited findings.

Palpation: Palpation of the nasal structures may be painful and may reveal indentation. Subcutaneous emphysema may indicate a maxillary fracture.

Rhinoscopy: There may be swelling, wounds, or bleeding in the nasal passage, or, very rarely, protruding bone or cartilage. Persistent epistaxis without deformity or clear rhinorrhea (CSF) must cause the ED to suspect a nasal, nasoethmoidal, or basilar cranial fracture!

Management: Management of uncomplicated acute nasal fracture includes the application of ice, the maintenance of head elevation, rest, and appropriate pain medication. If the nose is cosmetically unchanged, no reduction is required. Nasal X-rays have little use. X-ray and CT investigations are usually only indicated with a facial or sinus fracture. Once the bleeding has stopped (see Epistaxis below), the nose should be inspected to exclude a septal hematoma.

If the nose is deformed, a fracture may be presumed to be present and reduction is required. Most ENT specialists accept that fracture reduction can be performed 3–5 days after the injury.

Nasoethmoidal Fractures

These fractures may occur after a high-energy frontal blow to the face and nose. There may be collapse and telescoping of the nasal bones under the frontal bone, or laterally into the orbit potentially causing a naso-orbito-ethmoidal (NOE) fracture. Maxillofacial surgeons divide the face into many segments based on a complicated series of lines, and remembering these can be quite difficult. One measurement may have clinical significance for the ED. The distance between the center of each pupil (interpupillary distance) is usually twice that of the intercanthal distance (the canthus is the medial corner of the eye). With NOE fractures the interpupillary distance remains the same, but the intercanthal distance increases (traumatic telecanthus).

Fractures in this complex anatomical area may be difficult to diagnose due to swelling and bruising. Fractures may occur as isolated injuries or as part of more complex facial fractures involving the anterior cranium. Look for associated ocular injury if the eyelids are not too swollen. Fluid from the nose may be due to CSF leaks and may indicate a fracture of the anterior cranial fossa with an anterior dural tear.

Clinical Findings/Management NOE Fracture

Symptoms: The patient may be unconscious, or in pain, inability to breath through the nose, altered vision, double vision, epistaxis, dizziness, and anosmia.

Inspection: There may be deformity and bruising of the nose, intercanthal area, and periorbital structures. Look for traumatic telecanthus. There may be periorbital hematomas. Epistaxis may be present. The nose may be shortened (telescopic changes).

Palpation: Palpation of the nasal structures, intercanthal area, and lower frontal bone may be painful and reveal indentation or swelling.

Rhinoscopy: Not recommended if there is altered consciousness or threatened ABC. In a stable patient, there may be swelling, wounds, or bleeding in the nasal passage.

Management: These patients need stabilization of ABC and may have serious head and facial injuries. The ED should have a low threshold for referral to a specialist hospital with CT facilities with clinical findings indicative of injury to this region.

Septal Hematomas

After receiving a blow to the nose, an athlete may develop a septal hematoma. A hematoma may develop between the cartilaginous septum and the perichondrium/mucous plate. If allowed to develop, pressure from the hematoma may compress the blood vessels leading to cartilage necrosis, resulting in the "Popeye" or saddle deformity of the septum. In addition to being disfigured, this lesion can affect nasal respiration by obstructing the nares.

Clinical Findings/Management Septal Hematoma

Symptoms: Pain, inability to breath through the nose.

Inspection: There may be deformity of the nose, broadening of the septum (unilaterally or bilaterally), broadening of the columella, and septa may appear slightly discolored. There may be epistaxis, edema, and bruising of the nose, perinasal, and periorbital structures. The initial internal inspection may reveal the presence of large blood clots. A large clot may obstruct inspection of the septal wall, ask the patient to blow the nose gently, one nostril at a time (this is contraindicated if there is a maxillary or orbital fracture, particularly with a blowout fracture). Any mucosal lacerations should be noted because they may indicate an underlying fracture.

Palpation: Palpation of the nasal structures may be painful and reveal indentation. The swelling will initially be soft and fluctuant on palpation, unlike a normal septum which is hard.

Rhinoscopy: There may be swelling, smaller nasal passage (nares) on the injured side, with a swollen, red, medial septal wall.

Management: A patient with a suspected septum hematoma should be referred to a specialist that day. Hematomas may also become infected.

Epistaxis

In sport, nosebleeds usually occur after injury to vessels in the Kiesselbach plexus in the anterior nasal septum region (anterior nose bleeds). Occasionally, epistaxis can have a posterior origin and these bleedings, though rare, can be difficult to manage. Epistaxis is usually caused by local trauma or irritation but can be associated with systemic conditions such as a coagulation disorder or hypertension. When the medical team is called to a patient on the FoP, the ED must first conduct a primary survey and if the athlete's condition is stable, it is probably best to follow the ringside approach to manage nosebleeds (boxing doctors treat this condition often):

1. Decide if the bleed is venous or arterial in origin (venous blood seeps from the nose, and arterial blood spurts forwards and is thus easily recognized). Arterial bleeds should be compressed immediately using the doctor's thumb and index finger to compress both nares. The athlete should lie down and be stretchered from the FoP as physical exercise increases blood flow.
2. If there is a venous bleeding compress both nares and observe if the athlete winces with pain. If so, there is probably a fracture present and the athlete should be removed from the FoP for further examination in the athlete medical room.
3. If the athlete does not seem to be in pain, continue to exert pressure on the nares and inspect the mouth for blood. The presence of blood at the back of the mouth or behind the uvula and soft palate indicates significant, and possibly posterior, bleeding and the athlete should be removed from the FoP for further examination.
4. If the athlete is stable, then there is no sign of arterial bleeding, the athlete is not in pain, and the bleeding ceases after compression of the nares; it is wise to bring the athlete to the fieldside and conduct a concussion evaluation.

Fieldside evaluation of epistaxis – secondary survey This is preferably best conducted in the athlete medical room where facilities for examination and treatment are much better than at the fieldside. Conduct a secondary survey, including a basic neurological evaluation, usually a Glasgow Coma Score (GCS). The patient or other healthcare professional should compress the nares until the nose is examined – epistaxis usually requires a minimum of 5 min digital compression. Obviously, rhinoscopy is not recommended if there is altered consciousness or threatened ABC.

Clinical Findings/Management Epistaxis

Symptoms: Bleeding may be spontaneous (usually painless) or traumatic (painful), there may be difficulty breathing through the nose and the athlete may spit up blood.

Inspection: There may be deformity and bruising of the nose and face, indicating a more complex fracture (see above). Bleeding may be from one or both nares and must rapidly be defined as being arterial or venous. Inspect the mouth and oropharynx with a tongue depressor and light source for hematomas, deformities, and bleeding behind the uvula (possible posterior bleed). Similarly, examine the nose, with the patient in a sitting position, with a light source and speculum; if there is a clot blocking inspection, ask the patient (in the absence of facial fractures) to blow the nose gently, one nostril at a time. Inspect Little's area for injuries. Look for signs of septal deviation, septal hematoma, or swelling and bony deformity.

Palpation: Gently palpate the nose, including nasal bones, and the intercanthal/subfrontal area for tenderness and swelling. The rest of the face will be examined during the secondary survey.

Neurological Examination: Before considering an immediate return to play, a fieldside concussion evaluation should be made.

Management: If bleeding persists after examination in the medical room (or has not been stopped by the time the nose is examined), digital compression of the nares should be continued. At some stage, usually after 15 min of compression, if the bleeding does not subside, then the ED must consider packing the nose. Always recheck for postnasal drip (blood behind the uvula or soft palate) as this may indicate posterior bleeding and the need for hospital referral.

There are many ways of packing the nose and it is best to follow local guidelines and practices. Pack both nares to ensure bilateral compression with an anterior bleed. If no other tamponade equipment is available, then apply a small amount of Vaseline to an appropriately sized swab and pack the nares. Re-examine the patient after 15–20 min – bleeding may appear to have ceased anteriorly, but always check for postnasal drip. Some doctors use a topical anesthetic/vasoconstrictor fluid dripped onto the swab – however, be aware that epinephrine is currently on the WADA Prohibited List. If the anterior nasal pack does not stop bleeding, then refer the athlete to hospital. If a posterior nosebleed is suspected, then the patient should always be referred to hospital. If the anterior nasal pack does stop bleeding, then the patient may be discharged with advice on contacting a doctor on return home or to recontact a doctor if bleeding resumes. The pack can stay in place for at least 1 day.

Bibliography

Resident Manual of Trauma to the Face, Head and Neck, American Academy of Otolaryngology, Head and Neck Surgery Foundation.
http://www.entnet.org/mktplace/upload/ResidentTraumaFINALlowres.pdf

14 Eye Injuries and Other Ocular Emergencies

Sibel Kocabeyoglu,[1] Uğur Erdener [1] and David McDonagh [2,3,4]

[1]Department of Ophtalmology, Hacettepe University Faculty of Medicine, Ankara, Turkey
[2]Emeregency Deptartment, St. Olavs Hospital, Trondheim, Norway
[3]Faculty of Medicine, NTNU - National University of Science and Technology, Trondheim, Norway
[4]Medical Commission, AIBA - International Boxing Association, Lausanne, Switzerland.

Although, ocular injuries and emergencies are nowadays rare in sport, sport-related eye injuries can still result in the loss of function. Eye injuries caused by sport account for between 40,000 and 600,000 eye injuries each year in the United States (United States Consumer Product Safety Commission 2000) and approximately 42% of patients are admitted to hospital due to an ocular injury sustained as a result of sport-related trauma. However, estimation of the exact incidence of sport-related eye injuries is difficult as the types and patterns of the trauma vary from country to country. Data from The National Eye Trauma System in the United States found that sport-associated eye injuries account for 13% of all penetrating eye injuries. It is suggested that 90% of ocular injuries are preventable (Prevent Blindness America (1994)). In recent decades, the International Federations have had an increased emphasis on athlete safety and injury prevention with the resultant introduction of visors and protective goggles in alpine skiing, ice hockey, American football, and fencing. However, injuries such as superficial rifts, blowout fractures, or intraocular bleedings do still occur. Although most of the ocular injuries involve the external tissues, intraocular structures are affected in one-third of cases. The commonest injury to the ocular region is the periorbital hematoma or black eye, but this lesion can hide other injuries that are not immediately visible due to swelling and serious underlying ocular pathology may be missed.

The Ocular Trauma Classification Group defines the variables that affect visual outcome prognosis as being: "the mechanism of injury, the visual acuity at initial examination, the presence or absence of afferent papillary defect (pupillary reflex), and the location of the eye-wall opening".

There are a number of conditions, both traumatic and nontraumatic, the healthcare professional must be aware of and should refer to an ophthalmologist without delay. Primary among these traumatic conditions are the following:

1. Blunt trauma to the eye and periorbital structures
2. Penetrating injury to the orbit
3. Foreign bodies in the eye
4. Blowout and other fractures around the eye
5. Significant limitation of ocular motility
6. Cuts to the eyelids
7. Lacerations of periorbital structures including canalicular system
8. Proptosis (abnormal anterior bulging of the eye)

The IOC Manual of Emergency Sports Medicine, First Edition. Edited by David McDonagh and David Zideman.
2015 International Olympic Committee. Published 2015 by John Wiley & Sons, Ltd.

9. Enophthalmos (abnormal posterior displacement of the eye)
10. Irregular pupil
11. Blood in the anterior chamber

Nontraumatic emergencies include the following:

1. Acute loss of vision or visual field defects
2. Acute double vision
3. Light flashes or floaters (may also be traumatic)
4. Acute "red eye"
5. Acute eye pain

Fieldside Observation and Observations on Approaching the Athlete

The Emergency Doctor (ED) should follow the sporting event at all times if possible, in order to observe any incidents or accidents and to potentially gather important information regarding the type and severity of an injury. It will quickly become apparent if the athlete is unconscious, has reduced consciousness, or appears to be fully alert. It is recommended that the ED always follows the ABCDE mnemonic even though it may appear obvious that the ABC is normal. Disability (D) must always be tested with ocular injuries as patients may have concomitant facial, cranial, cerebral, or spinal injuries. By strictly adhering to the ABCDE regime other (more critical) conditions may be detected and correct treatment initiated in the proper order of priority. It is unlikely that an athlete will have to cease activity due to the acute onset of nontraumatic pain, red eye, or visual changes but if so, the athlete should be taken from the FoP to the fieldside and preferably to the more controlled environment of the athlete medical room for further evaluation.

FoP Management Eye Injury

Initiate the examination by conducting a primary survey to rapidly identify and treat life-threatening conditions. With ocular injuries, there will obviously be a focus on the neurological examination. Having excluded any life-threatening conditions, if the athlete complains of or has signs of ocular or periocular injury, remove the athlete to the fieldside for further evaluation. In the event of a major penetrating injury to the eye, the patient will require onfield ABCDE stabilization and local protection of the eyes. Penetrating foreign bodies that are implanted in the eye should not be removed. They should be stabilized, the eye should be covered if possible, and the athlete should be immediately transferred to an emergency neurological/ophthalmological unit by ambulance.

Fieldside Management Eye Injury

If an athlete is unconscious, it is difficult to evaluate an eye injury unless there are visible signs of damage to the orbit or periorbital region. In a patient with altered consciousness the situation is more difficult. Repeat the primary survey at the fieldside and then conduct a secondary survey that includes an examination of the GCS, pupillary light reflexes, eye movement, and gross visual acuity.

In the completely alert athlete, a systematic secondary survey should be performed. An athlete who has several injuries simultaneously may focus on the most painful rather than the most serious of these injuries, hence the importance of conducting a systematic secondary survey. This will only take a few minutes if all is well and most eye injuries do not require immediate intervention either on the FoP or at the fieldside.

Take a focused history; this and further evaluation is best conducted in the athlete medical room. If the patient has abnormal pupillary findings, a GCS of 14 or less or any findings that could indicate a facial, cranial, or spinal fracture then the ED should consider referring the athlete to hospital.

In the case of isolated eye injuries in conscious patients, it is usually not necessary to repeat the primary survey, though this is always a good routine. If the athlete has any abnormal visual symptoms or findings, then the athlete should be removed to the athlete medical treatment room for further evaluation. Ask the patient if they have any eye defects or abnormalities. This examination includes the following:

1. Gross inspection of the periorbital region and eyelids (ecchymosis, deformity, and cuts); conjunctiva, cornea, and sclera (foreign bodies, abrasions, or lacerations); anterior chamber (hyphema)
2. Inspection of the pupils for anisocoria (unequal pupil size) and any irregularities in shape
3. Pupillary light reaction should be checked for presence or absence of a relative afferent pupillary defect (RAPD). The pupils must be equal and round in shape and react equally to light. Any irregularity should be considered as a sign of a serious intracranial or intraocular trauma (an afferent pupillary defect may be suggestive of optic nerve damage)
4. A gross assessment of visual acuity by testing the ability to count fingers (or portable Snellen visual acuity cards) and confrontational visual field assessment
5. Eye movements should be checked by asking the patient to look in the four main directions of gaze (up, down, left, and right). Both eyes should have full motility in all positions of gaze. A limitation in eye movements may suggest an orbital floor fracture, which may cause double vision. In addition, significant periorbital edema, hemorrhage, or lack of patient cooperation often prohibits formal motility testing
6. Finally, fundoscopic examination should be performed to evaluate the red reflex
7. If there is a suspicion for globe rupture, a protective eye shield should be placed over the eye and the patient should be transferred to hospital without further manipulation

Eye – Blunt Trauma

Blunt trauma occurs when the eye is struck with a tennis ball, golf ball, a racquet, a thumb (gouging), a fist, or other solid object. Damage to ocular structures is due to sudden compression and indentation of the eye and may produce bleeding in the anterior chamber, scarring of the lens (traumatic cataract), lens subluxation/dislocation, retinal tears with bleeding into the vitreous gel (posterior chamber hemorrhage), retinal tears that may lead to retinal detachment, and even retrobulbar hemorrhage. If the external force is large enough, then a fracture or even a blowout fracture can also occur.

Depending on the scale of the injury, symptoms may vary from mild eye pain with or without blurred vision, to intense pain, loss of vision, or diplopia. The following conditions can occur after blunt trauma.

Hyphema – Anterior Chamber Hemorrhage

Hyphema is a common sports-related ocular injury. Direct blunt trauma to the eye, hockey stick, puck, tennis, or squash racquet, and so on may lead to rupture of blood vessels in the iris and results in bleeding into the anterior chamber. The blood settles and forms a fluid level, so the bottom of the iris appears red like a bloody half moon. The condition can take some hours to develop fully. Patients will complain of reduced vision, visual field defects, pain, and photosensitivity. The amount of blood is related to morbidity and poor visual prognosis and may result in increased intraocular pressure with secondary glaucoma in larger hyphemas (Figure 14.1).

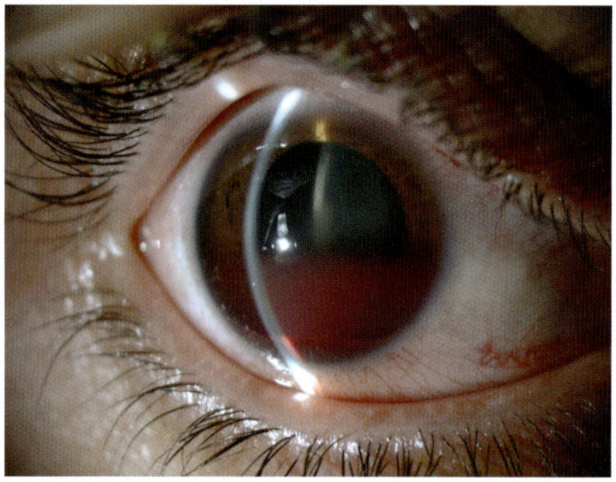

Figure 14.1 Traumatic hyphema. Fresh red blood layered in the anterior chamber (*Source:* Courtesy of Hacettepe University, Department of Ophthalmology.)

Clinical Findings/Management Hyphema

Symptoms: Pain, blurred vision, visual field defects, and photophobia.
Gross inspection of the periorbital region and eyelids: May be bruising, swelling, conjunctival and scleral damage, or bleeding. Gross layering of blood with a "fluid level" in the anterior chamber.
Inspection of the pupils: May be normal.
Pupillary light reaction: May be normal.
Gross assessment of visual acuity: May be reduced.
Eye movements: May be normal.
Fundoscopy: May be normal but limited due to the hyphema.
Management: Cover the eye with an eyeshield. Athletes should be hospitalized for further evaluation and treatment.

Lens Subluxation

Traumatic lens subluxation may occur secondary to tearing of the suspensory ligament. The lens may be luxated into the anterior chamber (Figure 14.2).

Clinical Findings/Management Lens Subluxation

Symptoms: Diplopia, decreased vision.
Gross inspection of the periorbital region and eyelids: There may be signs of trauma to the conjunctiva, sclera, and periorbitally.
Inspection of the pupils: The edge of subluxated lens may be visible.
Pupillary light reaction: May be normal or abnormal.
Visual acuity: There will be a gross disturbance in visual acuity.
Eye movements: Generally normal.
Fundoscopy: Will be abnormal and findings will depend on the mechanism of injury.
Management: Cover the eye with an eyeshield. Athletes should be hospitalized for further evaluation and treatment.

Posterior Chamber Hemorrhage

Direct trauma to the eye may cause bleeding into the vitreous gel due to damage to a retinal vessel (Figure 14.3). There may also be damage to the retina and there is an increased risk of retinal detachment.

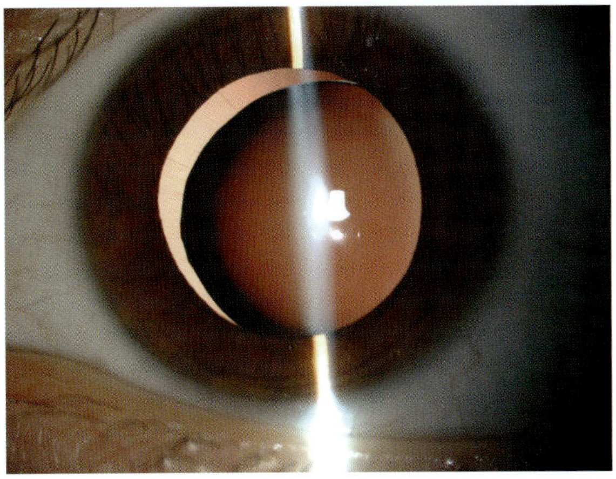

Figure 14.2 Inferior and temporal lens dislocation (*Source:* Courtesy of Hacettepe University, Department of Ophthalmology)

Figure 14.3 Traumatic posterior chamber hemorrhage (*Source:* Courtesy of Hacettepe University, Department of Ophthalmology)

Posterior Chamber Hemorrhage

Symptoms: Blurred vision or floaters.
Gross inspection of the periorbital region and eyelids: There may be signs of trauma to the conjunctiva, sclera, and periorbitally.
Inspection of the pupils: May be normal.
Pupillary light reflex: May be normal.
Visual acuity: May be reduced.
Eye movements: Generally normal.
Fundoscopy: The blood in the vitreus may obscure the red reflex.
Management: Cover the eye with an eyeshield. Athletes should be hospitalized for further evaluation and treatment.

Retinal Detachment

In sport, retinal detachments, where vitreous fluid seeps through a retinal tear, are usually caused by blunt trauma to the globe (Figure 14.4). Nontraumatic causes include diabetes, sickle cell disease, and central retinal vein occlusion. This can occur immediately or may develop over some days or even weeks. Referral to hospital is mandatory; if traumatic in nature, refer the athlete for a computed tomography (CT) of the brain and face. The retina can detach without any obvious or known trauma. An appropriate previous assessment is mandatory to identify prior conditions such as high myopia, previous history of retinal detachment or eye surgery, and family history of retinal tears. Athletes with any of these conditions are at increased risk of retinal detachment. Athletes with such risk factors should use an eye-protective device to reduce the severity of injury.

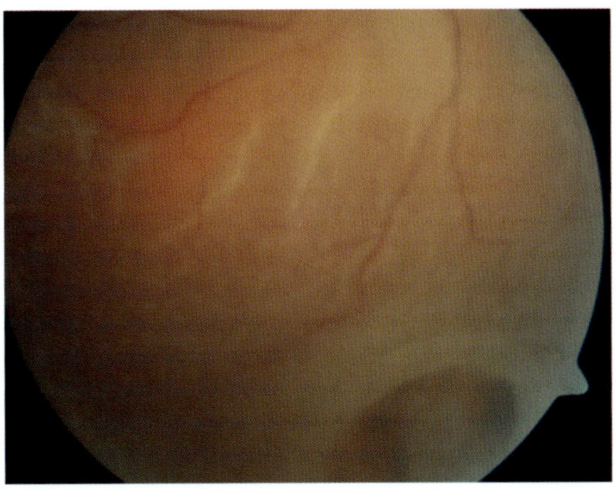

Figure 14.4 Appearance of retinal break in detached retina (*Source:* Courtesy of Hacettepe University, Department of Ophthalmology.)

Clinical Findings/Management Retinal Detachment

Symptoms: Floating spots, flashing lights, visual field defects perceiving as a "black curtain," and blurry vision.
Gross inspection of the periorbital region and eyelids: May be normal or there may be signs of trauma to the conjunctiva, sclera, and periorbitally.
Inspection of the pupils: May be normal.
Pupillary light reflex: May be normal, or there may be a relative afferent pupilllary defect (if the detachment is extensive).
Visual acuity: Visual acuity may be decreased.
Eye movements: Generally normal.
Fundoscopy: Blood in the vitreus may obscure the red reflex.
Management: Cover the eye with an eyeshield. Athletes should be hospitalized for further evaluation and treatment (Figure 14.4).

Blowout Fractures

A blowout fracture of the orbital floor is caused after orbital trauma, for example, a punch, a baseball bat, a tennis ball, a knee, or even a soccer ball in the face. There can be a sudden dramatic increase in intraorbital pressure that causes the eye to move backwards and then downwards through the weakest part of the orbit, the orbital floor.

The classical finding on investigation is that the damaged eye fails to elevate/rotate on testing (vertical dystopia). There is always the likelihood of concomitant intracranial injury, cranial fracture, and other trauma to the face, so the healthcare professional needs to be alert (Figure 14.5)

Clinical Findings/Management Blowout Fracture

Symptoms: Lid ecchymosis or edema, painful extraocular movements, diplopia, decreased sensation of the ipsilateral lower eyelid, cheek, and upper lip.
Gross inspection: Proptosis (abnormal protrusion of the eye) or enophthalmos (abnormal posterior displacement of the eye) or even rotation of the eye may be present along with ecchymosis, swelling, or black eye. Occasionally subcutaneous emphysema may be seen or palpated.
Pupil inspection: May be normal.
Pupillary reflex: May be normal.
Palpation: May reveal bony tenderness, subcutaneous emphysema, or numbness under the eye and on the cheek due to infraorbital nerve damage.
Gross visual acuity: May be double vision.
Eye movement: Classically, there may be restriction of the extraocular movement particularly upward gaze, as a result of entrapment of the extraocular muscles.
Fundoscopy: May be normal.
Management: Stabilize the patient and transfer to a hospital with CT facilities and an ophthalmologist.

Orbital Cavity Fractures

Fracture around the orbital cavity may be single or multiple. Multiple fractures in and around the orbit may lead to an "expanded orbit" with distinct deformity. Fractures may also be part of a Le Fort fracture line and may be associated with a cranial or facial fracture (See Chapter 13). Not all orbital fractures are "blowout" fractures. Blood under the superior conjunctiva may suggest an orbital roof fracture.

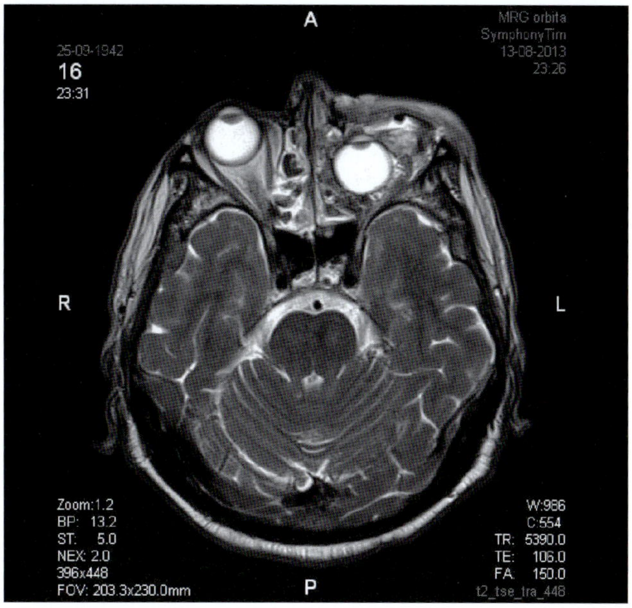

Figure 14.5 CT view of left orbital blowout fracture

(*Source:* Courtesy of Hacettepe University, Department of Ophthalmology.)

Clinical Findings/Management Orbital Fracture

As with a blowout fracture.

Rupture of the Globe

A globe rupture is the most serious result of ocular trauma and associated with significant visual morbidity. The rupture usually occurs at the weakest part of the eye and intraocular structures may prolapse causing an open globe injury. Rupture may be caused by blunt trauma or by penetrating foreign bodies. Removal of penetrating foreign bodies may cause prolapse.

Clinical Findings/Management Rupture of the Globe

Symptoms: Pain and decreased vision.

Ophthalmic examination: Deep eyelid lacerations, swelling of the cornea, subconjunctival hemorrhage, hyphema, shallow anterior chamber may be seen, irregular pupil (teardrop or D-shaped pupil), and intraocular contents visible outside the globe.

Management: Do not touch the eye. A rigid eye shield should be placed around the periorbital bone over the eye and the patient should be admitted to the hospital for surgical repair. The patient should avoid coughing, blowing the nose, and bending forwards. The patient should be kept fasting and will need IV analgesia.

Retrobulbar Hemorrhage

This condition may occur after trauma to the eye and is, of course, an ocular emergency as bleeding into the orbital cavity may lead to compression and ischemia of the eye and/or optic nerve. The patient needs urgent referral to an appropriate hospital.

Clinical Findings/Management Retrobulbar Hemorrhage

Symptoms: Severe pain and progressively decreasing vision.

Ophthalmic examination: There may be signs of trauma to the eyelid and eye with progressive loss of vision, progressive ophthalmoplegia and loss of eye movements, and forward bulging of the eye (proptosis).

Management: Do not touch the eye. A rigid eye shield should be placed around the periorbital bone over the eye and the patient should be admitted immediately to the hospital for surgical repair.

Periocular ecchymosis

Periocular ecchymosis (diffuse bruising) or "black eye" consisting of hematoma (focal collection of blood) (Figure 14.6) is a common result of blunt injury in most contact sports. The danger with this injury is that there may also be intraocular damage, so enquire about double vision, inspect the eye and periorbital structures, palpate for bony structure tenderness, test visual acuity and eye movements, and perform a fundoscopy to exclude intraorbital bleeding.

It is important to exclude some more serious conditions including orbital fracture and any open globe trauma. A periorbital hematoma may be associated with a fracture of the infraorbital region and blowout fracture, so these must be excluded when examining the athlete. Loss of sensation or parasthesia just below the eye in the distribution of the infraorbital nerve may indicate a fracture in the orbital floor or maxilla. If there is a bilateral ring hematoma (panda eyes), a basal skull fracture should be considered.

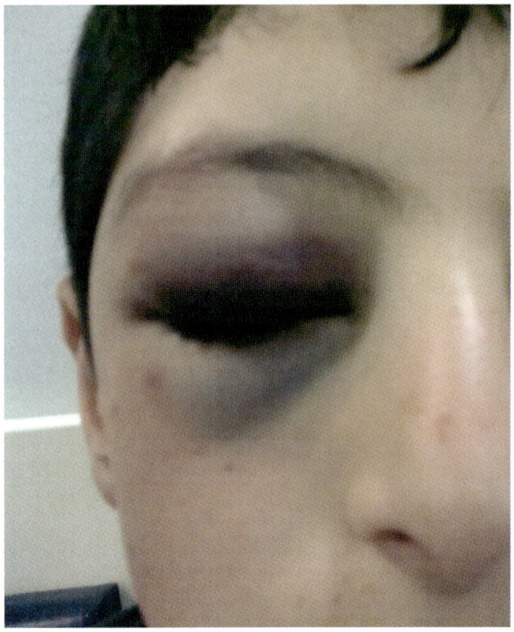

Figure 14.6 Periorbital hematoma and edema. (*Source:* Courtesy of Hacettepe University, Department of Ophthalmology.)

Clinical Findings/Management Periocular Ecchymosis

Symptoms: Pain, swelling, reduced vision due to swollen lids, and blurry vision.

Inspection: Swelling of the eyelids, limitation of eye movement due to eyelid congestion (especially during the acute period), and subconjunctival hemorrhage may be seen.

Pupil inspection/reflexes/eye movements and fundoscopy should be normal.

Eyelid Injuries

These injuries are potentially serious if the eyelids are damaged and may lead to drying of the eye, chronic infection, and corneal inflammation. Deep lacerations may penetrate the sclera or cornea, thus causing an open globe injury. These patients need referral. The most common external injuries of eyelids are contusions

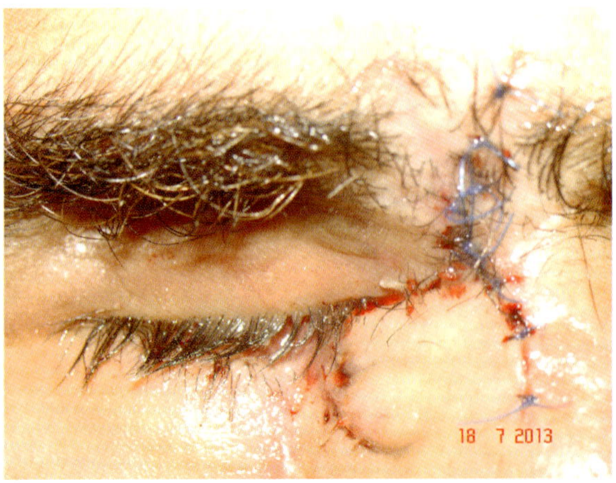

Figure 14.7 Repair of lid laceration following eyelid trauma

and lacerations (see Chapter 27). Small and uncomplicated eyelid lacerations can be repaired under local anesthesia, but if the lid margin or canalicular system is involved, (Figure 14.7) refer to an ophthalmic specialist. Special attention should be given to any injury involving the medial part of the eyelids.

Subconjunctival Hemorrhage

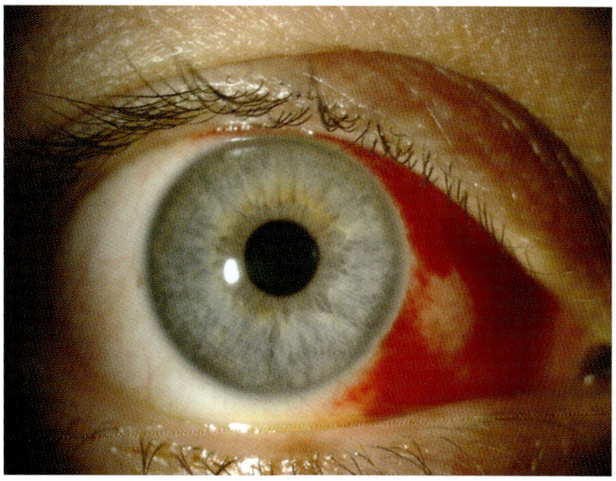

Figure 14.8 Subconjunctival hemorrhage (*Source:* Courtesy of Hacettepe University, Department of Ophthalmology.)

This is due to capillary bleeding between the sclera and conjunctiva – often creating a bright red hemorrhage (though they can also be dark) (Figure 14.8). The blood will always stay limited to the white sclera; it will not cross over into the clear cornea. They may be limited to a small sector of the eye or may be more extensive affecting most of the sclera. Hemorrhages can also occur after direct trauma to the eye, with orbital roof fractures or after lifting heavy weights or intense coughing episodes. Similarly hemorrhages can be associated with hypertension or bleeding disorders. Measure the athlete's blood pressure and enquire about bleeding tendencies. The benign variants are self-limiting, conditions which disappear after 1–2 weeks without treatment. A subconjunctival hemorrhage without any concomitant ocular pathology does not cause loss of vision.

Clinical Findings/Management Subconjunctival Hemorrhage

Symptoms: A painless, nondischarging, red patch on the white of the eye.

Ophthalmic examination: Macroscopic examination reveals hemorrhage between the conjunctiva and sclera. All other findings should be normal. If associated with trauma, then a detailed examination must be conducted.

Corneal Abrasions

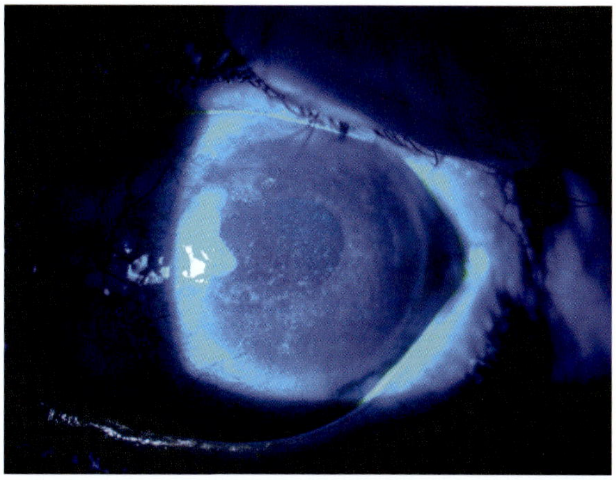

Figure 14.9 Corneal abrasion and punctate staining with fluorescein (*Source:* Courtesy of Hacettepe University, Department of Ophthalmology.)

A fingernail scratch can cause a corneal abrasion (Figure 14.9). Many athletes use contact lenses and these may scratch the cornea if not removed on time, or if removed roughly. Foreign bodies may also be introduced if lenses are carelessly inserted on the FoP. The primary symptom is one of pain and redness often followed by infection. Treatment involves removal of any foreign body, topical antibiotics, and applying an eyepatch.

Eye – Chemical Burns

Fortunately, these injuries are extremely rare in sport. Should they occur they must be urgently treated. Liquids and gases all have their own pH. Acidic agents attack ocular tissue, but their burning effect only lasts for some seconds. Alkaline agents, however, may burn for hours and patients require continuous ocular irrigation for up to 8 hours. When a chemical injury occurs, the eyes should be flooded immediately with fluid (e.g., water) to minimize burning for as long as it takes to get to hospital. Continuous irrigation can be difficult in an ambulance. It is possible to tape an infusion set over an open eyelid in such a way that it runs continuously during transport.

If there are visible chemical burns, always check the airway/respiration for inhalation injuries.

Eye – Nonpenetrating Ocular Foreign Bodies

In sport, the commonest agents are dust, dirt, grass, small stones, and small metal particles (when polishing/sharpening skates, blades, etc.) and the vast majority are nonpenetrating, though this possibility must not be forgotten. For dust and small particles, simply rinsing the eye may be enough. For other objects, inversion of the upper eyelid with a Q-tip swab stick is recommended to allow adequate inspection. Apply a local anesthetic first before gently wiping the foreign body away using a second Q-tip. However, the swab may leave behind small fibers so inspect carefully. Sometimes a corneal scraper may be needed. Dripping the eye with flourescein followed by an ophthalmoscopic inspection may reveal the foreign object or a conjunctival/scleral sore. This procedure is best conducted in the dark, so withdraw to the athlete medical room.

If the eye is very painful after treatment, apply chloramphenicol cream and cover the eye with a patch. Oral Per oral 500 mg paracetemol tablets can be taken if the pain is severe. Chloramphenicol drops can be used if the eye is more uncomfortable than painful. If the athlete has intense pain, then reconsider the diagnosis.

Eye – Penetrating Injuries

Deep penetrating foreign bodies should not be removed as the whole orbit may collapse. The patient should be sent urgently to hospital by ambulance. If the penetrating object is unstable, then endeavor to stabilize the foreign body as best as possible. If the foreign body is in the eye, cover the eye with a rigid eyeshield. Also cover the healthy eye to prevent unnecessary ocular movement. There may be a concomitant cerebral injury and the patient must be stabilized during the primary survey.

With smaller metal foreign bodies, the healthcare professional must always consider the possibility of an intraocular foreign body, if the foreign body had a high velocity and if a conjunctival rift is present. Try to ascertain what type of substance may have penetrated the eye – metal, plastic, and so on. A careful case history is recommended. Check the athlete's vision. Inspect the eye with an ophthalmoscope. If the combination of high-velocity metal foreign body and a conjunctival rift is present, then the possibility of an intraocular foreign body cannot be ruled out.

Treatment

Ensure that the patient is stabilized after the primary survey. Immobilize the foreign body if necessary. Cover the eye if possible with an eyeshield without causing further

	Red	Pain	Itchy	Blurred vision	Photophobia	Ciliary flush
Conjunctivitis	Yes	No	Maybe	Maybe	No	No
Foreign body	Maybe	Yes	Yes	Maybe	Maybe	No
Corneal abrasion	Yes	Yes	No	Maybe	No	No
Keratitis (Figure 14.10)	Yes	Yes	Maybe	Yes	Yes	Maybe
Iritis	Usually	Yes	No	Yes	Yes – maybe bilateral	Maybe
Scleritis (Figure 14.11)	Yes	Yes	No	Yes	Yes	Yes
Uveitis (Figure 14.12)	Yes	Yes	No	Yes	Direct and consensual	Yes
Subconjunctival hemorrhage	Yes	No	No	No	No	No

Table 14.1 Acute "red eye" – symptom and sign overview

damage. Do *not* give oral painkillers. The patient should be kept fasting until evaluated by a specialist – ingestion of food or fluids may delay surgical intervention.

Non-traumatic Ocular Emergencies

The following nontraumatic emergencies all require urgent referral to a specialist (Table 14.1) with the possible exception of some acute red eye causes. (Fig 14.1)

1. Acute loss of vision or visual field defects
2. Acute double vision
3. Light flashes or floaters (may also be traumatic)
4. Acute "red eye"
5. Acute eye pain (Figures 14.10–14.12)

It is beyond the scope of this manual to go into detail about all these conditions.

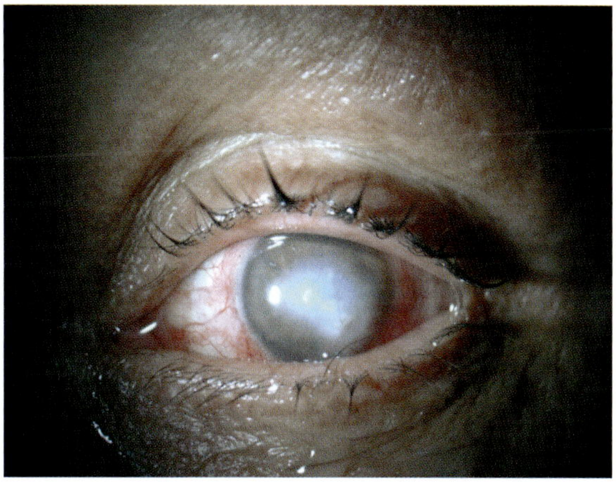

Figure 14.10 Herpetic keratitis
(*Source:* Courtesy of Hacettepe University, Department of Ophthalmology.)

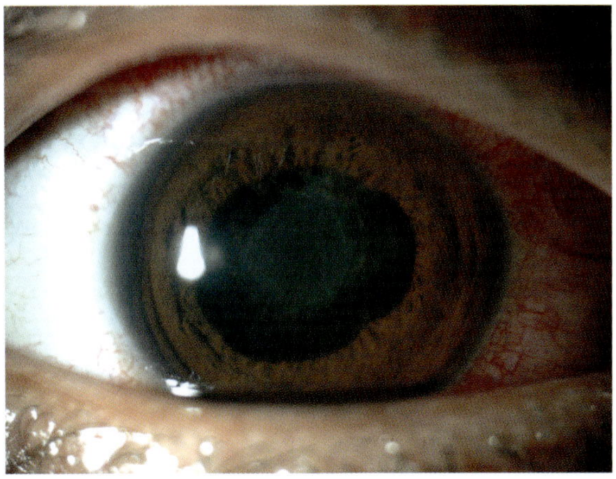

Figure 14.12 Signs of acute anterior uveitis; aqueous flare and fibrinous exudates
(*Source:* Courtesy of Hacettepe University, Department of Ophthalmology.)

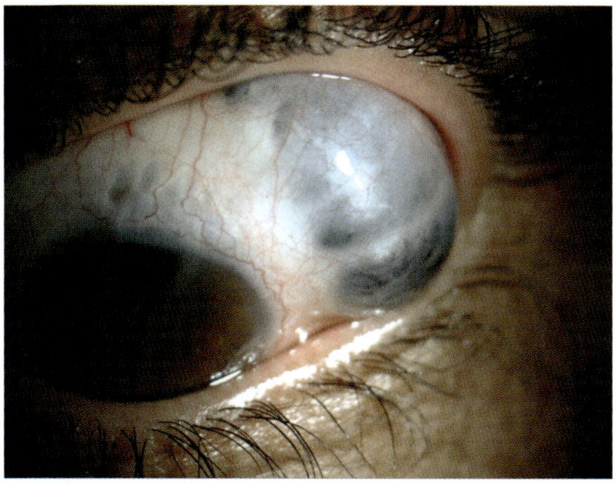

Figure 14.11 Scleritis
(*Source:* Courtesy of Hacettepe University, Department of Ophthalmology.)

Bibliography

Holck, D. (2005, ISBN-13: 978-0-7216-8756-8, ISBN-10: 0-7216-8756-3) *Evaluation and Treatment of Ocular Fractures*. Elsevier.

Kuhn, F. & Pieramici, D.J. (2002, ISBN-3-13-125771-7, ISBN 1-58890-075-4) *Ocular Trauma. Principles and Practice*.

Kim, T., Nunes, A.P., Mello, M.J. & Greenberg, P.B. (2010) Incidence of sport related eye injuries in the US: 2001-2009. *Grafe's Archive of Clinical and Experimental Ophthalmology*, **249**, 1743–1744.

MacEwen, C.J. (1986) Sport associated eye injuries: a causalty department survey. *British Journal of Ophthalmology*, **71**, 701–705.

Prevent Blindness America(Formerly National Society to Prevent Blindness): 1993 (1994) *Sports and Recreational Eye injuries*. Prevent Blindness America, Schaumberg, IL.

United States Consumer Product Safety Commission (2000) *Sports and recreational eye injuries*. Washington, DC. United States Consumer Product Safety Commission website. http//www.gov/library.html [accessed 6 February 2011].

15 Dental Injuries

Paul Piccinini[1] *and Anthony Clough*[2]

[1]*Dental Department, York University, Toronto, ON, Canada*
[2]*Eastman Dental Institute, University of London, London, UK*

There are very few sports injuries that are permanently debilitating. Fractured bones can heal, lacerations can be repaired, and ligaments can be surgically reconstructed. But orofacial injuries, especially to the anterior teeth, are disfiguring and require prosthetic repair for the lifetime of the athlete.

The incidence of these injuries is staggering. One North American-based injury prevention group estimated that more than 3 million orofacial injuries occur in sport on an annual basis in the United States alone.

These injuries can be costly to repair and maintain and are rarely part of any medical insurance plan. The lifetime cost for the repair and maintenance of one lost tooth in a young athlete can easily exceed 20,000 USD. Unfortunately, statistics confirm that up to 80% of all dental injuries occur in the four maxillary anterior incisors, making their damage even more significant.

Healthcare professionals must be comfortable in being able to identify athletes who are at risk, manage dental and orofacial injuries when they occur to minimize ongoing trauma and most importantly, recommend and reinforce the use of proper protective equipment to help reduce the incidence of these injuries.

Types of Injuries

Any discussion of orofacial injuries needs to address trauma to the teeth, the soft tissue and supporting structures, the facial bones, especially the maxilla and mandible and the temporomandibular joint (TMJ). High and rapid impacts (such as those from a ball or stick) often result in fractures of the teeth, while slower and milder forces can lead to tooth avulsion or luxation or TMJ subluxation.

While the incidence of dental injuries was once highest in ice hockey, field hockey, and American football, the increased use of facial and mouth protection in these sports has resulted in other sports such as basketball, baseball, and soccer taking over as the worst offenders for dental injuries. But no sport or athlete is immune and any fall in skating, sailing mast impact, or volleyball collision can result in a dental or jaw injury.

The IOC Manual of Emergency Sports Medicine, First Edition. Edited by David McDonagh and David Zideman.

Management of Dental and Orofacial Injuries

While dental injuries are often spectacular, hemorrhagic, and emotional, they are only life-threatening if they obstruct the airway. Foreign bodies in the airway must always be removed as a priority (see Chapter 4). Inspection of the teeth must be conducted and absence of a tooth or fragment should raise the doctor's level of alertness. An avulsed tooth or fragment if not identified could easily be lodged somewhere in the airway. Intraoral bleeding can readily obstruct the airway particularly in a compromised athlete.

Fractured Teeth

One of the most common dental injuries is a fractured tooth. These may vary from chipped small corners or edges (an injury which requires nothing more than simple polishing) to larger fractured segments that require restoration (although many of these fragments can be reattached if collected and delivered to the dentist). Fragment reattachment often results in an excellent aesthetic result.

Any tooth fracture beyond a simple one must be evaluated on the Field of Play (FoP) or fieldside to ensure that the sharp or unsupported edges are not putting the athlete at greater risk of further dental or soft tissue damage. In some cases, a fieldside dentist can do a quick repair to stabilize or smooth a small fracture and allow the athlete to safely return to play.

Tooth fractures become complex when the nerve is exposed. In this case, there will be a large piece of the tooth, which has been lost and care should be taken to try to find and safely store the fragment for transport. Nerve exposure necessitates removal from the competition because of both risk and pain. In most cases, this type of fracture will require both removal of the nerve and placement of a permanent crown.

After a solid blow to a tooth, the healthcare professional should consider referring the athlete to radiography as soon as reasonably possible, as many fractures can occur below the gum line and are only visible on radiograph. These teeth require careful monitoring and treatment if they are to be salvaged. It is also very important that the FoP doctor locate the fractured segment, to ensure that it is not in the impaled lip or other soft tissue, has not been aspirated, or is not in either the hand or head of another athlete after an altercation.

Dental Luxation

Any force delivered to a tooth will result in some reaction. As previously mentioned, high-impact forces will often fracture a tooth. Lesser forces can cause other problems.

The most common dental injury is a luxation. Following the blow, the athlete will often complain that the bite just does not feel like it did before and that something (usually the offending tooth) is "hitting" first. This is likely to be a luxation. Because the tooth is attached to the tooth socket only by a ligament (periodontal ligament or PDL), there is some reasonable potential for movement in any axis after a blow. In addition to the bite problem, the healthcare professional or the athlete may note that the tooth is sore or painful to touch, is slightly mobile, and may have a bit of bleeding around the collar of the tooth.

Immediate treatment for these injuries is removal from the FoP and, if possible, repositioning of the teeth to their original position. This is usually not a painful process, as the tooth will likely exhibit some pressure dysesthesia for some time after the blow. However, significant mobility or pain upon repositioning may be an indicator of a fracture below the gum line and repositioning should be delayed pending a radiograph. Luxated teeth will likely require some splinting (a nonrigid wire attached to the damaged and adjacent teeth) and careful follow-up to monitor the vitality of the nerve.

Intrusions

Teeth, especially the maxillary incisors, can also be intruded into the alveolar bone. These are particularly troublesome injuries because of the scraping of the root that takes place during the intrusion process.

The prognosis of these injuries is directly dependent on the degree of intrusion, but in all cases, the athlete must be removed from competition and referred for immediate radiographic assessment and treatment. Intrusions of up to 3 mm might spontaneously erupt or might require repositioning and splinting, while those with 3–6 mm of intrusion will usually require surgical repositioning and splinting. Over 6 mm of intrusion is very severe and the tooth may be lost as a result of trauma.

Avulsions

An avulsion is where the entire tooth is ejected from the socket. Research has changed the prognosis of these injuries related to the time that the tooth is outside of the socket. Current thinking dictates that these teeth must be replanted within 5 min in order to have any chance of reattachment and as such, the FoP ED, team doctor, therapist, or coach holds the key to success.

When a tooth is avulsed, the periodontal ligament, which holds the tooth to the socket walls, is torn. This allows the tooth to avulse. Management is based on preserving the integrity of this ligament. The tooth cannot be allowed to dry out or the potential for the ligament to reattach is lost. This is why immediate replantation is recommended.

The tooth should be identified and gently rinsed of any debris that might be on the root or crown area. Care must be taken to not remove or damage the PDL remnants on the root surface. The socket can be gently irrigated with saline to remove any clot or coagulum, and the tooth should simply be returned to the socket. Again, pressure dysesthesia will usually reduce discomfort, although some local anesthesia may be indicated. Once replanted, the tooth should be held in place with some damp gauze or simply closing the mouth on a gauze sponge while the athlete is transported for definitive treatment, including dental splinting.

When the athlete is concussed or facially damaged, the avulsed tooth cannot be replanted as there is a risk of aspiration of the tooth. In these cases or if the tooth is found at the FoP once the athlete has been transported, storage in an acceptable medium (Hanks balanced salt, Sav-a-Tooth, cold white milk or according to local/current guidelines) may help extend the lifetime of the PDL for up to 30 min.

Teeth, which are replanted with no chance of PDL healing, will likely ankylose and will be rejected later by the surrounding bone.

Trauma to the Alveolus

Jaw fractures are very common in high-impact and high-collision sports. Segmental fractures of the maxilla may mimic luxations, in that the teeth in the area will be out of position and the bite will not come together properly. However, these teeth will not reposition easily because the alveolus has fractured. These fractures require more extensive fixation and monitoring but usually have a good prognosis.

Mandibular fractures either to the body, ramus, or condyle are also quite common. Blows directly to the anterior aspect of the jaw can often result in a fracture in that immediate area, as well as a possible bilateral condylar fracture. Blows to either side of the jaw can cause a fracture at both the point of impact and in the contralateral condyle. In most cases, the athlete will report a significant malocclusion, with a possible crossbite that was not present prior to the trauma, or an open bite in one or both sides. Once identified, there is no course but removal from the FoP and definitive treatment by an oral and maxillofacial surgeon.

TMJ Trauma

While fractures and other severe injuries can occur to the TMJ complex, a much more common injury is a subluxation of the condyle. In most cases, the head of the condyle translates downward and forward around the articular eminence before becoming locked in an anterior position. As with many of the other injuries discussed, timely management is crucial. After a few minutes, the supporting muscles in the area will spasm and a simple reduction will no longer be possible without the use of sedation or muscle relaxants.

Once a fracture has been eliminated as the cause of the open bite, the practitioner should position themself behind the athlete who should be in a seated position. With two gloved hands, gentle pressure can be placed in downward and forward directions on the lower molars or the bone lateral to the molars. This will usually allow the condyle to pop back into position, often very quickly, so care should be taken to get one's fingers out of the mouth. Follow-up radiographs, minimal mouth opening, and a soft diet will be needed following successful reduction.

Soft Tissue Trauma

The FoP ED will play a key role in the management of soft tissue injuries. As many sports have rules about return to play while bleeding, it is important that these injuries can be treated quickly and effectively.

Lip lacerations must be assessed for both the presence of foreign bodies as well as the extent of the injury. Cuts that extend beyond the vermilion border of the lip are best be stabilized and referred for specialist treatment because of the greater potential for scarring. Deep lip lacerations should be closed in multiple layers, using an absorbable suture initially to minimize dead space and promote better healing.

Lip or other facial lacerations that fully penetrate the tissues must be closed from both sides. There is a very common misconception that the intraoral side of these lacerations should not be closed. Site sterilization may be a problem, but proper closure will promote healing, restore the damaged architecture, and reduce both scarring and discomfort. In most cases, the intraoral area should be closed first.

Another common fallacy is that a lacerated tongue should not be sutured, mainly because practitioners fear some postoperative swelling and possible airway compromise. Again, this is rarely the case. The tongue is easily anesthetized locally and lacerations can be easily closed with a few well-placed nonrigid sutures.

The frenulum under the tongue or midline of the upper lip can be torn following a blow to the lips or face. These injuries may bleed considerably but often do not require closure. However, a true degloving injury, where the labial tissues are torn away from the front of the teeth and alveolus, must be carefully cleaned, debrided, and repositioned to avoid permanent periodontal damage.

Injury Prevention

It has been said, with good justification, that a mouthguard may be the single most effective piece of equipment in sport. However, all mouthguards are not created equal and athletes must, with encouragement from team medical personnel, ensure that they have proper dental protection when competing or training.

Mouthguards are designed to prevent injuries caused by either direct or indirect impact to the teeth. As 80% of all injuries occur to the four maxillary incisors, the mouthguard is usually worn in the upper jaw.

Entry-level mouthguards are either stock (take out of the bag and wear, with no adjustment) or "boil-and-bite" (heat up and try to do some molding in the mouth). Neither of these offer acceptable levels of protection to most athletes, and are at high risk of being lost or not worn at the time of impact due to poor fit, breathing concerns, or phonetic compromise.

The current state-of-the-art of mouthguard is custom made from a plaster model of the athlete's upper jaw. Using both heat and pressure, layers of protective ethyl vinyl acetate (EVA) material can be built up to offer protection where the athlete most needs it as dictated by their sport, while retaining a level of comfort and retention, far exceeding those previously mentioned. Some feel that athletes returning to competition postconcussion should ensure that they are wearing the best possible custom-made mouthguard to reduce further impacts to the orofacial complex.

Facial protection (including a face mask and visor) is also useful in many sports to help reduce injury.

Team doctors should encourage athletes to complete a dental preparticipation examination (PPE) as a part of any preseason screening. A proper radiographic survey will show wisdom teeth, pathology, and carious teeth that may all increase the risk of dental trauma if not treated. Studies have shown that there is an up to a nine times greater incidence of jaw fracture when an impact occurs in the presence of an impacted wisdom tooth. A careful dental history and examination will identify crowns, orthodontic appliances, retainers, or dentures, which should either be protected or removed during competition.

16 Thoracic Injuries

David McDonagh[1,2,3] *and David Zideman*[4,5,6]

[1]*Emeregency Deptartment, St. Olavs Hospital, Trondheim, Norway*
[2]*Faculty of Medicine, NTNU - National University of Science and Technology, Trondheim, Norway*
[3]*Medical Commission, AIBA - International Boxing Association, Lausanne, Switzerland.*
[4]*Anaesthesia, Imperial College Healthcare NHS Trust, London, UK*
[5]*London Ambulance Service NHS Trust, London, UK*
[6]*Emergency Medical Services, London Organising Committee of the Olympic and Paralympic Games, London 2012, london*

The majority of thoracic injuries occur in high-energy sports (ice hockey, football, rugby, alpine skiing, etc.) and in sports with intrinsic penetration danger (javelin, fencing, ski pole, etc.). The commonest thoracic injury is the uncomplicated rib fracture. While serious chest injuries in sport are rare, the potential for injury is present in motorized sports, equestrian sports, and diving where the injuring forces are usually blunt. Penetrating injuries can occur in fencing and even during a pole vault or javelin event! Chest injuries pose a threat to the airway, respiration, and circulation. This chapter focuses on the emergency diagnosis and treatment of severe thoracic injuries in the prehospital sporting environment. It is important to able to diagnose and treat the following conditions, some of which may be potentially life threatening:

1. Tension pneumothorax
2. Pneumothorax
3. Hemothorax
4. Flail chest
5. Pulmonary contusion
6. Sternal fracture
7. Cardiac contusion and cardiac tamponade
8. Commotio cordis
9. Penetrating chest wounds
10. Costal and scapular fractures
11. Sternoclavicular (SC) joint injuries
12. Costochondral joint injuries
13. Muscle injuries

Fieldside Observation and Observations on Approaching the Athlete

During the competition, the doctor should visibly follow the event at all times if possible. This allows the doctor to observe the incident and gather important direct information.

The IOC Manual of Emergency Sports Medicine, First Edition. Edited by David McDonagh and David Zideman.
2015 International Olympic Committee. Published 2015 by John Wiley & Sons, Ltd.

Try to establish if the athlete is injured or has collapsed without any obvious trauma. Was there contact with another athlete or an object such as a goalpost or hard object? Is the athlete motionless?

If no trauma has occurred, then suspect more sinister causes such as syncope, hypoglycemia, a cardiac disorder, cerebral hemorrhage.

FoP Management Chest Injury

Initiate the FoP evaluation following the S-ABCDE mnemonic (see Chapter 3). The steps of onfield management are as follows.

Clinical Findings/Management Chest Injury

Rapidly evaluate the patient's condition to detect if a patient is critically ill. If the patient is standing and appears to be functioning adequately, then an examination should be undertaken and a decision made about return to play. If the athlete is standing but obviously compromised, lie the athlete down on the ground and then begin your evaluation. If the athlete is already lying down, test alert, verbal stimuli response, painful stimuli response, or unresponsive (AVPU). If conscious, take a focused history: "Are you in pain? Where is the pain? Can you breathe properly? What happened?" You will have already briefly inspected the patient noting if the patient is conscious, able to speak, in pain, cyanotic, or dyspneic. If unconscious, immediately initiate the ABCDE evaluation. Call for help. If there is any possibility of a cervical spine injury, carefully immobilize the neck while performing the primary survey.

General inspection: Is there cyanosis, breathing difficulty, noisy breathing, or stridor from a neck injury or any other obvious findings?

Inspection of the neck: All evaluations of chest injuries begin with an airway examination (see Chapter 3). Inspect the mouth for foreign bodies. Remove if they are found. Ensure airway patency using a head tilt and chin lift maneuver. If this is unsuccessful, perform a jaw thrust. Insert an oropharyngeal airway adjunct to assist in maintaining airway patency, particularly if the patient has reduced consciousness and is not vomiting or having a seizure. The establishment of an advanced medical airway by tracheal intubation, cricothyrotomy, or tracheostomy is unlikely to be necessary but must be performed if the airway is not well controlled with simple airway maneuvers or adjuncts and particularly if there is damage to the larynx. These procedures may be best performed off the FoP in a protected and quieter environment, especially if drug-assisted RSI is required.

Inspection of the chest: Count the respiratory rate. Inspect the chest wall for wounds, penetrating foreign bodies, and deformities. Evaluate chest wall movement; is it deep, shallow, or symmetric? Is there paradoxical respiration (part of the chest wall moving in the opposite direction to the rest of the chest wall)?

Palpation: Determine if there is pain on palpation of the thoracic cage or pain during respiration. Does palpation reveal abnormal chest wall movement? Attach a pulse oximeter and take a reading. Palpate the pulse – there is usually an increased pulse rate with mild-to-severe thoracic injury. The pulse rate may still be somewhat high due to the level of activity before the trauma but it may be maintained due to pain. Cardiac conditions or hemorrhage may also result in a raised pulse rate. A slower than normal rate may be found with cardiac arrhythmias, cardiac tamponade (both reduced rate and reduced pulse volume), and in deteriorating severely injured (often bleeding) patients. A low pulse volume may indicate major bleeding, cardiac tamponade, or myocardial infarction.

Percussion: Percussion of the unclothed chest may reveal dull (hemothorax) or tympanitic (pneumothorax) areas. Note any pain on percussion.

Auscultation: Auscultation of the traumatized chest may reveal normal or abnormal chest sounds. Absent or decreased chest sounds in part or all of a lung field may indicate the presence of a pneumothorax or hemothorax, atalectasis, or even a lung contusion if several hours have gone by since the incident. Wheezing sounds are typical of asthma or with airway infections.

It is recommended to auscultate the abdomen for normal bowel sounds. Bowel sounds can be auscultated in the thorax and their presence may indicate a diaphragmatic injury with parts of the stomach or intestines being trapped in the thorax. Bowel sounds may also be heard over a large pneumothorax due to the lack of lung tissue.

The back of the chest must also be inspected, palpated, and auscultated once the patient has been turned into the recovery position. Important information can be missed if this is not done.

Management:

- Open the airway, if necessary by head tilt/chin lift or a jaw thrust maneuver
- Check for breathing and administer 100% oxygen at 15 L/min by a simple nonrebreathing facemask
- If pulse oximeter readings are available, titrate the oxygen flow to keep oxygen saturation (SpO_2) between 94% and 98%
- If a pneumothorax is found, decompress it if the patient's vital signs are threatened. Insertion of a chest needle or drain is not likely to be necessary in the sporting environment. However, if a tension pneumothorax or cardiac tamponade is detected, then immediate decompression could be a life-saving intervention. This procedure may be better undertaken off-field in a protected environment, except where it may have been the primary cause of an immediate cardiac arrest
- If the patient is not breathing, commence bag/valve/mask ventilation immediately
- Consider a tension pneumothorax as one possible treatable cause of cardiac arrest
- Digitally compress any significant arterial bleeds
- Continue the primary survey
- Turn the patient into the recovery position and examine the back
- Immobilize the patient avoiding compression of the injured chest
- Remove from the FoP

Once the primary survey has been completed and the patient is stabilized, remove the athlete from the FoP to the fieldside and directly to an ambulance if necessary. If not necessary, conduct a fieldside evaluation.

Fieldside Management Chest Injury

Initiate monitoring of vital signs – respiratory rate, pulse rate, pulse oximetry, blood pressure, and Glasgow Coma Scale (GCS).

Blood pressure may be slightly elevated due to a high activity level at the time of trauma. This can still be the case initially even in the presence of severe internal bleeding. A low blood pressure may be present if the cause is syncopal or if the patient is about to go into shock.

Attach electrocardiogram (ECG) pads if there is a suspicion of a potential cardiac arrest or cardiac tamponade.

Repeat the primary survey and address any issues.

Decompress any pneumothorax if the patient's vital signs are threatened.

Establish IV access if not already done.

See the subsequent text for specific treatment guidelines for specific conditions.

Conduct a secondary survey (see Chapter 3).

Pneumothorax

A pneumothorax occurs when there is a collection of air in the pleural space between the parietal and visceral pleura. This air may have leaked internally from the lung parenchyma via a lesion in the visceral pleura injury (a closed pneumothorax) after a blunt injury to the chest or may have originated from a penetrating wound to the chest wall injury or diaphragm, thus allowing air to enter the pleura through a pathological opening in the parietal pleura (open pneumothorax). In a healthy athlete, there is a negative pressure in the pleural space. Inspiration increases negative intrathoracic pressure thus causing air to enter the lung. When air (or fluid) enters the pleural space, the pressure gradient is disturbed and normal lung expansion and therefore lung function is impeded. In a simple pneumothorax, this collection of air is nonexpanding and relatively static. In a tension pneumothorax, the volume of air increases continuously – air enters the pleural space on inspiration but does not exit on expiration – thus causing a dynamic, progressive pressure increase in the pleural space. At some stage, the pressure in the pleural space will be higher than that in the surrounding lung tissue, resulting in a failure lung tissue to expand during inspiration and its possible displacement. The ability to transfer gases is inhibited in this part of the lung. If pressure in the pleural space is allowed to increase, there will ultimately be a reduction in lung function leading to clinical deterioration, which if untreated can even lead to cardiac arrest and death. When a tension pneumothorax occurs, this pressure increase can occur within minutes and can lead to significant deterioration and death. This dynamic and potentially deadly condition must be diagnosed and treated immediately.

In athletes, primary spontaneous pneumothoraces occur when small air-filled sacs in an otherwise healthy lung rupture. This is usually related to exertion, in particular, during underwater or high-altitude activity in otherwise healthy people. A secondary or complicated spontaneous pneumothorax occurs when there is a similar rupture in a pathological lung. Olympic athletes are unlikely to have serious lung conditions. Patients with underlying lung conditions tend to be more distressed than the healthy simple spontaneous group. In the athletic population, spontaneous pneumothoraces, when they occur, are usually minor in nature and it is unusual to find major spontaneous pneumothoraces in the athletic population. The symptoms and findings with a spontaneous pneumothorax are similar to a traumatic pneumothorax – without the trauma symptoms.

Clinical Findings Traumatic Pneumothorax

Inspection:

- The patient will probably be conscious (if there is no hemorrhage or head injury)
- The patient may be in pain due to rib fracture and lung injury. The pain from the pneumothorax may be dull, sharp, or stabbing, of sudden onset, worsened with deep breathing or coughing
- There may be shortness of breath and the patient may have a cough
- There may be moderate cyanosis
- Chest movement is most likely be restricted but symmetrical due to pain but on occasions the chest movement may be slightly reduced on the injured side

Percussion: May reveal tympanitic sounds (absence does not exclude a pneumothorax as tympanitic percussion sounds are very difficult to elicit at the FoP or fieldside and may be first detected in the relative quiet of the medical room). Dull percussion sounds are more indicative of intrathoracic bleeding, as with a hemothorax (the patient is usually much more poorly if a hemothorax is present).

Palpation: Pain, indicating a possible costal fracture; abnormal movement, asymmetrical respiration.

Pulse oximetry may reveal slightly lower than normal but sustained saturation levels.

Auscultation: Reduced or absent breath sounds. Conducted bowel sounds may be auscultated in the chest.

Pulse rate is likely to be elevated.

Respiratory rate is likely to be elevated.

Blood pressure will vary, but lower pressures should cause one to suspect bleeding or an early tension pneumothorax.

If a major pneumothorax is present, it is often accompanied by other injuries such as hemothorax, multiple rib fracture, sternal fracture, cardiac or vessel damage, neck or abdominal damage, spinal injury, or head injury. There is always the possibility of a tension pneumothorax developing, so these patients must be monitored closely.

Inspect the chest wall for wounds. The presence of a large open wound usually indicates the presence of both an open pneumothorax and a hemothorax; the patient will often have severe respiratory difficulty and will probably have had a significant hemorrhage: this patient is in a life-threatening situation. If the wound diameter is greater than the tracheal diameter, then more air will enter through this pathological opening than through the trachea. If the wound creates a flap, then there is severe risk of developing a potentially lethal tension pneumothorax. During inspiration, air may enter through a chest wall opening and may or may not be expelled during expiration. Air entry or exit sounds from a wound should raise immediate concern. Always listen over a chest wound for small gushes of air: this may be indicative of a tension pneumothorax.

Open chest wounds should be covered and classically taped on three sides with one side of the wound untapped. This is supposed to allow air to exit from the pleural space, thus avoiding the creation of a tension pneumothorax, but may fail and the tension pneumothorax reoccur. Alternatively an commercial chest seal dressing can be used. Where possible a surgically introduced chest drain, with an underwater seal or flap valve, should be introduced on the same side but away from the chest wound to prevent the development of a tension pneumothorax. The patient's airway must be kept patent, oxygen administered, and respiration assisted if necessary, before volume replacement intravenous therapy is initiated. This patient will require rapid evacuation to hospital.

Clinical Findings Major Traumatic Pneumothorax

Inspection: For foreign body penetration, open or closed wounds, swellings, bleeding, bruising, and chest wall deformity.

The patient may be unconscious; however, if conscious, the patient may be in great pain with palpation tenderness over a fracture.

The patient will often be pale, cyanotic with clammy, moist skin.

There will be restricted and asymmetrical chest movements on the injured or both sides of the chest.

Palpation: There may be subcutaneous emphysema, fracture tenderness, and asymmetrical chest expansion while breathing.

Percussion: Tympanitic sounds over the pneumothorax, but may also have the percussion dullness of a hemothorax.

Auscultation: Findings may be normal, but there will probably be reduced respiratory sounds over the injured lung. Conducted bowel sounds may be heard. If there is an open wound, listen for air movement or a whistling wound flap, also indicating a tension status. Also auscultate the abdomen for abdominal sounds.

Pulse oximetry will probably reveal lower than normal saturation levels.

The *pulse rate* will probably been elevated.

The *respiratory rate* will be elevated: a fall in respiratory rate in an untreated patient is a significant finding and indicates major pulmonary dysfunction.

Low blood pressure may imply some level of bleeding or an early tension pneumothorax.

Clinical Findings Tension Pneumothorax

Inspection: Look for foreign body penetration and wounds, swellings, bleeding, bruising, and chest wall deformity.

There may be an open, noisy, chest wall wound.

There may be bloating of the face and neck due to large-scale subcutaneous emphysema – Michelin Man appearance.

The patient may be unconscious; however, if conscious, the patient may be in great pain.

The patient will be pale, cyanotic with clammy, moist skin.

There will be restricted and asymmetrical chest movements on the injured or both sides.

Palpation: There may be subcutaneous emphysema, fracture tenderness, and asymmetrical chest expansion.

Percussion: Tympanitic sounds over the pneumothorax, but may also have the percussion dullness of a hemothorax.

Auscultation: Findings may be normal, but there will probably be reduced respiratory sounds over the injured lung. If there is an open wound, listen for air movement or a whistling wound flap, also indicating a tension status. Auscultate the abdomen for abdominal sounds.

Pulse oximetry will reveal lower than normal saturation levels.
The *pulse rate* will be elevated.
The *respiratory rate* will initially be elevated; a fall in respiratory rate in an untreated chest trauma patient is a significant finding and indicates major pulmonary dysfunction.
Blood pressure may be raised immediately after the injury. It may fall after some time due to bleeding into the cavity or as a preemptive sign of imminent cardiac arrest.

Pneumothorax Treatment

In the prehospital environment, needle thoracostomy is the simplest treatment if a decision to decompress a pneumothorax has been made. There are two approaches to the prehospital management of a pneumothorax:

1. If a diagnosis of a pneumothorax is made (i.e., history, dyspnea, increased respiratory rate, tachycardia, tympanitic percussion sounds, absent respiratory sounds, etc.) in the noisy prehospital environment, then there is probably a relatively large pneumothorax present and needle thoracostomy should be attempted (see below).
2. If a diagnosis of a pneumothorax is made, needle thoracostomy should only be attempted if the patient has deteriorating vital signs and is becoming unstable. This latter approach is supported by the authors: the introduction of a needle into the chest cavity may puncture the healthy lung and actually cause a pneumothorax or worsen an existing pneumothorax.

Whether the pneumothorax is decompressed or not, the patient should receive immediate high-flow oxygen at 15 L/min by facemask to maintain the SaO_2 to between 94% and 98%. If the patient is unconscious, insert an oropharyngeal airway and be prepared to assist ventilation using a bag, valve, and mask. Be extremely careful if using continuous positive airway pressure (CPAP) or other end-expiratory pressure valves, as these can worsen the pneumothorax.

Tension Pneumothorax

A tension pneumothorax demonstrates the same findings as a pneumothorax with one major difference: the pneumothorax becomes progressively worse as each minute passes, findings become more pronounced with time, and the patient's condition deteriorates rapidly.

Thus, a tension pneumothorax is a dynamic condition that can lead to significant clinical deterioration, cardiac arrest, and death within minutes and must be diagnosed and treated immediately. Do not wait for an X-ray to confirm the diagnosis of a tension pneumothorax.

Tension Pneumothorax – Immediate Treatment

If a tension pneumothorax is detected, then thoracic decompression must be performed immediately or the patient may continue to deteriorate and eventually die. There are two possible decompression techniques: needle thoracostomy or surgical drain insertion.

Needle thoracostomy is the simplest procedure for the nonsurgically trained doctor, particularly in the prehospital environment. However, the procedure is often unsuccessful. There are several reasons for failure:

1. The needle may reach the pleural space
2. The soft plastic cannula while initially effective may kink and thus cease to function as a pressure release device

3. The cannula diameter may be too small and become blocked with tissue or fluid
4. The needle has been inserted into the healthy pleural space thereby inducing a pneumothorax

There is a serious issue of false security if the initial needle thoracostomy has been successful with an initial rush of trapped air through the cannula: the Emergency Doctor (ED) may falsely assume that the tension pneumothorax has been adequately treated. The improvement in the patient's condition may be temporary and the patient may then deteriorate rapidly despite this initial improvement. These patients must be continuously monitored. A new needle thoracostomy should be performed if the patient does not improve or if vital signs deteriorate. If after a second needle thoracostomy there is a failure to respond or deterioration occurs after an initial improvement, then the ED must consider performing a surgical thoracostomy. This technique requires training. If neither technique is attempted (due to lack of training), then insert a forceps into the skin flap covered wound and open the flap, thus allowing the free transfer of air.

All patients with chest injuries, but especially those who are unconscious, should be administered high-flow oxygen by face mask before leaving the FoP and their pulse oximetry monitored. Titrate the oxygen flow to maintain pulse oximetry saturation readings to between 94% and 98%. Intravenous access must be ensured.

Transport unconscious patients with a neck collar but in ambulatory chest injury patients with normal, painless neck movements, and absent neck spinal process tenderness, cervical collar application can be delayed.

Rapid transportation to hospital is mandatory. The patient will remain in a critical condition until a formal chest drain has been inserted and the tension pneumothorax has been shown to be definitively treated.

Surgical drain insertion for depressurization of a tension pneumothorax Though the treatment of choice, this technique requires training and should be conducted in a clean/sterile environment. Emergency chest drain kits are now supplied in small disposable packs.

The authors of this chapter recommend that at an Olympic Games, a medical officer attending a high-velocity sport or a sport with a definitive risk of penetrating chest injury should be trained in both needle and open thoracostomy procedures and chest drain insertion.

Needle Thoracostomy of Tension Pneumothorax

- Clean the skin with antiseptic cleaning fluid and use an aseptic technique
- Wear sterile gloves
- Insert a 14-gauge intravenous catheter with a syringe attached
  - Insertion site – insert the needle over the top of the second rib in the second intercostal space in the mid-clavicular line until air escapes
  - If in doubt aspirate air into the syringe – or remove the syringe and you may hear a gush of air
- Remove the needle trochar from the cannula and, holding it firmly in place, tape the cannula to the chest wall
- If available, attach the hub of the cannula to a Heimlich valve and tape firmly in place
- Once the needle thoracostomy has been performed, open the airway using chin lift or jaw thrust
- Respiration and ventilation should be supported if necessary
- Cardiopulmonary resuscitation (CPR) must be performed when necessary

Beware: the cannula may move and fail to continue to function as an exit for air; it may be necessary to repeat the procedure or to progress to a more definitive thoracostomy.

Hemothorax

A hemothorax occurs when there is a collection of blood in the pleural space. This occurs with blunt major trauma or when an object penetrates the chest wall, through the pleural space and into the lung damaging intercostal arteries en route, the internal mammary arteries (which can bleed profusely), or the pulmonary blood vessels and lung tissue. With an open (penetrating) hemothorax injury, both blood and air enter the pleural space increasing the pressure in the cavity and thus preventing the normal expansion of the lung during respiration. Both pneumothorax and hemothorax can also occur with closed injuries particularly if there has been rupture of lung tissue and/or a bronchus.

Damaged blood vessels may also bleed extensively ultimately leading to hypotension and shock. The patient has then both reduced respiratory and circulatory functions. The possibility of developing a tension pneumothorax is also present if there is an associated air leak without proper venting. It is important that these conditions are diagnosed and treated as quickly as possible. Hemothorax needs definitive surgical treatment.

A doctor's ability to diagnose a hemothorax in the prehospital environment is limited and unfortunately if the task becomes easier, the more serious the condition becomes. Always suspect a hemothorax with an open chest injury or with a penetrating injury. Classically, the patient has had a chest injury, is in respiratory difficulty, and is developing symptoms of shock – falling blood pressure, rising pulse and respiratory rate, and becoming cyanotic with moist, clammy skin.

Clinical Findings/Management Hemothorax

Always look for a tension pneumothorax.

Inspection: If conscious, the patient will most likely be in pain, will be dyspneic, and they will have speech difficulties due to pain and/or respiratory difficulties

There may be moderate or severe cyanosis

The patient will often be pale and have clammy, moist skin

There will be restricted and asymmetrical chest movements on the injured or both sides

There may be a wound – beware of open wounds and their association with a tension pneumothorax

Palpation: Will reveal tenderness over a fracture, there may be subcutaneous emphysema, chest wall deformities, or abnormal chest wall movement during respiration

Percussion: Percussion of the chest will reveal the percussion dullness of a hemothorax and possibly the tympanitic sounds of a pneumothorax

Auscultation: Findings may be normal, but there will probably be reduced respiratory sounds over the injured lung. Auscultate the abdomen for abdominal sounds

Pulse oximetry will reveal lower than normal saturation levels

The *pulse rate* will be elevated

The *respiratory rate* will be elevated: a fall in respiratory rate in an untreated patient can indicate serious life-threatening injury

The blood pressure may be normal initially. Low or falling blood pressure would indicate significant internal bleeding or the development of a tension pneumothorax

Management: The primary goal of prehospital treatment is fivefold:

- Administer enough oxygen to compensate for the reduced lung capacity and to maintain the SaO_2 to between 94% and 98%
- Assist ventilation if necessary
- Establish widebore IV access
- Correct any hypovolemia from bleeding into the pleural space and lung using 250ml boluses of fluid to a systolic blood pressure of 90mmHg.
- Treat any other life-threatening conditions found in the survey, for example, pneumothorax
- Transfer the patient to an appropriate hospital as quickly as possible

The patient will need repeated primary survey monitoring until they arrive at an appropriate hospital for definitive treatment. Do not be attempted to drain the hemothorax without the availability of replacement blood for transfusion.

Flail Chest

A flail chest occurs when a portion of the rib cage is separated from the rest of the chest wall due to multiple rib fractures. This condition occurs after a major blunt force trauma to the chest wall and may be combined with a pneumothorax, hemothorax, pulmonary contusion, sternal fracture, and mediastinal injury. Flail chest is rarely seen in sport.

The flail segment does not move in biomechanical harmony with the rest of the rib cage, thus lung expansion is inefficient. The segment moves inwards or does not move on inspiration and moves outwards when the rest of the chest moves inwards during expiration. Large or multiple flail segments will disrupt pulmonary mechanics and these patients will most likely require ventilation (even the use of a continuous positive airway pressure (CPAP) unit).

Inspect the chest wall for wounds. The presence of a large open wound usually indicates the presence of both a pneumothorax and hemothorax; these need to be treated first before covering the wound. The patient's airway must be kept patent at all times, oxygen administered and respiration assisted, if necessary, before volume replacement intravenous therapy is initiated. The patient will require rapid evacuation to hospital.

A patient with a flail chest may have several other life-threatening injuries.

Clinical Findings/Management Flail Chest

Inspection: Patient may be unconscious or in great pain.
There will be cyanosis, with pale, clammy, moist skin.
There will be restricted and asymmetrical chest movements on the injured or both sides, with paradoxical movement on respiration.
Palpation: Tenderness over the fracture. There may be paradoxical respiration and subcutaneous emphysema.
Percussion: May have tympanitic sounds of a pneumothorax and the percussion dullness of a hemothorax.
Auscultation: Probably reduced respiratory sounds over the injured lung.
Pulse oximetry will probably reveal lower than normal saturation levels.
A fall in *pulse volume* may occur with cardiac tamponade.
Pulse rate will be increased.
Respiratory rate will be elevated.
Blood pressure values may vary – a low pressure would imply shock or severe hemothorax.
Management: Conduct a primary survey and treat all life-threatening findings; however, expect to find a pneumothorax, a hemothorax, hypovolemia, an unstable chest, and other multiple injuries.

Transfer to hospital urgently.

This is about as serious as it can get in the prehospital environment. Stabilize the patient as best possible until help arrives. Effective pain control, without further compromising respiratory function is important if the patient is conscious.

Pulmonary Contusion

A pulmonary contusion occurs after lung parenchyma has been injured, leading to swelling of the lung tissue and bleeding into the alveolar spaces, thus causing a loss of normal lung function. Often occurring after blunt trauma to the chest, a pulmonary contusion normally develops over a 24-h period and results in poor gas exchange at the injured site, increased pulmonary vascular resistance, and decreased lung compliance. The presence of blood components in the alveolar spaces may cause a significant pulmonary inflammatory reaction with fluid filling up air sacs, leading to the potentially life-threatening acute (adult) respiratory distress syndrome (ARDS). ARDS can develop within hours of the injury and patients may even require intensive care unit (ICU) treatment. Patients become cyanotic, have difficulty breathing, the respiratory rate increases dramatically, blood pressure falls, and auscultation of the chest may reveal abnormal breath sounds due to fluid in the lungs (crackles). Often the blood pressure is low. Pulse oximetry will fall with SpO_2 values $<90\%$.

Pulmonary contusions are not necessarily as dramatic as described earlier and they are rarely diagnosed on physical examination in the prehospital environment. This condition must be suspected, however, with severe blunt chest trauma, particularly with obvious signs of chest wall trauma, hemoptysis, and dyspnea. Pulmonary contusions are often seen in combination with other thoracic injuries such as multiple costal fractures, flail chest, hemothorax, and pneumothorax. Signs are seldom present on initial examination but if present, look for bloodstained expectorate, dyspnea, and crackles on auscultation. This is one reason why an ED should be restrictive with any return to play decisions in an athletes with a chest injury.

Clinical Findings/Management Pulmonary Contusion

Inspection: Initially, there may be minimal findings.
After some hours, the patient may be cyanotic, dyspneic, with pale, clammy, moist skin. Chest movements will probably be normal.
Palpation: Tenderness over the chest wall segment where the initial injury occurred.
Percussion: May have tenderness over the chest wall and with some percussion dullness of a hemothorax.
Auscultation: Probably reduced respiratory sounds over the injured lung. Crackles may be heard.
Pulse oximetry will probably reveal lower than normal saturation levels.
Pulse rate will be increased.
Respiratory rate will be elevated.
Blood pressure values may vary, and low pressure may result if developing shock.
Management:

- If pulmonary contusion is suspected, then the patient should be sent to hospital for further evaluation – chest X-ray, CT scan, and blood gases.
- If the patient is dyspneic, complete a primary survey and ensure airway patency, administer supplemental oxygen, and transfer the patient to hospital with complete basic monitoring.
- If there are signs of ARDS with increasing dyspnea and signs of a falling oxygen saturation, tracheal intubation may be necessary. Hospitalization is obligatory.

Sternal Fracture

Sternal fractures result from severe mediastinal trauma and are most commonly seen with high-velocity high-energy motor vehicle incidents; they are otherwise rarely seen in Olympic sport. Sternal fractures can result from forceful hyperflexion injuries and can thus be associated with spinal column injuries. Sternal fractures are most often seen in deceleration injuries and/or direct blows to the anterior chest, with transverse midbody fractures predominating. Manubrial fractures can also occur. Some cases of sternal fractures have been reported in wrestlers.

Owing to the energy involved, other structures can often be injured concomitantly, in particular, the heart. Cardiac injuries can include myocardial contusion, pericardial injuries, cardiac tamponade, and there may be associated commotio cordis, dysrhythmias, and conduction disturbances or ST-segment changes. There is also a danger of damage to mediastinal and pulmonary vessels with resultant bleeding. Similarly, both the larynx and trachea can be injured or fractured with resultant airway impairment. The spleen, liver, and even kidneys may also be damaged with sternothoracic disruption if the area of impact is not restricted to the chest.

Clinical Findings/Management Sternal Fracture

Inspection: If conscious, the patient will have intense pain worsened by movement, respiration, or coughing.
Swelling, which can hide bony deformities, especially bone indentations.
The patient may be cyanotic or dyspneic.
Chest movement may appear normal though chest expansion is usually reduced due to deformity, the pain of respiration or to underlying lung damage.

Palpation: Tenderness over the fracture area. There may be costal disruption and swellings over the sternocostal and SC joints.

Percussion: May reveal dullness or tympanitic sounds if accompanied by a hemothorax or pneumothorax.

Auscultation: There may be abnormal sounds of bone movement during respiration.

The *pulse rate* may increase. A low pulse volume might indicate cardiac tamponade.

The *respiratory rate* will most likely be elevated due to insufficient ventilation. Pain will limit the respiratory rate and depth of respiration. This will ultimately affect oxygen saturation, so pulse oximetry values may fall.

Blood pressure may fall if there is bleeding.

Management: The main concerns are firstly the airway and secondly that of concomitant injury – pulmonary, vascular, cardiac, abdominal organ, and head and spine injuries. Conduct a primary survey, stabilize, and transfer to hospital as soon as possible. These injuries are extremely painful and may require intense analgesia or anesthesia to allow the athlete to breathe.

Cardiac Injury and Cardiac Tamponade

Myocardial contusion in blunt trauma is a common injury and this may lead to ECG changes and enzyme elevation. Trauma to a coronary artery can result in thrombosis and myocardial infarction. Acute atrial or ventricular rupture is usually rapidly fatal, though on some occasions, if the pericardium is intact, bleeding and leakage may be restricted. Aortic rupture is usually fatal.

Cardiac tamponade occurs when there is bleeding or effusion into the pericardial cavity, between the visceral and parietal layers of the pericardium. The normal level of pericardial fluid is 15–50 mL but with myocardial trauma this volume can increase several times over, thus restricting myocardial movement and cardiac expansion, reducing cardiac output and potentially initiating cardiogenic shock.

The first problem with cardiac tamponade is the difficulty of diagnosis. Beck's Triad of a low arterial blood pressure, distended neck veins, and distant, muffled heart sounds is not commonly found. To have any chance of making a diagnosis a 12-lead ECG must be recorded. The presence of cardiac arrest with pulseless electrical activity (PEA) in a patient with a sternal fracture, thoracic wall disruption, or major chest trauma should cause one to consider the additional diagnosis of tamponade.

There is only one life-saving procedure for tamponade, pericardiocentesis. The aspiration of small amounts of pericardial fluid can significantly improve the patient's hemodynamic status. This is a complex technique that can trigger cardiac arrhythmias; it should only be attempted if the operator has been specifically trained. Some authorities state that pericardiocentesis should only be attempted under ultrasound guidance and certainly never without electrocardiographic monitoring. Some emergency experts promote the use of portable ultrasonography devices in these cases, but this requires training to read and understand the results.

Treatment is based on inserting a large bore long cannula into the pericardium and aspirating blood. With the ECG leads still connected to the chest (or using ultrasonograhy guiding), place the patient in a semirecumbent position (lift the patient 30° up from a supine position) as this brings the heart nearer to the anterior chest wall and the pericardial fluid nearer to the diaphragm. If possible, insert a nasogastric tube to decompress the stomach.

There are at least two cannula insertion sites – the subxiphoid and the left sternocostal margin (fourth intercostal space). If using the subxiphoid approach use a cannula that is at least 8 cm long. A shorter cannula can be used with the sternocostal margin site. The lumen (bore) should be as large as possible to facilitate the aspiration of blood. Use a 60 mL syringe to aspirate the tamponaded fluid and the cannula should be removed when no more fluid can be aspirated. The cannula should definitely be removed before lifting or transferring when the patient is being transferred. This is a difficult technique and the operator often fails to enter the blood filled pericardial space or may inadvertently insert the needle into the (right) ventricle believing that the aspirated blood is from the pericardium.

In cardiac arrest, and especially when associated with penetrating chest wall injury, it may be worthwhile considering an emergency (clam shell) thoracotomy – this maneuver obviously requires training before performing, but there is published data to show that when carried out properly it can be life-saving.

Needle Pericardiocentesis

1. Use gloves (preferably sterile)
2. Clean the skin with an antiseptic solution
3. Use local anesthesia if the patient is conscious
4. Use a long cannula over needle attached to a three-way tap and a large syringe
5. Insert the cannula through the skin at a 45° angle to the abdominal wall and aim for the left shoulder (a 45° angle to the sagittal plane preferably under ultrasound guidance)
6. While inserting the cannula aspirate on the syringe so that fluid can be aspirated when contact with the tamponade space is made
7. The cannula should be inserted up to a depth of 5 cm and then withdrawn if no fluid is aspirated
8. If the syringe suddenly fills with fluid, then the cannula may be in the correct position
9. Withdraw the sharp needle, leaving the cannula in place and continue withdrawing fluid
10. When the syringe is full, close the three-way tap and change the syringe, leaving the cannula in place
11. Changes in ECG waveform may indicate that the cannula is in the correct place or that it has entered the myocardium. If in doubt remove the cannula
12. Remove the cannula when no more fluid can be aspirated
13. Transfer the patient immediately with full monitoring and an appropriately trained escort to a suitable hospital for definitive treatment

Commotio Cordis (See Chapter 4)

This poorly understood, rare but potentially life-threatening condition, typically affects young male athletes who receive a sudden blunt (and often innocent looking) nonpenetrating blow to the sternum or left anterior chest causing immediate collapse, ventricular fibrillation, and cardiac arrest. The timing of the blow in relation to the T-wave may be of consequence and current evidence suggests that the object must strike the chest within the cardiac silhouette with a velocity of at least 49 km/h and in the 20 ms window of the upstroke of the T-wave. Suffice it to say, that death is usually due to ventricular fibrillation and early FoP defibrillation is the only tool available to the doctor. Resuscitation survival rates are not good but have improved recently where FoP defibrillation has become available. Early resuscitation and defibrillation, within

1–3 min, seem to improve the survival rate, though treatment is often delayed by the sheer surprise of a patient with a relatively innocuous injury becoming so ill.

Management: CPR should be initiated immediately and defibrillation attempted as soon as an AED is available (see Chapter 4).

Scapular Fractures

Fractures of the scapula are also associated with high-energy or high-velocity trauma and are thus not common in sport. The body of the scapula is the commonest site of injury. Owing to the trauma forces involved, always look for associated pulmonary injuries, pneumothoraces, other fractures, and pulmonary contusions.

Management: Once again, there is not a lot that can be done with the fracture in the pre-hospital environment other than utilizing an arm sling. However, one must ensure that rib fractures, pneumothorax, and other thoracic and pulmonary injuries are also treated. Scapular fractures must be evaluated radiologically. Administer oxygen if indicated by pulse oximetry as the patient will probably have superficial breathing due to fracture pain.

Costal and Rib Stress Fractures

Always look for a pneumothorax, hemothorax, and tension pneumothorax. Isolated fractures of the ribs can impair breathing and there may be indications for giving analgesics.

Multiple rib fractures can lead to a flail chest and are associated with pneumothorax, hemothorax, and lung contusion.

A fracture of the first rib indicates significant force and the underlying brachial plexus and arteries may be damaged, resulting in a brachial plexus deficit, absent radial pulse, or even a pulsating supraclavicular mass.

Classical symptoms of a simple fracture are pain on coughing or laughing and on deep inspiration. There is tenderness with or without crepitus with palpation of the fracture site. In exceptional circumstances, pain-relieving taping of the fractured rib with sports tape may be considered but this may give temporary pain relief. However, taping is not generally recommended as it is purported that prolonged or exaggerated taping may cause atelectasis in the underlying lung. Many practitioners immobilize the arm on the affected side, while others use no form of bandaging or taping whatsoever.

Stress fractures can occur in the ribs and these have been reported in golfers, rowers, swimmers, and weightlifters.

Undislocated fractures are difficult to visualize on radiographs.

Management: The treatment of simple costal fractures is symptomatic – rest is advised, avoid painful motion, analgesics may be necessary initially.

Fractures of the first rib do require definitive investigation and treatment in hospital.

Penetrating Thorax Injuries

As with all major penetrating injuries, the foreign body should not be removed until the athlete is at a hospital. The removal of foreign bodies is often accompanied by extreme bleeding and a patient can rapidly deteriorate into shock without the provision of immediate surgery and blood transfusion. The ED does not have blood for transfusion readily available, so do not remove impaled objects.

When considering damage caused by penetrating objects, consider two things: blood loss and structural damage. In the case of the thorax, the lungs, heart, aorta, great veins, spinal cord, esophagus, and diaphragm are all at risk. One can therefore expect to find signs of pneumothorax, hemothorax, subcutaneous emphysema, pneumomediastinum, hemoptysis, vascular damage, and breathing difficulties. The abdomen must also be examined as puncture wounds in the chest may involve the upper abdominal organs such as liver, spleen, and stomach.

It is important to remember that any penetrating injury to the fourth intercostal space or below may well cause damage to the diaphragm and intraabdominal organs.

Primary Management of Penetrating Thoracic Injuries

1. Do not remove the impaled object
2. Support and if possible stabilize the impaled object
3. Initiate the primary survey, treating as necessary. Clinical examination will almost certainly reveal a hemothorax, probably a pneumothorax, and probably some organ injury
4. High-flow oxygen should be administered to help to maintain a viable SaO_2
5. Laceration of intercostal or internal mammary arteries can cause serious bleeding, compress these arteries if possible, to reduce blood loss
6. Administer enough intravenous fluid to maintain a systolic blood pressure of at least 90 mmHg
7. Stabilization and rapid transportation to hospital are the keys to success

Stabilizing the impaled object may be a difficult task. The deeper the object sits in the patient, the more stable the object. If the external length of the impaled object (that which is outside the patient) is more than a meter long, then this creates practical problems. It is not easy to move the patent without rocking the foreign body (thus potentially causing shearing injury to internal blood vessels, organs, etc.). It is also difficult to find a proper position in the ambulance. When a foreign body is over a certain length, a decision about cutting the foreign body must be made. Most modern fire services have powerful metal cutters that can cut through most objects quickly. There is a definite risk of shearing internal structures during this metal cutting process, so it is essential that maximal effort is put into stabilizing the foreign body during cutting. One person should have a dedicated role of stabilizing the impaled object and preventing any twisting or torque movements.

Sternoclavicular (SC) Joint Dislocation

Like any other joint, the SC joint can be contused, either by a direct force or by injuries to the shoulder joint. The SC joint is the least commonly injured joint of the shoulder girdle. The joint is stabilized by the costoclavicular ligaments, SC ligaments and capsule, intraarticular disk, and interclavicular ligament. The joint is injured and becomes unstable when the clavicle is dislocated anteriorly or posteriorly, usually after a blow to the shoulder. In the acute phase, a posterior SC joint dislocation can have serious consequences if mediastinal structures are compressed or if there is injury to the underlying lung. Anterior SC dislocation is painful and possibly disfiguring but has no real functional significance, except possibly in throwing sports.

The athlete may complain of local pain and tenderness at the SC joint and discomfort on shoulder movement. Occasionally, there may be breathing and swallowing difficulties with a posterior SC dislocation: these symptoms must be taken seriously and same day referral to a specialist unit is recommended. Reduction on the FoP or in the athlete medical room never recommended.

Management: Most injuries are mere contusions or moderate subluxations without full bone thickness dislocation and can thus be treated conservatively with ice, compression, and rest. Capsular and ligament injuries may take up to 6 weeks to heal. Anterior dislocations are rarely treated surgically. Posterior dislocations are potentially more serious and require further investigation. The athlete is not usually able to return to play on the same day of injury due to pain, even if the injury is a contusion. Return to play can occur when the athlete has a full range of motion and strength. Athletes under the age of 22 years with an SC injury are likely to have had an epiphyseal fracture and thus require a minimum of 4-week fracture healing time.

Costochondral Injuries

Costochondral injuries are most commonly seen in contact sports such as wrestling, rugby, American football, and ice hockey, but also in weightlifting. These injuries include costochondral joint subluxations or luxations but also small fractures to both bone and cartilage. Similar lesions can occur at the chondralosternal junction. It can be quite difficult or nigh impossible to clinically differentiate between these various conditions in the prehospital environment; however, the description of a popping-like sensation over the joint should alert one to a diagnosis. Further investigation does not always lead to a definitive diagnosis.

Management: Conservative treatment based on rest and pain-free movement is the usual recommended treatment. Temporary taping may give short-term symptomatic relief. The athlete should contact their own doctor for further ongoing investigation.

Muscle Injuries

Thoracic muscle injuries are not common but when they do occur they most commonly present as muscle contusions. Muscle tears are more seldom and total ruptures are extremely rare being mostly reported in weightlifting and powerlifting. Treatment is the same as for other muscle injuries – Protection, Rest, Ice, Compression, and Elevation (PRICES). Withdrawal from the FoP may be necessary and it is advised to use an ice bag over the injury site. There can be an array of costal, chondral, periosteal, and soft tissue injuries accompanying such injuries and definitive diagnosis can be difficult.

Bibliography

Bahr, R. (2012) *IOC Manual of Sports Injuries.* Wiley Blackwell.

McDonagh, D. (2011) *FIMS Sports Medicine Manual, Event Planning and Emergency Care* ISBN-10: 1582558736, ISBN-13: 978-1582558738.

Reichman, E. & Simon, R. (2004) Pericardiocentesis. In: *Emergency Medicine Procedures.* McGraw-Hill, USA, pp. 204–216 ISBN-13: 978-0071360326.

John Marx MD , Robert Hockberger MD , Ron Walls MD (2009) *Rosen's Emergency Medicine – Concepts and Clinical Practice.* Elsevier | ISBN-10: 0323054722 | ISBN-13: 978-0323054720 | Edition: 7.

17 Abdominal Injuries

David McDonagh[1,2,3] *and Dara Lundon*[4]

[1]*Emeregency Deptartment, St. Olavs Hospital, Trondheim, Norway*
[2]*Faculty of Medicine, NTNU - National University of Science and Technology, Trondheim, Norway*
[3]*Medical Commission, AIBA - International Boxing Association, Lausanne, Switzerland.*
[4]*Surgical Laboratory, School of Medicine and Medical Sciences, University College Dublin, Dublin, Ireland*

Abdominal injuries are fortunately rare in sports and are usually of minor significance. Occasionally, more serious conditions, notably splenic injuries, can occur particularly in high-velocity and high-energy sports such as skiing, snowboarding, equestrianism, American football, rugby, and mountain biking. In sport, the spleen is the most frequently injured abdominal organ; however, the liver is the most frequently injured abdominal organ when all trauma causes are summated. The kidney may also be injured from blunt abdominal trauma.

As injuries to these organs can be potentially fatal, it is important that the Emergency Doctor (ED) be able to recognize the early signs of sports-related intra- and extraabdominal injury.

While it is natural to assume that acute abdominal pain in an athlete may be due to a sports-related injury, pain may be due to other abdominal conditions or due to referred pain from adjacent anatomical structures. If pain is not due to trauma, then take a full medical history, assess the athlete's hemodynamic stability, and perform a systematic quadrantic abdominal examination. Be aware that some patients with evolving major intraabdominal injuries may be relatively asymptomatic initially with minimal physical signs.

Athletes who sustain a direct blow to the abdomen resulting in injury to the spleen, liver, or kidney may develop immediate severe pain and may rapidly develop signs of shock and peritonism. However, they may also continue to play despite having occult bleeding in an organ but collapse later on either the field, at the side-line, or at home. Patients will often be pale, sweaty, thirsty, with a rapid and weak pulse before collapsing. Therefore, an athlete should not return to play after blunt abdominal trauma if still in pain. The pulse and blood pressure should be checked regularly if there is a debilitating blow over the spleen, liver, or kidneys and the athlete should be kept fasting and refrain from taking medications or fluids by mouth. If the athlete collapses or has clinical peritonism, they should be placed in a recumbent position, with their legs elevated to assist venous return and arrangements made for immediate transfer to hospital.

The IOC Manual of Emergency Sports Medicine, First Edition. Edited by David McDonagh and David Zideman.
2015 International Olympic Committee. Published 2015 by John Wiley & Sons, Ltd.

This chapter focuses on the emergency diagnosis and treatment of severe and less severe abdominal injuries in the prehospital sporting environment. It is important to be able to diagnose and treat the following conditions:

1. Abdominal wall injuries
2. Winding
3. Penetrating injuries
4. Blunt injuries
5. Splenic injuries
6. Liver injuries
7. Kidney injuries
8. Gastrointestinal tract injuries
9. Acute abdomen

FoP Management of an Abdominal Injury

Initiate the Field of Play (FoP) evaluation following the ABCDE mnemonic. The steps of onfield management are as follows.

Clinical Findings/Management Abdominal Injury

Rapidly evaluate the patient's condition to detect if a patient is or is not critically ill. If the patient is standing and appears to be functioning adequately, it is advisable to take the patient off the FoP for a formal examination and particularly if the patient is dazed or unsteady.

Symptoms and signs of internal abdominal organ injury are often delayed.

If the patient is lying down on the ground, test alert, verbal stimuli response, painful stimuli response, or unresponsive (AVPU).

Assess the patient noting if the patient is conscious, able to speak, in pain, cyanotic, or dyspneic.

If conscious take a focused history – "Are you in pain? Where is the pain? Can you breathe properly? What happened?"

If unconscious, immediately initiate the ABCDE evaluation. Call for help. If there is any possibility of a cervical spine injury, carefully maintain inline immobilization of the head and neck while performing the primary survey.

General inspection: Is there cyanosis, is the patient pale, in pain, or has breathing difficulty?

Inspection of the abdomen: Examine the thorax, abdomen, and pelvis. Are there open wounds, bleeding, foreign bodies, bruising, swelling, and signs of bony deformity in the lower thorax or pelvis?

Palpation: Observe pain on palpation of the abdomen, including its bony borders at the lower rib cage and pelvis (see Chapter 18). Is there any subcutaneous emphysema?

Attach a pulse oximeter and take a reading.

Percussion: Percuss the unclothed abdomen chest for dull or hyperresonant sounds. Note any pain on percussion. Initial percussion findings are unlikely to reveal serious pathology in the timeframe immediately after the injury, though pain may be elicited.

Auscultation: Auscultation of the abdomen will probably reveal normal bowel sounds. Absent or decreased bowel sounds may be found with major intestinal damage. Bowel sounds can be auscultated in the thorax in the presence of a diaphragmatic injury or a large pneumothorax (see Chapter 16).

Remember: The back of the abdomen must also be inspected, palpated, and auscultated once the patient has been turned into the recovery position.

Management: This usually involves stabilizing the patient and transferring to the fieldside for further evaluation. A better examination can usually be conducted in the more secluded environs of the athlete medical room. Administer high-flow oxygen at 15 L/min by facemask if the athlete is hypoxic and titrate the oxygen to keep saturation (SpO_2) between 94% and 98% if a pulse oximeter is attached.

Digitally compress any significant arterial bleeds.

Continue the primary survey.

Turn the patient into the recovery position and examine the back.

Remove from the FoP.

Once the primary survey has been completed and the patient is stabilized, remove the athlete from the FoP to the fieldside and directly to an ambulance if necessary. If urgency is not critical, conduct a fieldside evaluation.

Abdominal Wall Injuries

Blows to the abdominal wall are not infrequent in sport and can be seen with "winding" or "solar plexus" punches. They may result in contusions in the abdominal wall muscles (usually the rectus abdominis muscle). Incidence statistics vary from sport to sport, with some of the highest incidence of torso injuries being reported in the English Premier League Football (Soccer) – 7% of all injuries. As with other contusions, early icing, nonsteroidal antiinflammatory drug (NSAID) treatment, and rest are the usual treatment modalities. Some athletes may need several days of rest, others several weeks. Other injuries, such as lateral and rotatory stretching injuries, sudden explosive weight lifting, and hyperextension of the spine can cause partial muscle tears and contusions. Tennis players often suffer from myalgia in the rectus and transversus muscles, usually due to the rotations during serving.

The diagnosis of myalgia is usually straightforward as the pain is often superficial and can be easily provoked by stretching the affected muscle. Tightening of the abdominal muscles will often cause discomfort in an abdominal wall lesion. Palpation will further enhance the discomfort. At times, it can be difficult to differentiate between abdominal wall injuries and underlying minor organ injury, so beware!

Some athletes, particularly unconditioned athletes or ones who have recently eaten, may experience lateral abdominal pain while running, so-called "side cramps" or "side stitches", or more precisely "exercise-related transient abdominal pain". The cause of this phenomenon is unknown and has previously assumed to be due to muscle cramping, though recent evidence seems to suggest that this is not the case. Diaphragmatic ischemia and rapid increase in hepatic venous flow have also been proposed as likely causes. Proper warming-up exercises can purportedly prevent stitches. There is no treatment for the condition, other than moral support and patience as the condition usually resolves itself within a few minutes.

Winding

Winding is a relatively common injury in contact sports resulting from a blow to the "solar plexus" of the abdomen. The exact pathophysiological mechanism is unknown; however, it is thought that external forces cause vagal stimulation and resultant temporary diaphragmatic spasm. Typically, the winded athlete doubles up and has difficulty breathing with short gasping breaths. As with "side cramps" the situation resolves itself quickly without any residual symptoms. If symptoms persist, then exclude an internal injury by further examination, observation, and on occasion even hospital referral.

Penetrating Abdominal Injuries

A penetrating injury occurs when the abdominal region abruptly comes into contact with a sharp object. These objects can be part of the sporting apparel as in fencing, hockey, or gymnastics but can also be by any kind of stationery object – from picket fences, camera equipment, stanchions, and so on. With all penetrating abdominal injuries, there is a risk of accompanying thoracic and diaphragmatic injury.

Most diaphragmatic lacerations occur on the left hemidiaphragm and usually occur after high-velocity automobile accidents. The stomach can herniate into the thorax and undergo volvulus dilatation and can even cause compression of the left lung, with a mediastinal shift to the right. Gastric distension can, in extreme cases, result in perforation and should be prevented by inserting a nasogastric tube to deflate the stomach of gas. Diaphragmatic injury is often associated with other severe thoracic-abdominal injuries. Spleen and liver injury is also common with penetrating diaphragmatic injuries.

Clinical Findings/Management Penetrating Abdominal Wound

Evaluate (A) airways and (B) breathing, and (C) circulation before examining the abdomen.

The patient may be unconscious, but if conscious, the athlete will be in pain, usually severe pain. There may be severe respiratory distress due to lung or diaphragmatic injury with dyspnea and cyanosis. The respiratory rate will most likely be elevated as a result of peritonism.

Inspection: The presence of a penetrating object must be noted and a presumption of internal organ injury made. There is always the possibility of a foreign body having entered the abdomen but this is unlikely in a sporting environment. The patient will be in intense pain and there may be increasing abdominal swelling and guarding.

Percussion: May be dull sounding due to internal bleeding or tympanitic with air from intestinal puncture.

Auscultation: Auscultation of the abdomen may reveal the absence of normal bowel sounds.

Pulse Oximetry may reveal normal or lower oxygen saturation values.

Pulse rate may be elevated and blood pressure may fall, particularly if there is intrathoracic or intraabdominal organ injury with severe internal bleeding and the patient may show symptoms of shock.

Management on the FoP involves ensuring airway patency and assisting respiration if required. Secure adequate oxygenation and ventilation and evaluate the need for endotracheal intubation. This will probably require drug-assisted RSI (see Chapter 4), which is best achieved in the ambulance or the athlete medical room.

Blood volume should be restored by establishing intravenous access and administering boluses of intravenous fluids. Rapid infusion is not advised as a sudden rise in blood pressure may disturb the natural wound hemostasis. Slower infusion is advised and the ED should endeavor to maintain the systolic blood pressure at around 90 mmHg. If possible use wide bore intravenous cannula with two IV sites being safer than one.

If the patient is becoming hemodynamically unstable, then rapid transportation to the nearest hospital is essential. Treatment throughout transfer may also be necessary, so a doctor capable of managing the patient's condition should accompany the athlete. Intravenous analgesia should be considered in conscious patients and Entonox (nitrous oxide and oxygen mix) should be avoided. The use of antishock trousers is contraindicated due to the risk of intraabdominal bleeding. Never remove a foreign body, as removal will almost always lead to increased bleeding. Penetrating foreign bodies should be left in place, but they must be supported and immobilized to prevent further shearing damage to internal organs (movement may cause a sawing-like effect) during transport. Open wounds should be covered with saline-dampened bandages.

Blunt Abdominal Injuries

Most blunt abdominal injuries in sport, while they can be temporarily incapacitating, are not of a serious nature. Athletes may suffer abdominal wall muscle contusions or strains and sometimes even winding. Occasionally, they may suffer abrasions or lacerations but these are usually minor in nature. The most common abdominal trauma mechanism in sport is when an athlete has a sudden rapid deceleration due to colliding with or being tackled by another athlete or after crashing into a stationary object. The greater the athlete's velocity and weight, the greater the potential for more serious intraabdominal organ injury. As most sports are relatively low velocity in nature, forced rapid deceleration rarely results in intraabdominal organ contusion, shearing, laceration, or hemorrhage, however, these may occur if there is underlying organ pathology or previous injury. The organs most commonly involved are the spleen, liver, and small intestine and if damaged, the patient will require immediate medical intervention, stabilization, and evacuation to a trauma hospital for ongoing treatment. In trauma patients, intraabdominal and pelvic hemorrhage can be misdiagnosed during the primary and secondary surveys either due to the patient being unconscious or due to the initial bleeding being moderate and occult.

Expect a higher incidence of more severe injury in high-velocity sports (e.g., alpine skiing, ski jumping, bicycling, motor sports, and equestrian), contact sports (e.g. rugby, American football, handball, ice hockey, and soccer), and the combat sports (e.g. boxing, judo, and taekwando).

After a blunt injury to the abdomen, the patient is unlikely to lose conscious unless there are high-energy forces involved. Look for other causes of unconsciousness and perform a primary survey, starting with airway, breathing, and circulation. If there is a suspicion that the cause of unconsciousness is due to intraabdominal organ injury, then it is extremely important to check the patient's hemodynamic status (pulse, blood pressure, SpO_2) in case there is internal abdominal bleeding.

The presence of signs of shock such as rapid pulse, low blood pressure, increased respiratory rate, pale sweaty skin, raised capillary refill time (CRT), constriction of peripheral vessels combined with pain, and guarding over the liver, spleen, or kidneys should give cause for concern. With major bleeding, abdominal distension may occur often requiring rapid cardiovascular stabilization, immediate transfer to hospital, and emergency surgical intervention.

Clinical Findings/Management Blunt Abdominal Injury

General inspection: Is the patient conscious or unconscious? Is the patient in great pain?
Primary survey: ABCDE.
History: The usual complaint is that of pain. The localization of the pain and its intensity can give vital clues as the severity and anatomical location of the injury.
Inspection: Look for abrasions, lacerations, contusions and swellings, and pain on breathing.
Palpation: Tenderness (superficial or deep), guarding, rigidity, and abdominal distension.
Tenderness over a lower rib fracture should alert one to the possibility of underlying organ injury.
Percussion: Tympanitic sounds often present with gastric distension and dull sounds with hemoperitoneum. Percussion tenderness may also be present.
Auscultation: Auscultation may reveal the presence or absence of normal bowel sounds.
Management Treatment starts with examining and ensuring the patency of the airway, followed by an evaluation of breathing and, if the athlete is unconscious, insertion of an oropharyngeal airway. Administer high-flow oxygen, aiming to maintain oxygen saturation at between 94% and 98%, with consideration of drug-assisted RSI and assisted ventilation if necessary. Establish IV access, preferably at two sites and administer an adequate amount of fluid to keep the systolic blood pressure See above at a minimum of 90 mmHg. Transfer the patient to the fieldside for further evaluation or arrange immediate transfer to hospital.

If the ED is unsure of the presence of organ injury and chooses not to refer the athlete for further investigation, then it is important to evaluate the athlete's initial hemodynamic status, observe the patient for a period of time, and reevaluate the patient's physiological signs regularly. Remember that athletes can appear to be in reasonably good form for some hours after injuring an organ (particularly the spleen) before there is a sudden rapid deterioration. The athlete or his coaching team should be informed of this possibility so that plans can be adapted, that is, cancellation of long air flights, or return to remote locations. Accompany the athlete to hospital if the medical staff in the ambulance does not have required emergency skills.

If there is a suspicion of minor organ injury, the athlete should be withdrawn from sporting activity, stabilized, and transferred to hospital for a computed tomography (CT)/ultrasound investigation. Ensure that the airway is patent, give high-flow oxygen, insert a venous catheter, and administer intravenous fluid to maintain the systolic blood pressure at 90 mmHg.

Splenic Injuries

Bruising, tearing, or even rupture of the spleen can occur after a direct blow to the upper left abdomen from either a knee, shoulder, or kick. Owing to the spleen's rich blood supply (10–15% of the total body blood volume is filtered every minute) trauma may cause varying degrees of bleeding. If the splenic capsule is intact, bleeding from splenic injuries may not present with classic peritonitic findings, though the intensity of pain should alert the ED to the possibility of significant organ damage. Thus, splenic injury may present with or without peritonitic findings and with or without immediate changes in the patient's hemodynamic status, depending on whether there is damage to the splenic blood vessels and the splenic capsule. With minor injuries, small subcapsular hematomas and small capsular tears can occur without significant splenic parenchymal damage, with limited and local bleeding. There is also concern regarding "return to play" issues, as undiagnosed capsular tears and contusions may worsen if reexposed to trauma, especially if there is an underlying mononucleosis. These minor lesions must also be investigated. Larger contusions may also occur with bruising and bleeding, affecting larger areas of the spleen.

The main challenge is to detect these serious splenic lacerations, stabilize the patient as best one can, and admit the patient urgently to hospital.

Splenic trauma is more common in children than in adults, probably due to the fact that they are more active than adults, but also because their abdominal organs are less protected by bone, muscle, and adipose tissue. In adults and adolescents, ruptured spleens are sometimes associated with splenomegaly caused by infections such as infectious mononucleosis, immune system disorders, malignancy, and other splenic diseases, which may be unknown to the FoP healthcare professional. Traumatic ruptures have been reported.

With penetrating injuries, the risk of splenic damage is obviously present. The foreign body should be stabilized and circulating volume substitution will become a priority once the airway and breathing functions have been assured. With penetrating splenic injuries, great care must be taken in avoiding infection as reduced splenic function may lead to decreased white blood cell production.

Clinical Findings Splenic Injury

General inspection: Is the patient conscious or unconscious. Is there pallor, cyanosis? Is the patient in pain?

Primary survey: ABC – are there symptoms/signs of shock or, more commonly in sport, the gradual onset of shock findings such as dizziness, vomiting, fainting, sweating, pale or clammy skin, rapid heartbeat and weak pulse, falling blood pressure, dyspnea, increased respiratory rate and generalized deterioration of vital signs, and eventually loss of consciousness.

History: A history of blunt trauma to the upper left abdomen should raise concern. The usual complaint is that of pain. The localization of the pain and its intensity can give vital clues as the severity and anatomical location of the injury.
Always ask about previous or current Epstein Barr Infections and other illnesses associated with splenomegaly such as malaria.
Inspection: Look for abrasions, lacerations, contusions, and swellings over the spleen, pain on breathing.
Palpation: Tenderness (superficial or deep), guarding, rigidity, and abdominal distension are always a possibility. Tenderness over a protective left rib should alert one to the possibility of splenic injury.
Percussion: There may be dull sounds with an enlarged spleen or with a hemoperitoneum. Percussion tenderness may also be present.
Auscultation: Findings will probably be normal.

Liver Injuries

Liver, bile duct, and pancreas injuries are once again rare in sport. However, like splenic injuries, they may pose significant diagnostic and therapeutic challenges to the sports doctor in the prehospital setting. The ED must have a high index of suspicion and any indication that the injury is more than just a local external contusion, should cause the ED to err on the side of safety, withdraw the athlete from the FoP, and refer for diagnostic tests and treatment at an appropriate hospital.

The liver is the most frequently injured intraabdominal organ despite being relatively well protected (though splenic injuries are more common in sport). For the ED, patients with injuries to the liver can be best classified as being hemodynamically stable or unstable. The hemodynamically stable patient with a probable liver injury should be administered high-flow oxygen via a facemask, provided with appropriate volumes of intravenous fluid and transferred urgently to hospital. The patient may require intravenous analgesia.

If the patient has a normal and stable pulse and blood pressure parameters but is dizzy, vomiting, fainting, feels unwell, is sweating, or has pale or clammy skin, then there is an increased possibility of intraabdominal bleeding. Again, rapid airway/circulation intervention and hospital transportation is required.

The patient with abdominal tenderness and any other symptoms (dizziness, vomiting, fainting, malaise, sweating, or has pale or clammy skin) should be withdrawn from the FoP and referred to hospital immediately. The need for referral of a patient with abdominal tenderness but no other symptoms or signs, (and who is of course hemodynamically stable) has to be made on an individual basis, but if the pain and tenderness are moderate and the case history does not suggest major impact trauma, then the patient can be observed and reevaluated after 10–15 min. Once again, the importance of taking an accurate and detailed case history cannot be emphasized enough.

Pancreatic trauma is rare but is seen with injury to other intraabdominal organs.

Clinical Findings Liver Injury

Will be similar to those found with splenic injury except that the pathological findings will be on the right-hand side of the abdomen and not the left
General inspection: Is the patient conscious or unconscious, in pain?
Primary survey: ABC – are there shock findings?

History: Is there a history of blunt trauma to the upper right abdomen? Is there pain and what is the localization and intensity?
Inspection: Look for abrasions, lacerations, contusions and swellings over the liver and surrounding areas (including the back), and pain on breathing.
Palpation: Deep tenderness, guarding, and rigidity under the right costal margin, possible abdominal distension. Tenderness over the protective ribs.
Percussion: There may be dull sounds with a damaged liver or hemoperitoneum. Percussion tenderness may also be present.
Auscultation: Findings will probably be normal.

Kidney Injuries

The kidneys are usually well protected by abdominal structures to the front and by the lower rib cage and back muscles to the side and back. Blunt trauma can, however, damage the kidneys and injuries have been recorded in rugby, American Football, ice hockey, rugby, soccer, lacrosse, cycle accidents, and in equestrian sports.

Once the physical examination had been completed and the decision made not to refer the patient to hospital but to observe in the medical room, it is appropriate to take a urine sample. Often blood is found, but not always immediately, after renal injury. Also, the absence of hematuria does not exclude kidney injury (as seen when there is disruption between the kidney and ureter). Bleeding can range from microscopic to macroscopic hematuria to profuse bleeding. In some cases, there is significant blood loss and hypovolemic shock can develop. The combination of macroscopic hematuria and hypotension is potentially serious. Severe renal trauma is often accompanied with injuries to intraabdominal organs. No athlete should be allowed to return to play until the urine sample is normal and without traces of blood. Most episodes of microscopic hematuria clear up within a week and require no further follow-up. Persistent or repetitive episodes do, however, need to be assessed.

If renal trauma is suspected, then the patient should be stabilized and transferred to hospital for CT examination; ultrasound examination alone is not sufficient. Most blunt renal injuries are treated conservatively with strict bed rest until the hematuria has resolved. Surgical repair is seldom needed after blunt sports trauma.

Penetrating trauma is, of course, much more serious. Stabilize the patient and the penetrating object, ensure that the patient's airway is patent, that there is optimal breathing, give highflow oxygen via a facemask, set up an intravenous line, stabilize the circulation, and transfer the patient to hospital as soon as possible for surgical evaluation. Once again the patient's hemodynamic stability is of major importance.

Clinical Findings Kidney Injury

Will be similar to those found with splenic and liver injuries except for anatomical location.
General inspection: Is the patient conscious or unconscious, in pain?
Primary survey: ABC – are there clinical symptoms and signs of shock?
History: Is there a history of blunt trauma over a kidney? Is there pain and what is the localization and intensity?
Inspection: Look for abrasions, lacerations, contusions, and swellings over the flanks and back, loss of loin contour, and pain on breathing.
Palpation: Deep tenderness or guarding over the kidneys or adjacent ribs.
Percussion: Will probably be normal as long as there is no intraabdominal injury. Percussion tenderness may also be present.
Auscultation: Findings will probably be normal.

Gastrointestinal Tract Rupture

In high-energy trauma injuries to the abdominal region, severe intraabdominal lesions must always be suspected. Rupture of the small intestine or colon can cause symptoms similar to those of peritonitis. Rupture of the colon causes pain and findings of tenderness, guarding, and rigidity and the patient may develop symptoms of shock. Precise fieldside diagnosis is difficult (even with sophisticated portable ultrasound devices) and patients should be transferred to hospital for further diagnostic investigation. Injuries of the pancreas are often overlooked due to lack of clinical findings in the initial phase.

Routine stabilization treatment is the goal; ensure that the patient's airway is patent, that there is optimal breathing, administer high-flow oxygen by facemask, and establish an intravenous infusion. Analgesia should be administered if necessary. If there is a gastrointestinal rupture, then the patient may deteriorate rapidly, so urgent transfer to hospital is advised. Owing to the risk of occult injury, all high-energy abdominal injuries should be referred to hospital for observation and or advanced diagnostic imaging.

Acute Abdomen

Rarely, an athlete may present with intense abdominal pain some hours after a sporting event, the athlete being uncertain if the pain was due to a blow or of nontraumatic origin. The athlete may well be surprised by the intensity of the discomfort considering the force of the blow. This is a potentially dangerous scenario as the doctor can be mislead into believing that the insignificant trauma was in fact the cause of the patient's pain and in reality the athlete may be presenting with an acute abdominal pain of nontraumatic origin. Undifferentiated abdominal pain remains the commonest diagnosis for patients admitted to hospital with acute abdominal pain (35–41%). Patients may also present with various forms of gastroenteritis, urinary tract, or gynecological infections. Acute appendicitis is always a potential diagnosis in the younger population and must always be considered. Amenorrheic athletes with abdominal pain may in fact be pregnant but the same symptoms could arise from a torted ovarian cyst or dysmenorrhea. The list of possible causes is long and it is not within the confines of this manual to discuss all the potential causes of abdominal pain.

Genital Injuries

Genital trauma is more common in men and includes injury to the testes, scrotum, and penis. Penetrating injuries can occur, though these are very rare. Minor lacerations can occur in the penis or scrotum, as well as bites, burns, and zipper injuries. Blunt trauma is the commonest cause of testicular injury and bleeding in and around the testicle can lead to testicular contusion. If there is major damage, then the protective tunica albuginea may be injured and may cause testicular rupture. In motorbike incidents, testicular dislocation has been described when the testicle has been forced out of the scrotum and into the abdomen.

Refer to hospital with swelling or acute pain.

Clinical Findings/Management Scrotal Trauma

Symptoms: The athlete describes a direct blow to the scrotum (often from a knee, fist, and foot). There is intense pain, nausea, and even scrotal swelling.

Inspection: The athlete may be lying curled up on the ground holding or protecting the groin region. The athlete usually resists all form of examination initially until the pain has lessened. Take the patient to the fieldside and ask the patient if he wishes to be examined. This may take place in the ambulance or athlete medical room. In the vast majority of cases, the situation is self-resolving and the athlete will often wish to return to play.

The scrotum may be discolored and tender. If there is bleeding in the scrotum, it may be possible to palpate a hard scrotal mass or hematocele – but examination is usually limited by pain. The scrotum may fail to transilluminate. In these cases, it is wise to refer the patient to scrotal ultrasound in case there is a need for surgical repair.

Palpation: If the patient gives consent, then there will be tenderness.

Management: Refer if pain persists or if swelling develops.

Penile injuries are rare, though zipper injuries can occur (uncommon in sport due to the lack of zippers in sporting pants and underwear). Using a wire cutter, injuries can be corrected by cutting the bar on the top of the zipper slider: the zipper usually comes apart. Injecting local anesthetic into the affected area and attempting to unzip the zipper is another option.

Lacerations to the female perineum may occur but are rare. Wounds should be evaluated by the ED, with a female assistant in attendance, in the athlete medical room.

Acute Testicular Pain

Acute nontraumatic testicular pain can occur at any age and time, the commonest causes being testicular torsion, acute epididymitis, and acute epididymoorchitis. The most important task is to suspect acute testicular torsion and refer the patient to a surgical unit. Differentiating between these entities is almost impossible and unnecessary in the prehospital environment. Testicular torsion is a surgical emergency. Failure to operate within an appropriate time may lead to reduced spermatogenesis (4 h) in the affected testicle or even infarction (6 h). There is usually a predisposing congenital abnormality (often called the "bell clapper" anomaly), which allows the testicle to rotate on the spermatic cord within the tunica vaginalis, causing venous and arterial occlusion, with subsequent ischemia and testicular infarction. A torsion may be categorized as complete, incomplete, or transient.

Torsions can occur after trauma.

Clinical Findings/Management Testicle Torsion

Symptoms: Sudden severe pain in one testicle, usually without a history of trauma. Enquire about possible trauma episodes, recent or past, mild or severe. Pain can occasionally build up slowly. Some patients have a previous history of intermittent testicular pain that resolved spontaneously (intermittent torsion and detorsion). The patient may be nauseous and feel dizzy.

Inspection and palpation: The patient may be vomiting and protecting the groin. There may be swelling around the affected testicle with tenderness. The tender testicle may be elevated and may have a horizontal lie. Scrotal erythema and ipsilateral, loss of the cremasteric reflex, and fever have been described.

Management: All patients with acute nontraumatic unilateral testicular pain should be referred to a specialist surgical unit. *Do not* refer suspected testicular torsions for ultrasonography at a radiological department – too much time may pass and the patient may sustain testicular ischemia and infarction if the torsion time approaches 6 h. Always take a good medical history to find out precisely when the pain started.

Abnormal Vaginal Bleeding

Abnormal vaginal bleeding may be described to be present if there is a heavy flow of dark colored clotted blood, usually accompanied by pain. In the absence of trauma this may be associated with spontaneous abortion or cystic rupture. In trauma cases, vaginal lacerations, uterine rupture, or pelvic fracture may be associated with vaginal bleeding.

Patients should be referred to a specialist if there is a suspicion of pelvic trauma, spontaneous abortion, or ectopic pregnancy.

Bibliography

Advanced Trauma Life Support (2008) *Advanced Trauma Life Support (A.T.L.S.)*, 8th edn. American College of Surgeons, Chicago, Illinois.

Flik, K. & Callahan, L.R. (1998) Delayed splenic rupture in amateur hockey player. *Clinical Journal of Sports Medicine*, **8**, 309–310.

Kim, P. (2006) Mountain biking injuries requiring trauma center admission: a10-year regional trauma system experience. *Journal of Trauma Injury Infection & Critical Care*, **60** (**2**), 312–318.

Marquirriain, J. (2007) Rectus abdominis muscle strains in tennis players. *British Journal of Sports Medicine*, **41**, 842–848. doi:10.1136/bjsm.2007.036129

McDonagh, D. (2011) *FIMS Event Physician*. Lippincott Williams Wilkins.

Rifat, S.F. & Gilvydis, R.P. (2003) Blunt abdominal trauma in sports. *Current Sports Medicine Reports*, **2** (**2**), 93–97.

Tsalkidis, A. *et al.* (2008) Acute abdomen in children due to extra-abdominal causes. *Pediatrics International*, **50**, 315–318. doi:10.1111/j.1442-200X.2008.02578.x

Walter, K.D. (2007) Radiographic evaluation of the patient with sport-related abdominal trauma. *Current Medicine Reports*, **6** (**2**), 115–119.

Waninger, K.N. & Harcke, H.T. (2005) Determination of safe return to play for athletes recovering from infectious mononucleosis: a review of the literature. *Clinical Journal of Sports Medicine*, **15**, 410–416.

18 Pelvic Injuries

Andy Smith[1] *and João Grangeiro Neto*[2,3]

[1]*Yorkshire Ambulance Services, Leeds Medical School, Leeds, UK*
[2]*Brazilian Olympic Committee and Olympic Games Rio 2016, Brazil*
[3]*Sports Medicine Department, INTO-MS, Rio de Janeiro, Brazil*

It is relatively uncommon for athletes to injure their pelvis. In English Premiership rugby union, there is a match day incidence of 2.61/1000 h (one injury every 10 matches) – there is the possibility of more frequent and more serious injuries in high-energy sports such as equestrian and motor sport activities. Pelvic fractures can be relatively minor or they can be life threatening with significant blood loss. It is important that an athlete with pelvic trauma is managed appropriately on the Field of Play (FoP) and transported correctly and safely to the appropriate hospital with the necessary facilities to manage such injuries. Preevent planning should identify the appropriate facility.

The pelvis is a bony ring made up of the sacrum, coccyx, and the two hipbones. They are jointed at the two sacro-iliac joints, the sacrococcygeal joint and anteriorly at the pubic symphysis. Disruptions of the pelvic ring at two or more sites may cause both hemodynamic and biomechanical instabilities. Major pelvic injuries are usually the result of significant forces being applied to the pelvis. The usual mechanisms of injury are falls directly onto the pelvis, heavy weights falling on the pelvis, or from external force transmission via the femoral shaft resulting in either anteroposterior, lateral, or vertical compression. The fracture pattern is dependent on the forces applied to the pelvis during the mechanism of injury. Fractures can be classified as follows:

1. *Type A*: Stable fractures not involving the complete pelvic ring, for example, iliac crest, anterior inferior iliac spine, or minimally displaced stable pelvic ring fractures, for example, superior pubic rami
2. *Type B*: Rotationally unstable, vertically stable fractures, for example, open book fractures
3. *Type C*: Rotationally and vertically unstable fractures involving major damage to two or more areas of the pelvic ring

Three major force vectors can act in isolation or in combination to produce pelvic fractures: side impact may cause lateral compression, leading to internal rotation of the hemipelvis; anterior posterior-compression leading to external rotation of the affected hemipelvis (seen with mechanical crush injuries) and vertical shear injuries leading to cephalic displacement of the hemipelvis (usually after falls from a height).

The IOC Manual of Emergency Sports Medicine, First Edition. Edited by David McDonagh and David Zideman.
2015 International Olympic Committee. Published 2015 by John Wiley & Sons, Ltd.

The pelvis could be considered a visceral organ that contains aspects of the urinary system, reproductive system, bowel system, soft tissues, arteries, veins, nerves, and bones. Major pelvic injury is often associated with other significant injuries. Pelvic trauma can result in significant hemorrhage due to the disruption of the pelvis, resulting in an expanded diameter of the pelvis and thus bigger potential space for fracture hematoma and/or disruption of the venous plexus. Neurological injuries can also occur with damage to the lumbosacral plexus and the femoral nerve.

Pelvic trauma may include the following:

1. Major pelvic fractures with intrapelvic complications
2. Hip fractures
3. Minor pelvic fractures
4. Hip dislocations and subluxations
5. Soft tissue injuries

FoP Management Pelvic Injuries

Athletes with pelvic injuries should be assessed and their treatment priorities established based on their injuries, vital signs, and the mechanism of injury. After scene safety, assessment and management should follow the ABCDE principles, as described in detail in Chapter 3, ensuring that life-threatening conditions are identified and treated in a timely manner.

S: Safe approach
A: Manage any airway problems and manual inline stabilization (MiLS) of the cervical spine (if appropriate)
B: Manage any breathing problems, including adequate ventilation
C: Circulation and hemorrhage control: this may be significant in pelvic trauma
D: Assess for any coexistent head injury and take measures to minimize secondary brain injury
E: Exposure, assessment, and management of other injuries as necessary to facilitate packaging and movement into a more appropriate environment

The management of potential life-threatening injuries involving airway or breathing must always take priority. The exception to this rule is in the presence of exsanguinating external hemorrhage. The recognition and management of most nonimmediately life-threatening external hemorrhages occur during the circulatory assessment. Less obvious bleeding and deformities will usually be recognized under the exposure component of the primary survey or during the secondary survey. In an athlete showing signs of shock, (raised heart rate, raised respiratory rate, pale, weak or absent peripheral pulses, confusion due to cerebral hypoperfusion, and prolonged capillary refill time) and complaining of pelvic pain, the pelvis should be splinted without further examination of the pelvis. If an athlete is showing signs of shock and not indicating a specific area of trauma, the source of hemorrhage should be sought externally, in the chest, abdomen, pelvis, long bones, or retroperitoneal space.

Clinical Findings/Management Pelvic Injury

The clinical findings of circulatory shock, indicating major internal hemorrhage, if present, may be minimal and not immediately apparent. It is therefore essential to undertake a thorough primary survey. If pelvic trauma is suspected, immobilize the pelvis with a splint and tie the patient's feet together to reduce pelvic volume. Do not palpate the pelvis.

General inspection: The patient may be unresponsive. There may be gross lower extremity deformity. If responsive, the patient may be in severe pain with pelvic trauma.

Inspection: Is there shortening of one leg in comparison to the other, pelvic deformity, blood stains in the pelvic region from the urethra or rectum? If so, it should be assumed that there is pelvic trauma and no palpation of the pelvis should take place (as palpation may cause further damage). Keep monitoring the primary survey; package and evacuate the patient to hospital at the earliest opportunity.

Palpation: In the absence of clear signs of pelvic trauma, crepitus in the groin or pelvic region may indicate pelvic fracture. Crepitus in the presence of groin pain is indicative of pelvic injury. Bony tenderness may be detected by gently palpating the superior rami and symphysis for deformity or pain. Palpation should be performed once only.

Stability: In the absence of the above-mentioned findings, continue the examination by gently pressing on the anterior superior iliac crests to illicit pain or increased mobility with an inward pressure (no outward "springing" pressure should be applied due to the risk of clot displacement, further hemorrhage, and opening up of the pelvic volume).

Examination of the pelvis should be only undertaken once.

Positive findings should inhibit further examination and the pelvis should be immobilized.

Management: Should the patient's vital signs deteriorate or there is a cause for concern at any stage, return to the primary survey. If the patient is unresponsive and there is a suspicion of pelvic injury, ABC must be stabilized and the patient should be securely immobilized and rapidly transferred to hospital. If conscious, conduct a rapid history, there will be pain in the pelvic or groin region with pain on hip movement. If a patient shows signs of shock combined with pain in the pelvic region, it should be assumed that there is major pelvic trauma and no palpation of the pelvis should take place.

The injured athlete should be administered high-flow oxygen at 15 L/min via a nonrebreathing mask titrating the oxygen dose aiming for a target saturation within the range of 94–98% and transported to an appropriate resourced hospital at the earliest opportunity by a paramedic crew. If the athlete is not showing signs of shock, IV access can be delayed until the patient is reexamined on the fieldside while awaiting emergency transport. IV crystalloid fluid is only administered to maintain end organ perfusion guided by the presence/absence of the radial pulse or a systolic blood pressure of 90 mmHg. Fluids should be administered in 250 mL aliquots to maintain a systolic blood pressure of 90 mmHg.

Splinting of the pelvis can be achieved using either a bespoke commercial sling, for example, SAM sling (See Fig 18.1) or a sheet/triangular bandage. It is essential that these pelvic splints are not used as a belt but that pressure applied to the pelvis is *across the intertrochanteric* line to ensure the pelvis volume is reduced and not being opened up.

In addition to wrapping the pelvis, the athlete's legs should be tied together with a degree of internal rotation. It is essential to check distal neurovascular status pre- and postapplication of any pelvic sling/splint.

Adequate analgesia is often forgotten (but not by the patient!) or left late. It should be given as soon as it is safe to do so (after life-threatening conditions have been managed in the primary survey). Traditionally, morphine has been the drug of choice. However, with the restrictions now placed on the storage and use of morphine, together with its respiratory depression and induced nausea, other intravenous alternatives tramadol or paracetamol, depending on local preferences, may be considered. If the pain is very severe, neither of these agents will be strong enough and the onset of morphine may be too slow to be truly effective. Another option is the usage of low-dose intravenous ketamine (0.1 mg/kg) if the practitioner is trained in its use. Ketamine has the advantages of rapid onset and profound analgesia without associated respiratory depression.

Following recent Faculty of Pre Hospital Care, Royal College of Surgeons of Edinburgh consensus meetings and publications, it is now recommended that the transport of patients with a spinal injury should be undertaken using split scoop devices rather than the traditional long spinal board to promote hemostasis. The introduction of split long board devices/scoop stretchers that require a minimum tilt of the patient to allow insertion of the blades under the patient, reduces patient movement and hence the potential for exacerbation of internal hemorrhage. There is increasing evidence that log rolling pelvic trauma patients into the recovery position on traditional long spinal boards may promote further hemorrhage. The use of second-generation thermoplastic scoops allows for radiological imaging and hence further reducing patient movements once in the emergency department. Some disadvantages do remain with these new devices, for example, width of only ~47 cm, weight limits over aluminum extensions, and cost, but with the release of bespoke head block systems for scoop devices, they are now the preferred device for immobilization, transfer, and transportation to definitive care. Scoop devices should be regarded as lifting devices: the casualty should be lifted into a nearby basket stretcher or vacuum mattress for carrying.

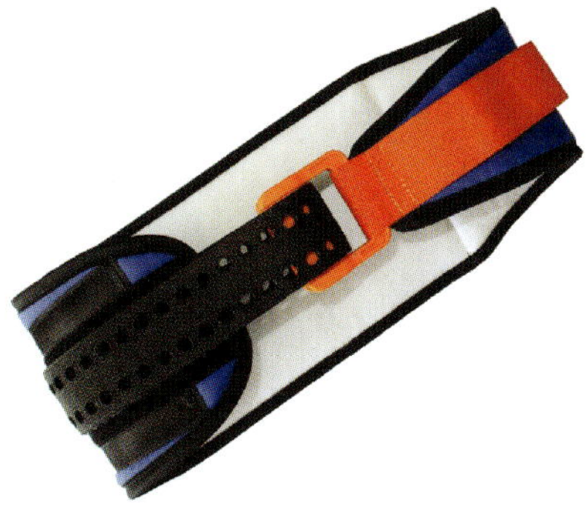

Figure 18.1 Pelvic SAM sling

Fieldside Management Pelvic Injury

On arrival at the fieldside, repeat the primary survey. In the early phase of hypovolemic shock, there may be minimal vital sign changes. Neurological changes can develop slowly. If the patient is unresponsive or if there are obvious signs of shock or deformity, conduct a rapid top-to-toe survey and establish basic physiological monitoring, then evacuate to hospital. If responsive and no signs of shock or deformity, initiate monitoring and if there is a delay before transfer, commence the secondary survey. This must include a sensory and motor neurological assessment of the lower extremities (the nerve roots most commonly affected are L5 and S1, as well as the femoral nerve, which is composed of L2, L3, and L4). On arrival at the fieldside, it may be appropriate to transfer the athlete directly into an ambulance as a proper examination of the pelvis requires exposure of the pelvis and this may be a more appropriate place to unclothe the athlete.

Clinical Findings Pelvic Injury at the Fieldside

Symptoms: If conscious, conduct a focused history, asking the patient about the extent and location of pain. "Did you hear any cracking sound from your neck or back? Is there any shooting pain, pins, and needles?"

Inspection: Exposure of the pelvic region may reveal the extent of deformity and the possible site of injury. Look for open wounds or the presence of ecchymosis in the groin, peroneal, scrotal, and surrounding areas. Blood at the urethral meatus may be indicative of pelvic trauma. Avoid unnecessary movement of the patient. Rectal examination is not necessary in this prehospital environment where there is suspicion of pelvic instability. Look for deformity of the extremities, rotation of an extremity, or limb length discrepancy.

Palpation: Palpation may reveal crepitus or bony tenderness in the pelvis or lower extremities. Test for sensation while palpating the extremities.

Sensory testing: Most doctors struggle to remember which nerves supply which dermatomes. A rough guide to lower extremity dermatomes: sensation to the anterior and medial aspect of the thighs, legs and feet is lumbar, sensation to the posterior aspect of the thighs, and legs is sacral, as is the lateral aspect of the foot and perineum. Therefore, sensory changes in the lower extremity may be indicative of pelvic ring fracture.

Motor function testing: If the patient has severe hip or pelvic pain do not test active or passive range of motion (ROM) in the hip or knee joint. Ask the patient to dorsiflex (L4 nerve) and plantarflex (S1 nerve) ankle joints; inability may indicate a neurological injury in the lumbopelvic region.

All documentation, including a SAMPLE history (Signs and Symptoms, Allergies, Medications, Past medical history, injuries, illnesses, Last oral intake and menstruation, Events leading up to the injury and/or illness) and patient's observations should accompany the athlete to hospital.

Hip Fractures

Hip fractures can be categorized into acetabular fractures, femoral head fractures, and femoral neck fractures. These injuries are fortunately rare in the majority of sports due to the high-energy forces required to fracture these bones.

Acetabular Fractures

Fractures of the acetabulum usually occur when forces are transmitted indirectly from the femoral shaft, for example, a fall from a height. The injury pattern is often dependent on the position of the femur at the time of injury. If the hip is flexed or extended, then it will usually dislocate with the potential to fracture the rim of the acetabulum. If the hip is in neutral, then the force is transmitted directly to the acetabulum with the potential to result in fracture.

The athlete will be in pain and any movement of the leg will exacerbate the pain. There may be shortening, adduction, and external internal rotation. If there is disruption of the acetabulum, there may be extensive hemorrhage and the athlete may show signs of shock. The athlete should be assessed by the ABCDE approach treating life-threatening injuries, administering high-flow oxygen, and transported by an emergency ambulance to a suitable hospital as soon as possible. Intravenous access should be gained before transfer but this should not delay the transfer. Intravenous fluids can be administered to maintain a systolic blood pressure of 90 mmHg and distal neurovascular assessment is essential.

Fractures of the Pubic Ramus

Pubic rami fractures are usually caused by a fall. Anteroposterior compression may produce isolated ipsilateral superior and inferior pubic rami fractures. Following significant falls (e.g., fall from a horse) the athlete may sustain both superior and inferior pubic rami fractures, thus causing the pelvis to be unstable.

The athlete will usually complain of pain in the hip, but careful examination of the site of pain will reveal that there is groin pain, with tenderness to palpation over the fracture site. There is no external rotation or shortening of the leg, but the athlete will find walking very painful. Hip movements tend to be painful due to the proximity of the fracture to the femoral head but usually the athlete will manage a straight leg raise. Anterior and lateral pelvic compression is usually painful.

Prehospital management includes providing the athlete with required supportive treatment including adequate analgesia, appropriate pelvic stabilization with the legs splinted together, and transfer to the hospital for further assessment, investigation, and management.

Avulsion Fractures of the Pelvis

Many power muscle groups have attachments with the pelvis, for example, hamstring muscles at the ischial tuberosity, sartorius at the superior iliac spine and rectus Femoris at the inferior iliac spine. Forceful contractions of these muscle groups during sporting activity can lead to avulsion fractures. The athlete experiences acute pain after muscle effort at the site of the avulsion with impeded functionality. The athlete should be provided with suitable analgesia and transferred to a medical facility for further investigation and management.

Hip Dislocation and Subluxation

Dislocation of the hip is a rare injury in sports, but could occur in, for example, rugby, cycling, gymnastics, water skiing, wrestling, soccer, snow skiing, and basketball. A physical examination should be carried out to rule out concomitant injuries.

The direction of dislocation is dependent on of the position of the hip and the direction of force applied at the time of injury. A forward fall on a knee with the hip flexed and being struck from behind when down on all four limbs is the most common mechanism of injury. An anterior dislocation is much less common and results from abduction and external rotation forces. Athletes who suffered a hip dislocation commonly report significant pain and are unable to move the affected limb, rise from the ground, or bear weight. The position of the lower limb is the key to diagnosis. The lower extremity is usually shortened, flexed, internally rotated, and adducted in posterior dislocations. In anterior dislocations, the lower extremity is externally rotated with varying amounts of flexion and abduction.

Closed reduction after radiological investigation is recommended. Athletes should be referred to hospital. If the distal vascular status is challenged or the patient has a gross deformity that prevents adequate immobilization during transfer, a FoP or field-side reduction may be necessary but is often difficult. Analgesia is usually necessary. Reduction techniques vary depending on the direction of dislocation.

Similarly to hip dislocation, hip subluxation usually occurs after a fall on a flexed knee with the hip adducted. The resulting force pushes the femoral head posteriorly onto, but not over, the rim of the acetabulum as in a hip dislocation. Hip subluxation can also occur after the athlete stops abruptly and pivots over a weight-bearing extremity to change direction. This places the extremity in the vulnerable position of hip flexion and adduction. The presentation is subtle, and the athlete who sustains a hip subluxation may be able to get up and walk immediately after the injury. The athlete may report only groin soreness and persistent pain with weight bearing. Once the diagnosis has been suspected, the athlete should be removed from competition, given crutches, and referred for further image studies.

Soft Tissue Injuries

Contusions are the most common sporting injury to the hip and pelvis and are usually caused by collisions with other athletes or falls to the ground. Contusions can be superficial (limited to subcutaneous tissues) or deep, with intramuscular or intramuscular hemorrhage and significant hematoma formation. Depending on the extent of contusion, pain, disability, and localized edema may occur immediately or after a 24–48 h interval. FoP evaluation should exclude fractures, significant muscle ruptures, and significant bleeding. Rest, Ice, Compression, and Elevation (RICE) treatment should be administered.

Ultrasonography or radiological evaluation may be necessary to exclude significant injury.

Labral Injuries

The acetabular labrum is a ring of fibro cartilage that lines the border of acetabulum and is continuous with the transverse acetabular ligament. These lesions have been reported as the most common cause of intraarticular hip pain in sports activities. Usually, athletes complain of pain in the groin in certain positions, usually with a twisting or pivoting motion. Athletes may have a clicking or a catching sensation. Anterior labral tears may be detected by moving the hip from a position of full flexion, through external rotation and abduction to a position of extension, internal rotation, and adduction. These athletes should be treated with analgesics, further imaging evaluation, and physical therapy.

Ligamentum Teres Tear

This ligament is an intraarticular structure that can be torn with acute trauma. Usually, a complete rupture is associated with hip subluxation or a sudden twisting injury. A partial or total tear may cause mechanical hip pain and dysfunction. Following a positive diagnostic examination, the athlete should be presented for arthroscopic surgery of the hip.

Trochanteric bursitis

Trochanteric bursitis causes pain on the lateral aspect of greater trochanter. This bursa can become inflamed mainly from trauma or repetitive trauma. Trochanteric bursitis occurs more often in females than males. In athletes, causes include an iliotibial band, excessive foot pronation, and leg-length discrepancies. This pain usually increases gradually and can sometimes radiate distally and must be distinguished from a neurologic disorder. The patient may limp or have difficulty walking. Pain is exaggerated by resisted abduction and external rotation. The athlete should rest with the application of ice packs, undertaking stretching exercises, and the administration of oral nonsteroid antiinflammatory drug (NSAID) medication.

Ischial bursitis

Ischial bursitis causes pain at the level of the ischial tuberosity and radiates down the posterior aspect of the thigh. Pain is exacerbated by hip flexion or sitting and can be confused with sciatica. Treatment is similar to the other types of bursitis.

Iliopsoas bursitis

The iliopsoas bursa is the largest synovial bursa in humans. Aggravation of the bursa occurs with rapid lengthening and contracting of the iliopsoas muscle over the pelvic brim. It occurs in track and field athletes and rowers. Patients present with inguinal pain, tenderness to palpation, weakness in external rotation strength in hip flexion, and a positive Thomas test. Treatment should begin with conservative measures, rest, physical therapy, and oral NSAIDs.

Iliopectineal bursitis

Iliopectineal bursitis is related to snapping of the iliopsoas over the iliopectineal eminence. Stretching of the iliopsoas tendon in hip extension will usually worsen this discomfort. Treatment consists of rest, oral NSAIDs, and possible steroid injection.

Summary

Pelvic injuries in athletes are uncommon but may be seen in contact/collision and high-energy sports. They should always be suspected if the mechanism of injury is appropriate. Pelvic fractures can be minor, requiring conservative treatment, or major life-threatening events which will require rapid stabilization, intravenous fluid resuscitation, and transfer to hospital.

Bibliography

England Professional Rugby Injury Surveillance Project Steering Group (2014). *England Professional Rugby Injury Surveillance Project 2012–2013 season report.*

Prehospital Emergency Care Course. Faculty of Pre Hospital Care, Royal College of Surgeons of Edinburgh.

Graves, I. & Porter, K. (2007) *Oxford Handbook of Pre-Hospital Care.* Oxford University Press.

Greaves, I., Porter, K. & Smith, J. (2011) *Practical Prehospital Care: The Principles and Practice of Immediate Care.* Churchill Livingstone.

Greaves, I., Porter, K. & Ryan, J. (eds) (2001) *Trauma Care Manual.* Hodder Arnold.

Sports Injuries, Their Prevention and Treatment. Lars Peterson and Per Renstrom, (2001), Martin Dunitz. ISBN 1-85317-1190.

Higgins, R., Brunker, P. & English, B. (eds) (2006) *Essential. Sports Medicine.* Blackwell Publishing.

Safran, M. (2002) Hip injuries in the athlete. *Sports Medicine and Arthroscopy Review*, **10** (**2**).

Scott, I., Porter, K., Laird, C., Greaves, I. & Bloch, M. (2013) The prehospital management of pelvic fractures: initial consensus statement. *Emergency Medicine Journal*, **30** (**12**), 1070–1072.

The Orthopaedic Clinics of North America (2002) *Management of acute athletic trauma.*

19 Spinal Injuries

Éanna Falvey [1,2] *and Craig Roberts* [3]

[1]*Ireland Rugby Team, Dublin, Ireland*
[2]*Sports Surgery Clinic, Dublin, Ireland*
[3]*South Africa Rugby Team, Cape Town, South Africa*

Spinal injuries are unfortunately not uncommon in the sporting setting. Spinal cord trauma is caused by contusion or tearing (partial or complete) of the cord. A partial tear may, depending on its location and severity, result in a partial or total loss of sensation, movement, or organ function below the level of injury. A complete transection of the cord will lead to immediate and complete loss of sensation, flaccid paralysis, and a loss of reflex activity below the level of injury. Both partial and complete spinal cord injuries may lead to autonomic dysfunction resulting in bradycardia and hypotension (neurogenic shock). These changes may occur within a few minutes of the injury, but may take several hours before the full extent of the injury is apparent.

Spinal injuries constitute about 10% of all the sports injuries. The effects of these injuries are many, ranging from missed competition 6% of professional cyclists in one study to chronic pain 33% of golfers, functional disability, and permanent neurologic deficit. Rugby Union players suffer cervical spine injuries with associated spinal cord injury between 0.8 and 13 times per 100,000 players per year (Quarrie and Hopkins (AJSM) 2008).

Measures to prevent spinal injury have proven difficult to implement. The most common patterns of injury are compression of the spine, compression-flexion of the spine, and flexion of the spine.

The use of protective equipment, rules, and supervision is limited. It is, however, possible to arrange sporting activities so as to reduce the number of spinal injuries, mostly to rules changes and proper officiating. The Emergency Doctor (ED) must be prepared to optimally manage any event that occurs on the Field of Play (FoP). EDs at a high-velocity sport or a sport with a definitive risk of traumatic cord injury should be trained in acute airway management and spinal cord immobilization. The medical response team should rehearse this management process regularly. It is preferable to have preexisting access to a Level I or II trauma center for immediate transfer of high-risk patients. This chapter focuses on the emergency diagnosis and treatment of severe and potentially severe spinal injuries in the prehospital sporting environment.

It is important to able to diagnose and treat the following acute injuries and conditions:

1. Cervical spinal cord trauma
2. Vertebral fractures
3. Facet Joint injuries

The IOC Manual of Emergency Sports Medicine, First Edition. Edited by David McDonagh and David Zideman.

History	Findings
Pain on hyperextension of the spine	Facet joint injury, spondylolysis
Pain on flexion of the spine	Disc pathology
Relief of pain on flexion	Facet joint
Relief of pain in neutral or extension	Disc pathology
Constant nocturnal pain	Suspect systemic cause, neoplasia
Fever, weight loss, and malaise	Systemic conditions
Bowel or bladder dysfunction	Central disc herniation
Pain radiating to limbs	Nerve root entrapment
Leg pain with activity	Vascular claudication (spinal stenosis)
Adolescent athlete	Always consider Traumatic spondylolysis
Older athlete	Be aware of neoplasm

Table 19.1 Differential diagnosis – acute back pain

4. Transient quadriplegia
5. Spinal cord neurapraxia (stingers/burners)
6. Disc herniation
7. Spondylolysis and spondylolisthesis
8. Soft tissue injuries

It is often difficult to find the cause of acute back pain. A list of common diagnosis and specific confirmatory tests can be found in Table 19.1. There is an array of other possible medical causes of back pain, but to deal with these goes beyond the scope of this manual.

Preparation for Onfield Management

All staff involved in the FoP management of spine-related injury should be adequately trained and should have performed recovery simulations together as a team prior to the event using all the available equipment such as spinal boards, cervical collars, immobilization devices, and scoop/basket stretchers. The Team Leader should be identified early and team members must follow the leader's instructions. In an ideal situation, all team members are adequately trained and any individual member should be capable of directing and managing immobilization and extraction. It is important that the medical team and paramedics onsite, are familiar with each other, their skills and deficiencies.

FoP Management Potential Spinal Injury

Ensure that it is safe for the medical response team to enter the FoP. It is important to know that the integrity of the cervical spine is not compromised.

The steps of onfield management are as follows.

Primary Survey Potential Spinal Injury

Try to approach the conscious athlete from the front so that they may see and hear you.

Where the patient is unconscious, verbalize using his/her name where possible in an effort to rouse/awaken them.

If the athlete is prone, it is best to carefully log roll into a supine position maintaining inline immobilization of the spine, removing the mouthpiece (if present) and evaluate the breathing pattern. If the FoP team is well trained, this is not a difficult task, but if not done properly, it is possible to convert an unstable spinal injury into a permanent neurologic deficit.

The head and neck should be immediately immobilized in a neutral position using MILS (Manual In Line Stabilisation). Firmly grasp the player's head and hold it in its relative position as the player is rolled into the supine position. Do not cover the athlete's ears so they can hear what you are saying. The head should remain at the same angle and in the same position in relation to the neck, shoulders, and pelvis throughout the logrolling process. Once secured, the head should at no point be released until the patient has been securely transferred to a definitive management setting.

If the athlete is not breathing spontaneously, open the airway using the jaw thrust maneuver and maintain inline stabilization of the cervical spine as best you can. If breathing is still abnormal or absent and the patient is unresponsive, initiate cardiopulmonary resuscitation (CPR). If spontaneous breathing returns in the unconscious patient, it is usual practice to carefully insert an oropharyngeal (Guedel) airway. Once the airway is secured and the patient is breathing normally, a cervical collar can be sized and then fitted. If the athlete is wearing a helmet (or face mask), remove this without flexing or extending the neck and firmly support the head to keep the head in line with body during the helmet removal process. (American Football has a different practice.) The helmet removal procedure should also be practiced by the FoP team prior to the event.

Continue on with the Breathing (B) evaluation. Possible (B) complications with a spinal injury are as follows:

Thoracic movement is dependent on muscular activity, primarily the diaphragm and intercostal muscles. Damage to the spinal cord at the C3 vertebrae and above may result in the loss of diaphragm function. (Diaphragm innovation is C3,4,5.) If the cord injury is complete, then CPR must be initiated. If the cord is partial, the patient will need to be ventilated. Damage to cord at the thoracic level may result in dysfunction of the intercostal nerves at that level and below – so the patient may require ventilation support. Inspection of the chest during inspiration may reveal reduced chest movement and reduced depth of respiration. The respiratory rate may increase. Oxygen saturation will fall.

Possible Circulation (C) complications with a spinal injury. Disruption of sympathetic outflow may lead to unopposed vagal stimulation, cardiac arrhythmias, bradycardia, hypotension, and subsequent possible circulatory collapse. This may be a life-threatening emergency that commonly occurs with severe spinal cord lesions at T6 or higher. A slowed pulse (50–60 bpm) must be considered as being pathological (possibly due to a spinal cord lesion and autonomic dysfunction) and not the physiologically low resting pulse seen in top athletes. Such a pulse is quite inappropriate for an athlete on the FoP who has been actively participating in sport. Blood pressure must also be assessed, an IV line must be established and circulatory support given in the form of IV fluids.

Patients with spinal cord injuries are at risk for deep venous thrombosis (DVT) and pulmonary embolism because of the loss of mobility and, potentially, abnormal platelet function and altered hemostatic and fibrinolytic activity.

Next, Disability (D), assess the athlete's level of consciousness (LOC). As described in other chapters, this is usually done using the AVPU scale. In rugby union, as opposed to most other sports, the doctor is allowed to examine the patient on the FoP and thus can conduct the secondary survey on the FoP. If the patient is alert, has normal ABC, but obviously has pain in the neck or spine, a cervical collar should be fitted and supported until the athlete can be safely transferred onto a scoop stretcher. An athlete with altered consciousness may not be capable of maintaining the integrity of their cervical spine and must be managed as a spinal injury until proven otherwise.

Exposure (E): Expose the patient to exclude other life-threatening injuries maintaining patient privacy and confidentiality.

FoP Management of a Patient with Findings Indicative of a Spinal Cord Injury

It is difficult to proscribe when a spinal injury casualty should be removed from the FoP. Where the FoP remains live, it may be necessary to remove the casualty quickly but safely. However, where a spinal injury is suspected, it may be better to be cautious and safe, but not necessarily slow.

Removal must be a practiced technique that is performed smoothly and with confidence and should not be compromised by FoP technical officials demands.

Transfer of the Patient onto the Spinal Board/Lifting Device

In practice it is most likely that the FoP team comprises four members. The leader of the medical team should apply gentle inline immobilization of the cervical spine. The second healthcare professional is responsible for the torso, pelvis, and hips. The third team member is responsible for the pelvis and legs. The fourth individual moves the spinal board or scoop stretcher into place. Some authorities recommend the use of a fifth person for a full spinal immobilization roll – leader at the head, three members positioned down the body at chest, pelvis, and legs and a fifth member to manage the equipment.

Follow local guidelines for choice and use of lifting device.

On the Team Leader's command, the athlete should be rolled onto the spinal board or scoop stretcher. Current practice is moving in favor of using a scoop stretcher as a lifting/transfer device because of the limited roll movement to position the device. Having positioned the patient on the scoop they can be easily strapped securely and lifted onto a spinal board or preferably a basket stretcher or vacuum mattress.

If a spinal board, ensure the patient is carefully positioned in the center of the spinal board and secure the patient with the straps and apply the head blocks to avoid cervical spine movement. The straps must be tight enough to prevent any movement or twisting of the spine on the smooth surface of the board. One of the more effective means of securing the player on their board is a spider harness. Do not leave the patient secured on a spinal board for a prolonged period of time as this can lead to pressure necrosis.

If a scoop stretcher is used, carefully roll the patient 10^0 from side to side to position each half of the scoop and then snap the two halves of the device together. Secure the patient with the scoop straps and head blocks and lift the patient carefully into a basket stretcher or onto a vacuum mattress. Finally, secure the basket/mattress belts and transfer the patient to the fieldside.

Transfer from the FoP to the Fieldside

When lifting the athlete, position at least two first responders on either side of the lifting device. If the athlete is heavy, it may be necessary to have more responders to lift and carry. Ensure that all responders have a firm grasp on the handles and understand the procedure. Brief the athlete about the lift. On the Team Leader's command (ready, steady, lift), all team members should lift the trauma device with the athlete together a comfortable carrying height. Team members should keep their backs upright when lifting and lift with the knees and legs. If the athlete vomits while immobilized, it is relatively easy the turn the device with the athlete attached, onto its side and to clear the airway without compromising the spine. When walking off the FoP, the team should always face the direction of travel, walking carefully forwards to avoid tripping. It will be necessary to preplan the evacuation route prior to movement so that the entire team is aware of the proposed direction of travel.

Fieldside Management Potential Spinal Injury

On arrival at the fieldside, repeat the primary survey. If the FoP athlete medical room is near, then continue to the room without further delay.

Check the pupillary response and examine ocular movement. Initiate monitoring and commence the secondary survey with due concern for the casualty's privacy. This should include checking for priapism (request permission to do this from the player first and explain the request). Careful examination of extremities should be performed.

Neurological examination: Initiate the examination with the Glasgow Coma Scale (GCS). A lower GCS may be indicative of both a head injury and/or spinal injury. Examine for cranial nerve abnormalities, abnormal papillary responses, and focal neurological findings.

Clinical Findings with a Potential Spinal Injury

In the early phase of a spinal cord injury, there may be minimal findings. Neurological changes can develop slowly as inflammation of the cord increases.

If the patient is unresponsive, immobilize the neck with a collar, check SABCDE, and do not evaluate range of motion (ROM).

Symptoms: If conscious, conduct a focused history, asking the patient to speak and avoid nodding or shaking the head: "Do you have any pain in your neck, thorax, back, pelvis, and legs? Is there any shooting pain? Did you hear any cracking sound from your neck or back? Can you feel your body? Do you have pins and needles anywhere? Is it difficult to breathe?"

Inspection: Is the airway patent? Is the patient breathing normally? Evaluate chest wall movement and the respiratory rate and oxygen saturation. Is there abdominal breathing (accessory breathing seen with thoracic spinal cord lesions)? Are there signs of bleeding? Check the pulse rate. Is the patient alert, responding to verbal stimulus, pain stimulus, or unresponsive? Is the patient in pain? Does the athlete appear to have muscle control in his/her arms or legs?

Palpation: Palpate for midline spinal pain tenderness. Test for sensation while palpating the extremities: "Can you feel your body? Can you feel the sensation in your hands and feet?" (test all using stimuli).

ROM testing: If the patient has severe-to-moderate neck pain do not test active or passive ROM. If the patient has moderate neck pain, then carefully examine both active and passive movements of the neck noting the ROM. If there is an increase in pain or resistance during ROM testing, then testing must cease and a cervical collar should be fitted while supporting the head.

"Can you move your arms and hands?" (ask the athlete to move each hand) "Can you move your legs and feet?" (ask the athlete to move each foot).

Test that strength is equal in both arms and both legs. Start with small movements of the arms and legs. Allow the player to move the body *very* slowly from one side to the other, then forwards, and backwards. Allow the player to stand up, offering support and being prepared to assist if required. If at any time, there is any pain, tingling, lack of sensation, or signs and symptoms of a fracture or spinal injury, *stop* and immobilize the player.

Return to Play After a Fieldside Evaluation of a Neck Injury

The ED may consider that it is safe for an athlete to return to play if, after a thorough examination and assessment, the results of the primary, secondary surveys and subsequent monitoring and examinations are normal. Specifically, the ED must have excluded a significant head injury (no LOC, GCS 15 – normal). There should be normal neurological findings, vision, and pupillary reflexes. The athlete should have passed a sideline concussion evaluation. There should be no severe pain or discomfort or deformity in the neck or back.

Cervical Spinal Fractures

If a fracture is suspected, then the ED must always suspect a spinal cord injury. In the acute FoP setting, it is very difficult to evaluate the level of spinal cord injury. The medical team must therefore err on the side of caution and manage any potential spinal column injury as a spinal cord injury.

Clinical Findings with a Potential Cervical Spinal Fracture

It is common practice to immediately support the neck before conducting the primary survey.

Symptoms: If conscious, is there neck pain, shooting pain, and midline spinal tenderness.

Inspection: Is the patient in pain? Holding their neck? Is there bruising or deformity to the neck region? Is the patient in pain? Does the athlete appear to have muscle control in their arms or legs?
The second team member can conduct the rest of the examination.

Palpation: Examine for midline spinal tenderness, sensation in the torso, and extremities.

Movement: If the patient has significant neck pain, immobilize the neck, apply a cervical collar if the neck is in a neutral position, and continue to support the neck (a cervical collar does not immobilize all of the cervical spine). If the neck is in a fixed nonneutral position, it is better to support the neck manually or with a vacuum splint. Applying a rigid cervical collar to a patient with a fixed fracture dislocation is not recommended. If the patient has mild-to-moderate neck pain, ask the patient to gently move the neck while the Team Leader supports the neck manually. The Team Leader must decide if movement is normal or restricted, painful, or painfree. If movement is normal and painfree and if there are normal neurological findings, it is reasonable to assume that there is no significant neck injury. Depending on the setting, it may be advisable to remove the patient to the fieldside for further examination.

All suspected cervical spine injuries must be fully immobilized from the outset and transferred to hospital for full examination and treatment.

Thoracolumbar Vertebral Fractures

Major fractures causing spinal instability are relatively uncommon except in high-speed sports such as motorsports. The spinal cord usually ends at the L1/2 interspace, hence damage to the thoracic spine tends to be associated with neurological deficit, whereas only 3% of lumbar spine dislocations have a neurological deficit (this is usually at a root level and is hence less debilitating). Fractures to the transverse process, spinus process, facets, vertebral bodies, and endplates, as well as traumatic spondylolisthesis may occur. A past history of any spinal problem should always be obtained. It is important to be aware that due to the large forces involved in a vertebral fracture, severe fractures may be associated with other injuries to the head, chest trauma, abdomen, pelvis, and extremities.

Athletes will often report severe pain; it is also important to ask about neurological symptoms related to compression of neural structures (pain, paraesthesia, weakness, and loss of sensation) and if present to accurately document the level and regions involved.

Management of suspected thoracolumbar fractures: The vast majority of injuries are minor, requiring rest, ice, and compression. In the more severe injuries, the athlete needs to the follow the SABCDE triage system and needs spinal immobilization before transport to hospital.

Facet Joint Injuries

These may include fractures or dislocations. Fractures usually present with unilateral pain and pain on extension. In young athletes, it may be associated with an epidural hematoma caused by bleeding at the fracture site; this in turn can lead to radicular symptoms. This is a stable fracture and once recognized can be treated conservatively.

Facet dislocations occur mostly in joints that have been exposed to repetitive loading, with resultant degeneration of the disc spaces, posterior subluxation, and intervertebral foramen impingement on the nerve. These conditions may be unilateral (combined flexion and rotation) and may be associated with an articular fracture and neurological compromise. Bilateral facet dislocation occurs when all of the interosseus ligaments are disrupted. The affected vertebra lies anterior to the vertebra below and may thus compromise existing nerves or the patency of the spinal canal. Ligamentous strain due to hyperextension/hyperflexion injury is painful and initially debilitating but usually results in neither abnormal alignment nor neurological compromise.

Clinical Findings/Management Facet Joint Injuries

Symptoms: Pain with prolonged standing, walking, or running or pain exacerbated with extension or rotation. Athletes may describe an acute sharp catching in the back: relief of pain with flexion of the spine. There is usually an absence of an acute precipitating event.
Inspection: Hyperlordosis.
Palpation: Tenderness over the facet joints on palpation.
Movement: Increased muscle spasm in intervertebral muscles. Back hyperextension or rotation is painful, relieved with flexion.
Management: Any athlete with acute pain and neurological findings should be referred to a specialist unit. Analgesia may be required.

Transient Quadraplegia and Paraplegia

Bilateral motor and or sensory neurological symptoms after an athlete receives a blow to the head or whiplash neck injury, suggests cervical spinal cord injury. Fortunately not all such episodes result in permanent injury; transient paresis and parasthesia in sport have been reported as occurring in 1.3 per 10,000 participants in college American football.

The initial FoP and fieldside management is the same as for a suspected spinal cord injury with full immobilization and rapid transport to hospital. It is impossible to distinguish between bony or ligamentous damage based on clinical findings on the FoP or fieldside. Radiographic investigations (X-ray, computed tomography (CT), and magnetic resonance imaging (MRI)) are required to rule out spinal column, spinal cord, or nerve root impingement.

Neuropraxia: Stingers or Burners

A "stinger" or "burner" is a common athletic injury usually occurring after a high-energy collision with another athlete and is most often seen in American Football where up to 65% of college football players have reported suffering from at least one stinger during their college careers. These injuries are also seen in rugby, wrestling, ice hockey, basketball, and boxing. It is reported that stingers may occur in as many as 50% of athletes involved in contact/collision sports. In this type of injury brachial plexus or the nerve roots suffer severe trauma, the C5 and C6 nerve roots of the upper trunk of the brachial plexus being most commonly involved. The athlete experiences burning pain and numbness in the affected limb and may attempt to "shake it off "or is seen supporting the arm with the contralateral hand. Weakness in shoulder abduction, external rotation, and arm flexion are reliable indicators that a stinger may have occurred. In most cases, symptoms resolve in a few minutes but in some cases, motor weakness may develop later on.

Injury may occur after a direct blow or traction injury to the brachial plexus, often with the neck laterally flexed neck away from the side of the blow and the shoulder depressed.

Stingers may be graded as follows:

1. Grade 1 neuropraxia (transient motor or sensory deficit without structural axonal disruption). Full recovery, usually occurs within 2 weeks, can be expected.
2. *Grade 2 injuries*: Axonotmesis (axonal disruption occurs with intact outer supporting connective tissue known as the epineurium). The neural deficit is present for at least 2 weeks following the injury.
3. *Grade 3 injuries*: Neurotmesis (total structural disruption of axons and epineurium). It persists for at least 1 year, with little to no clinical improvement.

Clinical Findings/Management Stinger Injury

Symptoms: Upper extremity weakness and burning pain. To alleviate the pain, the neck is kept in flexed position and the affected limb is raised with the help of the opposite hand. In this way, the athlete tries to alleviate the compression and stretch of the nerve.

Inspection: Looking for deformity of cervical spine, neck, and shoulder.

Palpation: Tenderness and deformity in the neck, clavicle, and shoulder.

Movement: Examination should include strength testing of all muscle groups and sensory evaluation of all dermatomes, and assessment of deep-tendon reflexes. Actively rotate, laterally bend, forward flex, and extend the neck within limits of comfort. In stringer syndrome weakness in the deltoid, supraspinatus, infraspinatus, and biceps muscles may be seen. A shoulder examination should include the clavicle, acromioclavicular joint, and supraclavicular and glenohumeral regions. An unstable shoulder may predispose to a stinger and weakness related to neural damage may in turn result in shoulder instability. Erb's point should be percussed to elicit any radiations.

Special test: Spurling maneuver is a confirmatory test and is positive in 70% of the cases. It is performed by asking the patient to bend the cervical spine to one side, while the examiner applies an axial load, thus applying a compressive force at the neural foramen. The test is positive if pain radiates into the ipsilateral arm, indicating nerve root compression/irritation.

Management: The management of stinger syndrome is mainly supportive. The player should be removed from play. If bilateral upper extremity symptoms are present, the athlete should be immediately immobilized and transported from the FoP to the nearest trauma center for full physical and radiographic evaluation. No athlete should return to play until symptoms have disappeared and there is full physiological resolvement.

Muscle Injuries (Sprains and Strains)/Soft Tissue Injuries

Muscle strains and ligament sprains are the most common form of injury sustained by athletes in the thoracolumbar spine. Athletes will have back pain that is exacerbated by rotation, lateral flexion, or extension (and on resisted movement). Significant contusion or hematoma should raise the suspicion of a transverse process fracture.

Management is the same as for other muscle injuries – protect, rest, ice, compression, elevation, support (PRICES). Withdrawal from the FoP may be necessary if there is functional impairment. If more severe injury is suspected such as a transverse process fracture, then X-rays are required as appropriate. Temporary sports taping may give short-term symptomatic relief.

Acute Disc Herniation

Most acute disc herniations arise during weight training or collision sports particularly after a pivot or twisting motion. The condition is most often seen in 30–50-year-olds, the L5-S1 being the most common site in 90% of cases. In adolescent and young adults, neurological symptoms are often less severe or absent due to the more supple ligamentous composition and generally more viscous nature of the disc.

Clinical Findings/Management Acute Prolapsed Disc

Symptoms: Pain is caused by nerve root compression or muscle spasm. There is usually a history of back pain. There may be numbness in the extremities, exacerbated by sitting, bending, or twisting. There may be loss of sensation and or weakness. Younger athletes may present with unilateral hamstring stiffness. Bowel or bladder symptoms may suggest cauda equina syndrome, which is a surgical emergency (0.24–2% of cases).

Testing for cervical herniation:

C4/5 (C5 nerve root) – shoulder pain and weakness of deltoid – numbness unusual

C5/6 (C6 nerve root) – this is the most commonly involved level, weakness of biceps and wrist extensors is seen, numbness may be seen into the thumb of the hand.

C6/7 (C7 nerve root) – weakness of the triceps or finger extensors may be seen, numbness in the posterior arm radiating to the middle finger may accompany any weakness.

C7/T1 (C8 nerve root) – weakness of finger flexors (hand grip) may be seen with numbness into fifth finger.

Testing for thoracolumbar herniation:

Decreased range of motion especially flexion.

Positive straight leg raise test with paraesthesia *or* radiating pain below level of the knee.

Passive plantar flexion may relieve symptoms.

Positive bowstring test (modification of the straight leg raise test).

Positive reverse Lasegue test – used to assess femoral nerve root impingement.

Increased pain with flexion, coughing, sneezing, or sitting.

Numbness and or weakness will give an indication of the nerve root involved.

Management: Remove from FoP if there is a functional disability or neurological symptoms.

Offer analgesia. Placing the athlete on his/her back with hips and knees flexed and supported at 90° may relieve symptoms: referral for appropriate specialist.

Management: Any athlete with acute pain and neurological findings should be referred to a specialist unit. Indications for surgical intervention are as follows:

1. Progressive neurological deficit
2. Bowel or bladder symptoms are present
3. Recurrent radiculopathy with neurological symptoms
4. Failed conservative treatment

Spondylolysis and Spondylolisthesis

Spondylolysis and spondylolisthesis are not uncommon injuries particularly in young athletes involved in sports that require repetitive hyperextension and axial loading such as football, gymnastics, and ice skating. The incidence of spondylolysis in adolescents with back pain has been found to be almost 40%. It is considered as a stress fracture of the pars interarticularis caused by repetitive hyperextension (85% occurs at L5 level). Spondylolisthesis is the forward slippage of the vertebra relative to the vertebral body usually due to the loss of the stabilizing effect of the pars interarticularis (bilateral spondylolysis) – it is graded radiologically into five grades, according to the percentage of the vertebral body that is displaced: 25%, 25–50%, 50–75%, 75–100%, and 100%.

Clinical Findings Spondylolysis and Spondylolisthesis

Symptoms: Back pain at site, usually gradual onset, although they may have acute onset. Pain made worse by extension and rotation activities (back walk over in gymnastics, throw-in in soccer or rugby, and cricket bowling). Severe spondylosisthesis may result in neurological symptoms.

Findings:

Athletes may compensate with knee and hip flexion on walking. In the case of a severe spondylolisthesis, the slip may be palpable.

Positive provocative single leg hyperextension test.

If spondylolisthesis is severe, there may be neurological symptoms appropriate to the level of involvement.

Management: Initial treatment is symptomatic, removal from the FoP if there is a functional disability or neurological symptoms. Refer to specialist examination.

Bibliography

Anderson, J., Reid, J. & Steinweg, J. (1998) *Atlas of Imaging in Sports Medicine*. McGraw-Hill Book Company Australia PTY Ltd. ISBN:0-07-470497-4.

Bahr, R. (2012) *IOC Manual of Sports Injuries*. Wiley Blackwell.

Clarsen, B., Krosshaug, T. & Bahr, R. (2010) Overuse injuries in professional road cyclists. *American Journal of Sports Medicine*, **38** (**12**), 2494–2501.

Cantu, R. (1997) Stingers, transient quadriplegia and cervical spinal stenosis: return to play criteria. *Medicine & Science in Sports and Exercise*, **29**, S233–S235.

Dunn, F., Proctor, M. & Day, A. (2006) Lumbar spine injuries in athletes. *Neurosurgical Focus*, **21** (4), e4.

Klopper I., deWet R. Boksmart (2010) *Acute on field injury management* www.boksmart.com [accessed on 6 September 2014]

Mitchell, L. (2013) *FIMS Team Physician Manual*. Routledge. ISBN:978-0-415-50532-1.

Lewkonia, P., Paolucci, E.O. & Thomas, K. (2012) Reliability of the thoracolumbar injury classification and severity score and comparison with the Denis classification for injury to the thoracic and lumbar spine in spine, Spine **37** (**26**), 2161–2167.

Robert, S. & Massimino, F. (1997) *ACSM's Essentials of Sports Medicine*. Mosby. ISBN:0-8151-0157-0.

Quarrie, K. & Hopkins, W. (2008) Tackle injuries in professional rugby union. *American Journal of Sports Medicine*, **36**, 1705–1716. doi:10.1177/0363546508316768

Vad, V.B., Bhat, A.L., Basrai, D., Gebeh, A., Aspergren, D.D. & Andrews, J.R. (2004) Low back pain in professional golfers: the role of associated hip and low back range-of-motion deficits. *American Journal of Sports Medicine*, 32, 494. doi:10.1177/0363546503261729

Vaccaro, A.R., Klein, G.R., Ciccoti, M. *et al.* (2002) Return to play criteria for the athlete with cervical spine injuries resulting in stinger and transient quadriplegia/paresis. *Spine Journal*, **2** (5), 351–356. Review

20 Extremity Injuries

Michael R Carmont[1,2] *and David McDonagh*[1,2,3]

[1]*Emeregency Deptartment, St. Olavs Hospital, Trondheim, Norway*
[2]*Faculty of Medicine, NTNU - National University of Science and Technology, Trondheim, Norway*
[3]*Medical Commission, AIBA - International Boxing Association, Lausanne, Switzerland.*

The majority of limb injuries in sport are simple soft tissue injuries consisting of strains, sprains, and contusions and are familiar to event medical providers. Injury surveillance programs of soccer and Rugby Union World Cup competitions have revealed that ankle sprains and muscular contusions are the most frequent injuries. In the 2012 Olympic Games in London, 59% of the Field of Play (FoP) injuries were designated musculoskeletal. Most players and athletes are capable of limping or walking with assistance from the FoP to the fieldside or athlete medical room for further assessment and management. FoP interventions by team doctors are infrequent (average 1.6 actions per match in professional soccer leagues), and the likelihood of being called to perform life and limb-saving procedures is minimal. Joint sprains and ligament injuries may require longer term recovery and rehabilitation but they do not pose any immediate management problems other than immobilizing the injured joint and the administration of adequate analgesia.

This chapter presents a safe management pathway to approach the athlete with life- or limb-threatening extremity injuries on the FoP and at the fieldside.

Fieldside Observation and Observations on Approaching the Athlete

Fieldside observers have the advantage of being close to the FoP for easy access, though this is frequently not the best position to witness the mechanism of injury. Some sporting organizers specifically place trained medical observers in the spectator areas in order to allow for optimal observation of the mechanism of injury and then transfer accurate information via radio to the fieldside team of care providers.

Observation of the mechanism of injury also offers information about the need to carry extra equipment onto the FoP, for example, stretcher, splints, analgesics, spinal board, cervical collar.

Providers must always ensure their own safety before entering a FoP (equestrian sports, skating sports, sliding sports, etc.) and be properly clothed and equipped with protective equipment, for example, gloves, nonslip footwear, boots, torches.

The IOC Manual of Emergency Sports Medicine, First Edition. Edited by David McDonagh and David Zideman.

Pitch or courtside providers are usually on the scene within a matter of seconds of the injury occurring, though for other outdoor sports in larger arenas, minutes may pass before the rescue team reaches the injured athlete, for example, alpine skiing and cross country events. On reaching the athlete, providers have to act quickly and efficiently to triage and stabilize the athlete before transfer from the FoP. In certain sports, permission to enter the FoP may have to be given by referees or other officials: procedures should be checked beforehand as rules vary between sports.

FoP Management - Limb Injury

The medical response team's approach to any medical or traumatic incident on the FoP should be standardized. The athlete should be evaluated according to the sequential priorities of a primary survey: airway (with consideration for cervical spine injury), breathing, circulation, disability, and exposure.

This rapid initial assessment should be performed for all injuries no matter how minor they appear, but should be adapted given the mechanism of injury as, for example, with a potential spinal injury. In rugby, players may fall to the ground after a tackle. Because of the frequency of spinal injuries, medical staff are always encouraged to support the head and neck (manual in line stabilization, MILS) before initiating the primary survey. The majority of athletes with isolated limb fractures and joint sprains will be found lying on the ground, alert, in pain, often holding or pointing to the injured part, thus indicating that the airway is patent (A), that there is adequate breathing (B), and that there is physiologically functioning circulation (C). The unconscious athlete will require special consideration, but in the obtunded or confused casualty, direct head injury or the cerebral effects of injury-associated hypotension and/or hypoxia should be considered.

Extremity injuries are associated with arterial damage and blood loss and thus form part of the circulation evaluation in the primary survey. These injuries include lacerations, penetrating wounds, crush injuries, and open or closed fractures. As part of the circulation (C) primary survey, external arterial bleeding must be stopped immediately by first applying direct digital pressure onto the bleeding site using a sterile dressing or packs and later bandages, followed by the safe elevation of the immobilized extremity (See Chapter 6).

Clinical Findings Limb Injury

Primary survey: The patient may be unconscious. However, if alert, may have great pain and may indicate the injury site. The patient may be pale, cyanotic with clammy, moist skin. If there is no injury other than the extremity fracture, the airway will probably be normal, breathing (B) will also probably be normal but there may be an elevated respiratory rate (due to the level of activity before the injury or the amount of pain) and pulse (C) for the same reasons. Pulse oximeter values should be normal.

Local inspection: Look for wounds, bleeding, swelling, bruising, and deformity. Look at the extremity distal to the fracture: is there distal pallor?

Palpation: Expose the injured limb. With both hands, gently palpate for bony deformity or fracture tenderness and decide if the injury is to a long bone or joint: this may be unnecessary with gross midshaft deformities. The skin temperature and tactile sensation above and below the fracture should be noted. Always palpate pulses distal to the fracture site and check the Capillary Refill Time (CRT) at the toes or fingers. Compare pulses in the contralateral extremity.

Note: Distal lower extremity pulses are not always easy to palpate and the foot may be adequately perfused despite the inability to find a pulse.

Palpation may reveal sensory neural injury, though athletes who are in great pain or distress may give an inaccurate response.

Movement: The athlete will usually avoid moving the fractured extremity, particularly the joint immediately distal to the fracture. A gross assessment of motor function can be made by asking the patient to move their fingers and toes. If active movements are very restricted, it may not be appropriate to proceed to passive movement testing as this may cause further soft tissue injury.

Onfield Management Limb Injury

The majority of limb injuries will not have long-term sequela. On occasions, injuries arise which require rapid recognition and emergency action on the FoP. These include gross fracture dislocations and joint dislocations, especially with loss of distal perfusion.

Fracture dislocations are not uncommon injuries in sport; however, long bone fractures of the humerus or femur are relatively rare. As mentioned earlier, bleeding from the bone or adjacent arteries and veins is a potentially serious complication. If the distal fragment is displaced at the time of injury, bone may cut into or compress arteries or veins. There are therefore two main major risks: systemic hypovolemia and distal tissue ischemia. Once the hypovolemia issue has been addressed (local compression of open hemorrhaging and initiating fluid replacement), the ED has two major decisions to make: should the fracture/dislocation be reduced and must this reduction take place on or off the FoP.

There is much discussion, both medical and medicolegal, around this topic. A more practical approach to this situation is to address the following issues:

1. *Is there a normal pulse distal to the fracture site?*
   If no, then an immediate onfield reduction or realignment must be considered. If there is a normal distal pulse, then consider the next problem.
2. *Is it possible to safely immobilize the patient without reducing the extremity fracture?*
   If the distal fragment of a fractured femur is externally rotated at a 45° angle it will be impossible to safely immobilize the extremity during FoP extrication without having reduced (or at least realigned) the fracture. A backboard or spinal board is often no more than 40 cm wide, so it would be impossible to adequately stabilize a grossly deformed fractured lower extremity and therefore not recommended. A vacuum mattress offers more width, usually around 80 cm, which may or may not be sufficient. An ambulance stretcher is usually only 60 cm wide as are most basket stretchers. The conclusion therefore is that a reduction should be considered if safe immobilization during extrication is not possible.
3. *Do you have the ability to give adequate analgesia on the FoP?*
   For the Emergency Doctor (ED), analgesia can be administered by two routes: inhaled or intravenous. Inhaled analgesia is easy to administer, but not readily accessible or approved for fracture reduction in all countries. As there is also a potential danger of hypovolemia with major fracture dislocations, an intravenous line should be established routinely, thereby providing a portal for intravenous medication.

Realignment of Fracture/Dislocations

Ensure that you have the appropriate splintage device available before commencing realignment. Some fractures will be required to be held firmly following realignment to prevent redisplacement.

Having administered adequate analgesia, hold the limb firmly above the fracture with one hand and place the other hand below the injury typically cupping the heel. Midshaft fractures are typically unstable and can often be realigned with minimum or moderate force. Apply traction by pulling the limb distally, while maintaining force to hold the proximal limb in position. Maintaining traction throughout, correct the deformity. In distal leg fracture/dislocations, this is usually achieved by traction, adduction and internal rotation of the cupped ankle and foot to the anatomically correct position.

Following any maneuver, the neurovascular state of the limb must be reassessed and compared with the original findings. If there is deterioration the limb should be repositioned until normal pulse and neurological activity is restored. The likeliest scenario is that perfusion will be restored to an ischemic limb, thus realignment is a potentially limb-saving maneuver.

As a general rule, extremity joint dislocations are not life-threatening conditions and thus form part of the secondary survey.

Transfer from the FoP

Swift, safe, and timely removal from the FoP is an essential part of patient care. Athletes with stable upper limb injuries may choose to walk from the FoP especially if they have a shoulder injury, which is often more painful when lying down. Athletes with unstable limb injuries may want to sit down and hold their limb to prevent further movement. Clearly they require further assessment, limb support, and splinting. Unstable lower extremity injuries should be splinted on the FoP.

Athletes may feel faint either due to pain, fear, or other emotion following injury particularly with the sight of blood. A vasovagal syncope can be avoided by encouraging players to lie down and/or be transferred from the FoP on a basket stretcher. Offer supplementary oxygen therapy but avoid oral fluids.

It is important to select the correct transfer equipment. The use of a spinal board where there is no spine injury is inappropriate and wheelchairs may not be the best choice in an outdoor sport arena. Many sports favor a basket stretcher or vacuum mattress using a split scoop stretcher for the initial lift transfer. The transfer wheelchair should be considered for sitting casualties if the surface is appropriate for their use.

Fieldside Management Limb Injury

Having performed the primary survey on the FoP, the ED performs a secondary assessment at the fieldside or in the athlete medical room (depending on the setting and the sport). Examination off the FoP allows the ED more time and privacy to perform a general physical and local examination of the injured extremity. Detailed joint examination should therefore be performed at the fieldside or in the athlete medical room.

Fieldside examination of an extremity injury during the secondary survey includes testing of active and passive movements, as well as ligamentous stability involving varus, valgus, and laxity testing for all involved joints. The validity of tests for each joint varies, but the decision to allow a return to play will in most cases be based on the player's subjective assessment of function following injury. In some sports, e.g., rugby, this secondary survey is often performed on the FoP during play.

Dislocated and Subluxated Joints

Traumatic dislocations of the hip can be easily misdiagnosed on the FoP and findings may represent pelvic or proximal femur fractures. Exercise extreme caution before reducing a hip or any other joint in the prehospital environment in the absence of radiological confirmation. Most doctors agree that dislocated shoulder, elbow, and ankle joint reductions should be performed after radiography to ensure correct diagnosis and address possible medicolegal issues. Control radiography after reduction is also advised. There are exceptions to this recommendation.

Joints such as the shoulder and hip are surrounded by large muscles, which make the identification of the full extent of the injury difficult. A considerable amount of traction may also be required to distract the joint adequately to allow correct reduction. These "ball and socket" joints have considerable stability in their dislocated position. The presence of an additional fracture, for example, Hill–Sachs lesion or greater tuberosity fracture will not be recognized without radiographs. Subsequent problems such as avascular necrosis may lead to undefendable allegations of iatrogenic injury at the time of initial management and accordingly prereduction radiographs are recommended. In addition, the direction of dislocation may not be apparent without imaging, and dislocations in different directions require different reduction techniques. Proper anesthesia/analgesia is important in order to achieve effective reduction and the ED needs to be experienced in safe reduction maneuvers. Postreduction radiographs should be taken.

Many joints may, however, be only subluxated and spontaneous relocation may occur during the process of gentle examination. Atraumatic techniques should always be used. Axillary nerve traction injury leading to altered function occurs in up to 8% of anterior shoulder dislocations.

Players are unlikely to be able to return to play and perform satisfactorily immediately after a successful major joint reduction and should be advised not to do so. Athletes may, however, return after having small nonweight bearing joints realigned, for example, proximal interphalangeal/distal interphalangeal (PIP/DIP) finger joints, if they have no bony tenderness. Verbal consent after informing the player of potential risks should be obtained. Written consent would be ideal but this may be impractical at the fieldside. The injured finger can be taped to the neighboring finger. A reexamination of the joint must be made after the event.

Splint Selection and Application (See Chapter 30)

The application of a splint has several benefits including the provision of analgesia and the protection of blood vessels and soft tissue by preventing unnecessary movement of the injured limb.

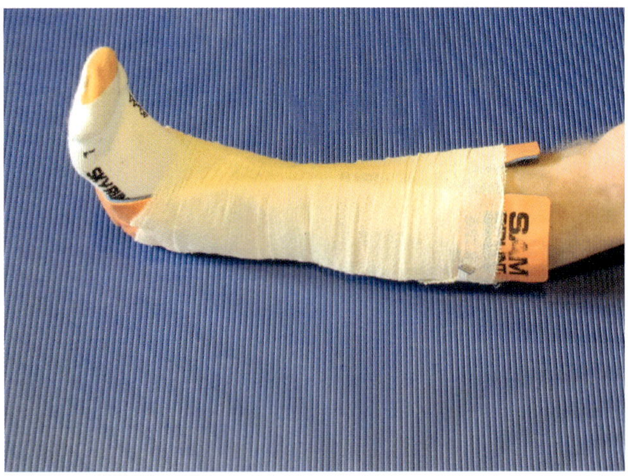

Figure 20.1 Malleable splint

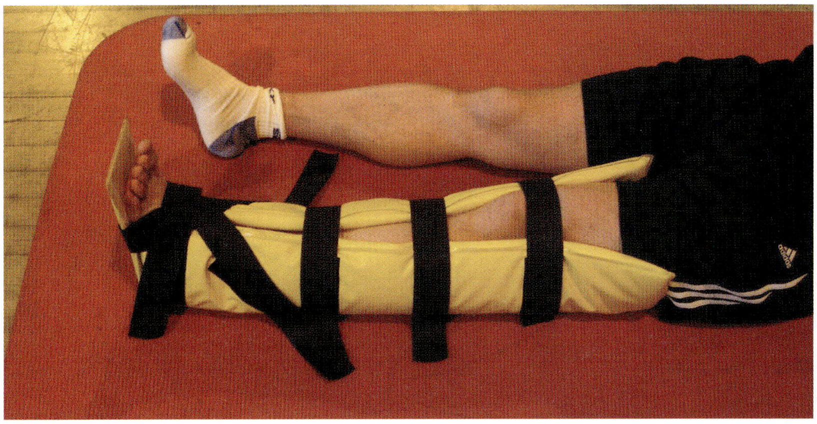

Figure 20.2 Box splint

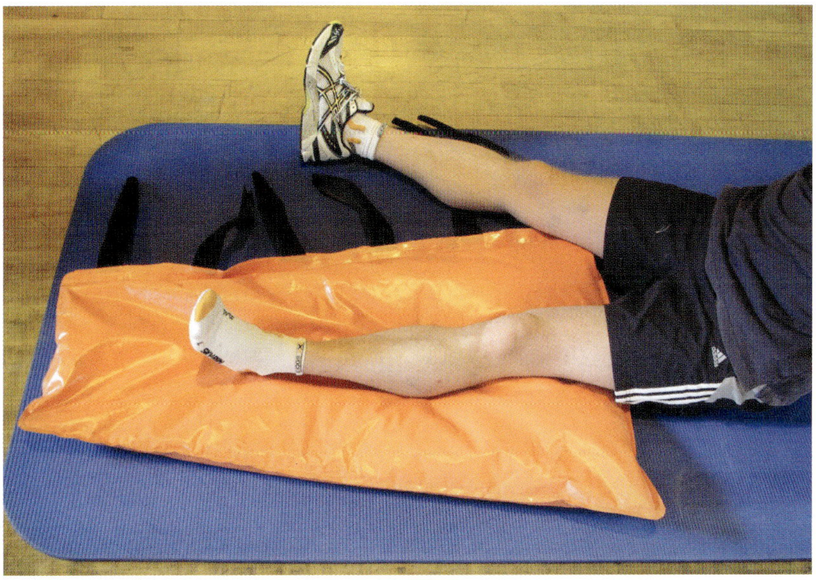

Figure 20.3 Vacuum splint before air extraction

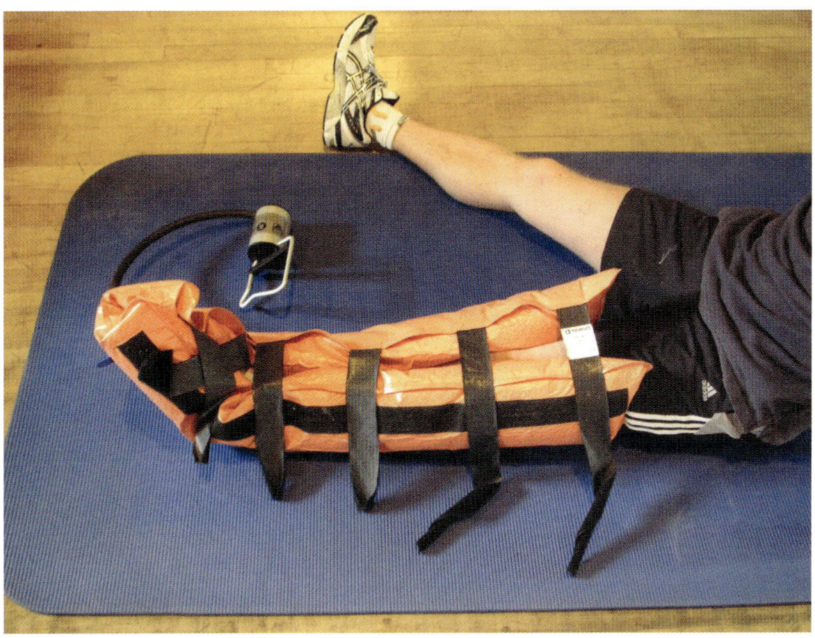

Figure 20.4 Vacuum splint after air extraction.

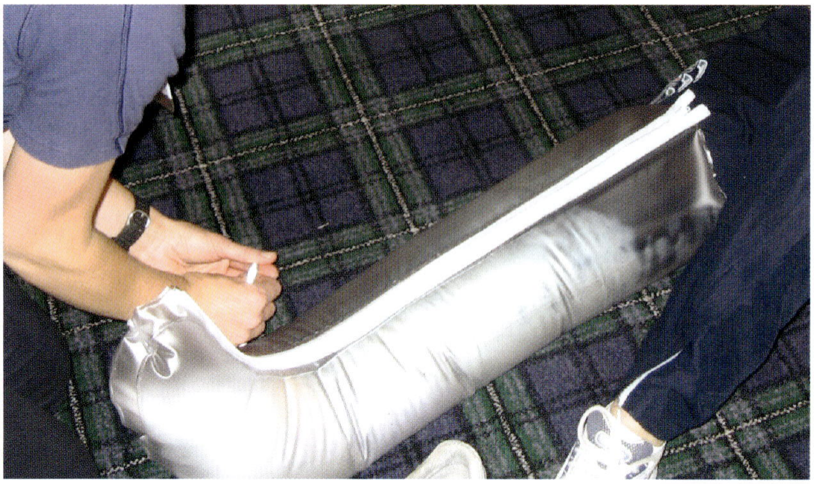

Figure 20.5 Inflatable splint.

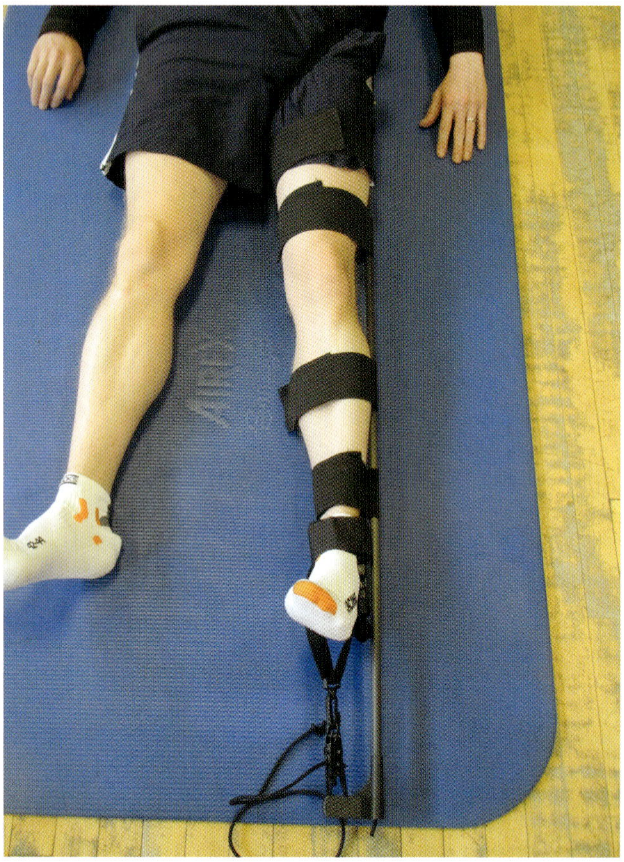

Figure 20.6 Traction splint

When choosing a splint, select one that is large enough to immobilize both the proximal and distal joints to the fractured bone. The splint should also be adjustable, nonconstrictive, well padded, and allow HCPs to make repeated neurovascular assessment of the injured extremity.

There are several different types of splints available and their characteristics are tabulated as follows:

Type	Description	Advantages	Disadvantages
Malleable (Figure 20.1)	Sheets of malleable aluminum covered by closed cell foam	Cheap, compact, and allows support for deformed limbs	Aluminum may become sharp with repeated flexing Difficult to immobilize whole lower limb
Box (Figure 20.2)	Open cell foam strips covered by tough plastic with nylon straps, allows the formation of a box	Long life time Cheap	Some models are bulky, do not allow support for limbs in a deformed position
Vacuum (Figures 20.3 and 20.4)	Tough plastic sealed section of plastic spheres, once air is removed it molds itself to the shape of the limb	Allows support for deformed limbs	Expensive, useless if punctured and without vacuum pump
Inflatable (Figure 20.5)	Plastic sealed unit, which when inflated adopts a preformed shape	Cheap, compact, and light	May not allow distal neurovascular assessment
Traction splints (Figure 20.6)	Have a pulley system to apply traction from a strap around the ankle against the ischial tuberosity, used for fractured femurs	Immobilizes all of the limb and provides good analgesia	These can be difficult to attach and must be placed correctly. Training is required

The above-mentioned splints are generally used for lower limb injuries. In the upper limb, the malleable splints are excellent for providing long bone splinting for humerus, radius, and ulna injuries. Further immobilization, support, and elevation may be provided by the use of a triangular sling.

As a general rule, shoulder injuries benefit from support beneath the elbow provided by a broad arm sling. Hand and wrist injuries require elevation offered by a high arm sling (elevation sling) to minimize swelling. Long bone injuries to the arm, forearm, and elbow typically require a combination of a splint supported by a crepe bandage and a broad arm sling.

As with all realignment maneuvers, neurovascular function must be reassessed following splint application.

Analgesia

Significant pain relief is often achieved after splint application. However, the procedure of realigning any limb is uncomfortable and can be excruciatingly painful. In some countries, inhaled analgesics, for example (nitrous oxide or methoxyflurane) are used to provide rapid onset analgesia during the reduction/realignment procedures, whereas in other countries intravenous analgesia is preferred. Low-dose intravenous ketamine (0.1 mg/kg) is a very effective and quick-acting analgesic. Morphine is the drug of choice in many countries due to the availability of naloxone, which can effectively reverse opiate-induced respiratory depression. Follow your local guidelines and practice when choosing prehospital analgesia. An experienced anesthesiologist may choose to perform a field block but be aware that such blocks may mask early compartment syndrome symptoms.

Local anesthesia is usually not recommended in the unsterile FoP environment due to the risk of infection.

Compartment Syndrome

Compartment syndrome is the increase in pressure within an osseofascial compartment so that the pressure occludes intracompartmental arterial flow, leading to increased muscular anaerobic metabolism. If unrecognized, this process may lead to muscular cell death and ultimately fibrotic contractures and limb dysfunction. The commonest cause of compartment syndrome is a hematoma formation within a compartment usually due to a nearby fracture or contusion. Other causes include crush injuries and burns, though these are unlikely to be seen in competing athletes. The syndrome is rarely so acute that it is seen at the fieldside or even in the athlete medical room but the clinical features of worsening pain following the injury despite oral analgesia, elevation, ice application, and compression should trigger immediate transfer to an emergency department for ongoing care and intracompartmental pressure measurement.

Amputation Injuries

These injuries are extremely rare in sport. There have been incidences in luge where fingers have been amputated by sleds. In the unlikely event of a finger amputation, the amputated part should be retained and placed in a saltwater container in case reimplantation is possible. The distal end of the stump may bleed profusely, so manual compression may be needed for several minutes before hemostatic bandages can be applied. Occasionally, a hemostatic ligature may need to be used to stop bleeding. The patient should be referred to hospital for further care. Avoid using loose noncompressing bandages as many finger amputations bleed for several hours.

For larger total or partial amputations, the main danger is that of extensive bleeding. In the military environment, tourniquets are used. There is an ongoing debate about the use of tourniquets in the civilian environment where rapid sophisticated care is usually more accessible. Tourniquets may be indicated where manual compression fails to stop life-threatening limb hemorrhage. The risks of causing distal limb ischemia are outweighed by the imminent risk of death due to hypovolemic shock. The CAT tourniquet is a simple device that can be quickly applied to the amputated stump. Compression must be applied until bleeding stops and not released until full surgical hemostasis is available (See Chapter 6).

Immediate emergency referral to hospital is required and the amputated extremity should accompany the casualty. Amputations may be extremely painful and the use of a tourniquet will exacerbate this. Adequate analgesia is necessary.

Ski Boot Removal

Another topic that is somewhat controversial relates to whether or not one should remove an alpine ski boot if there is a suspected leg fracture. The argument for removing the ski boot is that after removing it, the healthcare professional will expose the injury, which is a part of the (obligatory) FoP primary survey examination (E). This will allow for assessment of bleeding (C), the presence or absence of a distal pulse (C), and to inspect for an open fracture. The unbooted extremity is easier to immobilize than a booted extremity.

Many experts do not remove the boot in situ as the boot removal technique is usually extremely painful and may worsen any fracture dislocation and worsen circulatory problems. It may be better to postpone removal until full analgesia can be provided. As the ski boot is relatively tight, space in the boot is limited so it is likely that significant hemorrhage will cause blood to seep over the top of the boot and thus be visible. The healthcare professional will then have to make a specific decision regarding the need to remove the boot.

The best advice here is to be aware of and follow local guidelines.

Paralympic Sport

Paralympic athletes may have severe extremity injuries and not be aware of the extent of the physical damage. These athletes need careful and constant observation on the FoP so that any extremity injuries can be diagnosed and treated rapidly and effectively.

Documentation

Despite there seeming to be little time to complete notes for the acutely injured athlete on the FoP or fieldside, an accurate record of the mechanism of injury and the treatment provided including the neurovascular state of the limb before and after realignment maneuvers and splint application is mandatory. It provides a baseline for continuing assessment and further treatment.

Bibliography

American College of Surgeons (2008) *Advanced Trauma Life Support Manual*, 8th edn. American College of Surgeons, Chicago.

Junge, A., Engebretsen, L., Mountjoy, M.L. *et al.* (2009) Sports injuries during the summer Olympic Games 2008. *American Journal of Sports Medicine*, **37** (**11**), 2165–2172.

McDonagh, D.O. (2012) *FIMS Sports Medicine Manual: Event Planning and Emergency Care.* Wolters Kluwer Lippincott Williams & Wilkins, Philadelphia.

O'Brien, M.D. (2000) *Aids to the Examination of the Peripheral Nervous system*, 4th edn. Medical Research Council, London.

xxxx (2009) *Resuscitation and Emergency Management On-Field Manual.* REMO, Stoke.

21 Aquatic Athlete Injuries and Emergencies

Margo Mountjoy[1] and Saul Marks[2]

[1]M.G. DeGroote School of Medicine, McMaster University, Kitchener, ON, Canada
[2]Department of Psychiatry, University of Toronto, Toronto, ON, Canada

Introduction

Swimming is a sport which is enjoyed by many at a recreational level. At the elite level, the disciplines of swimming, diving, water polo, synchronized swimming, open water swimming, and the newest event of high diving, are part of the FINA competition schedule. At the London Olympic Games, approximately 631 athletes from 166 member federation countries competed for medals in their respective discipline. The Paralympics had 600 athletes from 66 nations.

This chapter focuses on the practical aspects of the tasks of the aquatic team doctor. The safety preparation as well as the poolside/beachside approach, Field of Play (FoP) management, and extraction for the athlete in trouble, will be reviewed along with the common illness and injury presentations in the respective aquatic disciplines. Guidelines for treatment are included in addition to advice for prevention.

Swimming

Preparation and Safety

Adequate preparation of the team doctor for a swimming event requires the doctor to be cognizant of the common presentations of injuries and illnesses. Injury and illness surveillance research from the FINA World Championships in 2009 and 2013 and the Olympic Games in 2008 and 2012 reveals that swimming has a very low incidence of acute new onset injuries and illnesses. As such, it is unlikely that the team doctor at a swimming event will have to manage traumatic injuries. It is imperative, however, that the team doctor ensures that the swimming event is appropriately supervised with lifeguards who are trained in removal of the submerged athlete, together with a fully functional, trained medical FoP team to manage the medical care on land.

Fieldside Observation

Observe the swimmers from the FoP sidelines for any change in expected performance behavior. A significant and unexpected change in performance could be a sign of the athlete in difficulty. Drowning is often silent and without warning. Constant vigilance

The IOC Manual of Emergency Sports Medicine, First Edition. Edited by David McDonagh and David Zideman.

to notice an athlete who is sinking is imperative. Observation of the FoP for environmental risks is another role of the team doctor.

In the Olympic and Paralympic Games the team doctor may not have direct access to the FoP or Poolside. The rescue and immediate treatment of a sick or injured athlete is then in the hands of the OCOG Life guards and the Medical FoP Team.

Approach to the Swimmer in Difficulty

In full competition (both competition and practice venues), there should be fully trained and practiced lifeguards in place who can effectively and efficiently remove a casualty from the water.

FoP Management

Team doctors should also be familiar with extraction techniques of the submerged athlete by the venue lifeguard team and FoP medical team. They should also be aware of acceptable methods of removal from the water in case of inadequate lifeguard supervision or skill.

If the athlete is conscious, he/she can hold onto a flotation device and be towed to the side. Should he/she be unconscious, the athlete can be stabilized on a flotation device with one arm and carried to the pool side using the other arm and legs for swimming. Should artificial respiration be required, it can be performed in the water by supporting the athlete on the flotation device. Removal of the unconscious or injured athlete from the water is best completed as a team with at least three individuals, either by raising the athlete horizontally on a spinal board, or by lifting the athlete out of the water by his/her arms while protecting the head. Full cardiopulmonary resuscitation can occur at the poolside. In order to ensure an efficient and safe response, lifeguards and the FoP medical team must practice these methods daily.

For the swimmer who has hit his/her head on the bottom of the pool when diving in, a cervical spine stabilization removal should occur to protect the spinal cord. Details of this technique can be found in the Diving Section of this chapter.

Common Injuries and Illnesses in Swimming

The team doctor will most often be called upon to treat chronic overuse injuries of the shoulder, lumbar spine, and the knee. Tendonosis of the rotator cuff is the most common shoulder injury seen in swimming. Lumbar spine pathologies, including spondylolysis, facet inflammation, and acute disc protrusions, are most often seen in swimmers who specialize in backstroke and butterfly. Breast strokers are particularly prone to knee pathologies including patellar femoral syndrome, medial collateral ligament strains, and meniscal degeneration. Treatment of these overuse injuries requires the involvement of a physiotherapist and stroke analysis to correct abnormal stroke biomechanics.

Unpublished Therapeutic Use Exemption data from the 2008 Olympic Games reveals that swimming had the third highest incidence of asthma of all summer Olympic sports with an incidence of 19.2%. Asthma is common in swimmers and is thought to be due to the inhalation of chloramines in the pool environment coupled with the effects of increased prolonged aerobic training. Nonasthmatic athletes may develop asthma as they increase their training volumes at the elite level. Symptoms include cough, dyspnea, decreased performance, and occasionally wheezing. Treatment includes the use of long-acting and/or short-acting beta-2 agonists coupled with maintenance inhaled glucocorticosteroids. Exercise-induced asthma is treated with inhaled beta 2 agonists taken 10–15 min prior to exercise. The diagnosis of asthma in the swimmer is made by clinical history and examination, spirometry, and/or broncho-provocation testing (see Chapter 8). The team doctor should be aware of the current recommendations on the World Anti-Doping Association's Prohibited List with respect to asthma medications to ensure that appropriate permission or Therapeutic Use Exemption rules are followed to prevent the triggering of an adverse analytical finding during doping control in the asthmatic swimmer (See Chapter 31).

Synchronized Swimming

Research from FINA World Championships and Olympic Games shows that synchronized swimming also has a relatively low rate of acute new onset injuries during competition. The majority of the injuries are from overuse with minimal time loss from training and competition expected.

Preparation and Safety, Fieldside Observation, Approach, FoP Management

A similar protocol can be taken in the management of the synchronized swimmer in acute distress as for the swimmer.

Common Injuries and Illnesses in Synchronized Swimming

Despite the relatively low rate of acute injuries during competition, traumatic injuries from high-risk acrobatic moves may occur during training. Prevention strategies including adequate supervision and graduated skill development will reduce this incidence. Conversely, synchronized swimming had one of the highest rates of illness at the London Olympic Games relative to all other sports at 12.5%. The majority of these illnesses were infectious in nature affecting the respiratory and gastrointestinal systems. As such, the team doctor should be prepared to educate illness prevention strategies in synchronized swimming including frequent and appropriate hand washing technique. They should also be prepared to treat viral and bacterial infectious diseases during competition events.

While unlikely to be an issue during competition at poolside, one of the major issues facing the synchronized swimming team doctor relates to body image issues. Being an aesthetic judged sport, synchronized swimmers like divers are prone to the development of the female athlete triad and/or eating disorders. Careful and sensitive monitoring of weight and body composition will assist the team doctor in the early diagnosis of these disorders. Implementation of prevention strategies has been shown to help minimize the prevalence of eating disorders in sport. Prevention videos raising awareness of the subject can be found at www.olympic.org/hbi. Early intervention with a multidisciplinary team including a psychiatrist, nutritionist, psychologist, sports doctor, and a physiologist as a means of secondary prevention has been proven helpful in decreasing the physical and psychological consequences of these disorders. Return to play guidelines for the athlete with an eating disorder should include close supervision and contractual goal setting.

Synchronized swimming, similar to swimming, has a high incidence of asthma – as high as 21.2% was recorded at the 2008 Olympic Games. The management of asthma in the synchronized swimmer is the same as that of the swimmer.

Diving and High Diving

Preparation and Safety

Preparation for a diving event varies from the swimming and synchro events. As there are significant heights (3 and 10 m in diving and up to 27 m in high diving) and fixed hard obstacles such as diving boards involved, an environmental survey and risk analysis of the facilities is essential. Attention to the structure and stair access of the diving boards and platform is essential to prevent falls from unsafe equipment. Assurance of adequate water depth for the particular height of diving platform is recommended. Prior to any diving event, the team doctor should ensure that an extrication device is readily available, as well as a team of lifeguards or other medical FoP medical personnel who are knowledgeable and skilled in the removal of an athlete with a suspected cervical spine fracture from deep water. There should also be a dedicated ambulance available during all diving events.

Fieldside Observation

The doctor should observe all diving events from the side of the pool, which provides the best opportunity to assess the risk of hitting the diving boards. Occasionally, divers may land horizontally "flat" on the water or hit their upper, lower, extremities or head on the board.

Approach and FoP Management

A team of at least three experienced and properly trained lifeguards plus the medical FoP Team is needed to manage the diver with a suspected cervical spine injury from deep water safely. Primary emergency care in diving follows the same principles of traumatic care for all victims including the primary and secondary surveys (see Chapter 3). Maintenance of the airway while in the water requires specific skill and practice. If the diver is unconscious and not breathing, then basic life support optimally should begin while the athlete is still in the water. Should the diver with a suspected cervical spine fracture be found face down, the athlete should be log rolled using a technique which stabilizes the head while rolling the athlete to the face up position. A second rescuer can then raise the legs slowly to the horizontal position maintaining the immobility of the spine while the third rescuer places the water rescue board under the athlete and secures the neck brace. Protection of the spinal cord through immobilization of the cervical spine during the FoP management and extraction is imperative.

The athlete is removed from the water by raising the athlete horizontally on a water rescue board, or alternatively by lifting the athlete out of the water by his/her arms while protecting the head. During removal from the water, the cervical spine and head can be protected by one of three techniques: the vice grip, body hug, or the extended arm grip.

Cervical spine immobilization must be maintained throughout transportation, first to the emergency vehicle an ambulance, then to the hospital, and throughout the assessment in hospital until the spine has been cleared.

All deep water removals must be practiced regularly by the water removal team (lifeguards) and coordinated by the poolside (land) FoP medical team. It should be remembered that the team doctor may not have immediate access to the FoP and will therefore rely on the FoP medical team to undertake the safe extrication and initial treatment of an injured athlete.

Common Injuries and Illnesses in Diving

Although very few catastrophic accidents occur in elite competitive diving, the trauma from hitting the diving board, or landing flat on the water can cause a myriad of injuries including orthopedic and nonorthopedic injuries as outlined in Table 21.1. Concussions, lacerations, loss of consciousness, cervical spine trauma, and/or transient dyspnea of the diver necessitate the extraction of the diver from the water with a special technique to protect the cervical spine.

Anatomical locations of orthopedic injuries	Nonorthopedic injuries
Shoulder Rotator cuff tendonosis Dislocation/subluxation Acromial-clavicular sprain	Perforation of tympanic membrane
Lumbar spine Spondylosis/spondylolisthesis Disc protrusion Facet inflammation	Retinal detachment
Wrist and hand Fracture Tendon rupture Sprain, contusion	Concussion
Ankle/foot Fracture Sprain (ankle) Sprain/strains (foot) Contusion	Lung perforation (pneumothorax)
Knee/thigh Subluxation Sprain Contusion Tendonosis	Brain or spinal cord injury
Elbow Sprain Strain Tendonosis	Lacerations

Table 21.1 Injuries sustained in the sport of diving

Research from the FINA World Aquatic Championships shows that diving has a high incidence of acute injuries relative to swimming and synchronized swimming and data from the London 2012 Olympic Games shows that diving has a high incidence of injury caused by overuse. Most injuries in the sport of competitive diving take place during the entry to the water and occur more commonly in the older elite, experienced divers performing difficult dives. Several potential areas for injury exist as the diver enters the water. As with all aquatic sports, the shoulder injury is the most common injury. Injuries to the lumbar spine, wrist, and neck are also common.

Shoulder injuries have increased in incidence over the past 30 years. Since the early 1980s, after the flight phase, the diver "lines up" prior to entering the water, in an attempt to complete the dive with the least amount of splash, known as a "rip" entry. This action involves bringing the hands together overhead and grasping one hand over the other, with the palms braced outward to take the impact. The hips extend so that the body is straight and the head is lined up between the shoulders, which are pressed tightly into the ears, in elevation and internal rotation. Limited shoulder flexibility could cause lumbar hyperextension when adjusting for the angle of water entry. As the diver can be traveling at over 64 km/h as they enter the water, the impact on the wrists and neck makes them susceptible to injury as well. Because of the force of impact, chronic overuse injuries can often become acute with one dive.

Water Polo

Water polo is a fast paced contact game with significant potential for traumatic injury. In addition to the contact, the emotions of the players as the game becomes closer in score, also factors into the injury risk. The team doctor should be aware of this added injury risk. In this sport the Team Doctor is usually on the FoP on the team bench. It is essential that the Team Doctor coordinates his actions with the Life guards and FoP medical team for effective an efficient FoP rescue and care.

Preparation

Given the high incidence of contact traumatic injuries in water polo, the team doctor should have access to a well-equipped poolside medical kit to manage traumatic injuries, which should include suture material and/or skin glue, as a bleeding athlete will not be allowed back in the water (see Chapter 27). Ready-access to ice packs during matches is highly recommended. At water polo tournaments, there should be an easily accessible athlete medical treatment room that is staffed with a trained FoP team including a trauma doctor with appropriate trauma equipment. A dental surgeon should be part of the FoP team at large water polo events. An efficient evacuation route to a local athlete medical room should be established and operational during all water polo events. Lifeguards and a FoP medical team trained in trauma recognition and deep water extractions are mandatory at all water polo tournaments for competition, warmup, and practice venues and should be practiced in water extrication procedures on a daily basis.

Fieldside Observation, Approach, FoP Management

Given the action and speed of play, it is essential that the team doctor observe the game closely from the team bench beside the FoP. Water polo is one of the few sports where the team doctor is present on the FoP. A fully equipped medisac and ice supply should be readily accessible. The FoP approach, treatment, and extraction is the same as for swimming described earlier and an satisfactory approach as to how the athlete will be removed from the water and FoP should be agreed between the team doctor and the FoP medical team. Special attention in water polo must be given during the primary and secondary surveys to the potential for blunt trauma to the chest, abdomen, and head.

Common Injuries and Illnesses in Water Polo

Research from Olympic Games and World Championships shows that the main cause of injuries in water polo is from trauma during competition. Of all the aquatic disciplines, water polo has the highest injury rate at 56% and the highest rate for time lost from sport. Women's water polo injuries in particular are increasing over time. In comparison with all team sports at the Olympic Games, water polo had the highest incidence of head injuries. As such, the team doctor should be trained to manage concussion and other traumatic injuries including lacerations, hematomas, contusions, fractures, tympanic membrane ruptures, and dislocations. Other injuries common in water polo include overuse shoulder tendonosis and a variety of overuse knee pathologies from egg beater kick including meniscal tears, medial collateral ligament injury, and patellar femoral syndrome.

As per the Zurich 2012 Guidelines for Concussion in sport, no athlete with a head injury should return to play on the same day as the head injury. A detailed concussion assessment of the athlete and close observation should occur to rule out more serious head injuries. The cornerstone of concussion management is rest from all physical and cognitive activities. Once symptom free, the athlete should return to play following a graduated water-polo-specific return to play protocol. Pressure to return an athlete to play prior to full recovery should be avoided as early return to play may result in a second impact to the head which compounds the seriousness of the concussion and significantly increases complications and recovery time (see Chapter 11).

Open Water Swimming

While swimming in open water has been practiced for centuries, open water swimming as a sport, is a relatively new competitive discipline coming under the umbrella of FINA in 1992 and becoming an Olympic event (10k marathon) in 2008. The swimming distances for FINA events typically are 5, 10, and 25 km; however, the FINA Grand prix circuit ranges from 15 to 88 km. Open water swimming attracts not only elite swimmers but also a unique athlete who enjoys the challenges of the unpredictable environment of the open water that are not found in the controlled environment of the swimming pool.

Preparation and Safety

For the team doctor, there are many factors that should be evaluated prior to a competitive open water swimming event. Environmental factors that team doctors must take into account when performing a safety screen of the FoP are described in Table 21.2. Other safety factors include athlete crowding which can lead to traumatic injury and/or athlete panic.

Water temperature
Cold water (=/>16 °C – lower safety limit)
Warm water (=/<31 °C – upper safety limit)
Currents
Tides
Weather
Flora + fauna
Water pollution
Algae
Air pollution

Table 21.2 Environmental factors in open water swimming

First aid equipment, blankets, water and automated external defibrillators (AEDs) should be available on the rescue craft if possible, or quickly accessible. The FoP medical team should have an agreed plan for the landing of sick or injured athletes from the rescue craft and this should be practiced on a daily basis.

The team doctor can prepare an athlete for the open water environment by ensuring that the athlete has undergone a periodic health examination and has had adequate training and preparation for the particular event and appropriate environmental acclimatization. Race day nutrition and hydration plans should be developed and rehearsed.

Prior to the event, in addition to ensuring adequate knowledge of the environmental factors of the FoP, the team doctor should familiarize himself/herself with the Safety Action Plan for the event including the numbers and location of the safety crafts, the qualifications of the safety personnel, the location and provision of the FoP medical teams and their equipment, the onsite athlete medical facility, and the evacuation plans to the local hospital. The team doctor should also review the water purity certificate provided by the event organizers to ensure that water safety standards are met for the FoP. Athletes should be carefully numbered prior to the race and wear electronic tracking safety devices. Rescue landing points for safety craft should be identified. Finally, the team doctor should familiarize himself/herself with the course evacuation plan and be satisfied that it has been successfully practiced by the local safety personnel.

Fieldside Observation

Adequate visual supervision in open water swimming can be challenging given the environmental obstacles that exist. Direct observation of the swimmers must be maintained at all times either from a watercraft or from the shore depending on the design of the race course. The athletes should be observed for an unexpected or erratic change in athletic performance, as this could be an indicator of the athlete in distress.

Approach and FoP Management

The open water swimmer should be approached via water craft (surfboard, dinghy, small boat, and kayak). An evaluation of the environmental risks is required to ensure safety of the athlete and the rescuers. This includes evaluation of the weather in addition to any risks posed by the flora, fauna, or water temperature. The primary and secondary surveys of the open water swimmer are the same as for the swimmer already described.

A speedy extraction from the FoP is recommended, especially if extremes in water temperature are suspected factors. Extraction of the athlete from the open water can be challenging depending on the environmental conditions on the FoP. Evacuation of the athlete from the water should be done by personnel trained in extrication from the water environment. Care must be taken to ensure that the watercraft does not capsize as the athlete is brought on board. It is advisable to have a suitably trained doctor on the rescue launch who can perform a primary survey and initiate life-saving treatment as soon as rescue has been completed and while the athlete is being transported to the landing point.

Common Injuries and Illnesses in Open Water Swimming

Heat-related illness is a serious medical concern in open water swimming. It is important that the team doctor and FoP medical team are able to recognize and manage the signs of the athlete in heat distress. In the hot environment, the warmup should be limited in intensity and duration and adequate recovery time be provided before the start of competition to rehydrate and restore the body's core temperature. Precooling with ice vests or cold water immersion may be beneficial. Other strategies to prevent heath-related illness in open water swimming include the provision for adequate acclimatization, the use of cooling facilities, modification of event scheduling to avoid peak hours of heat, and ongoing monitoring of the environmental temperature. The team doctor should have a predetermined medical action plan in coordination with the local organizing medical staff to manage hyperthermia.

Hypothermia in the open water environment can be caused by cool ambient temperatures, wind, currents, and cold water temperature. Exercise-induced asthma (EIA) can be exacerbated by cold temperatures. While on the FoP, the FoP team and the team doctor should have inhaled beta 2 agonist rescue medication available in case of the need for emergency treatment. The combination of cold water exposure, voluntary apnea, and face immersion (diving bradycardia) may result in increased sympathetic and parasympathetic activities, possibly causing ventricular premature beats. Cold water itself could be a contributing factor to fatal events in open water swimming. The FoP team should be prepared for this eventuality and ensure that all training and competitive environments are equipped with AEDs and have Advanced Life Support skills.

Swimming-induced pulmonary edema (SIPE) can be seen in endurance open water swimming. The athlete will present with severe dyspnea, cough, and sputum production. Hemoptysis occurs in 50% of the cases. There is usually no associated chest pain. The pathophysiology is thought to be overperfusion caused by the increase in ambient pressure, peripheral vasoconstriction from ambient cold, and increased pulmonary blood flow resulting from exercise. High pulmonary capillary pressures lead to extravasation of fluid into the interstitium resulting in hypoxemia and secondary pulmonary edema. Risk factors for SIPE are unclear; however, older individuals may be at higher risk. There is a 29% recurrence rate. Presentation of these symptoms requires FoP monitoring and oxygen administration with immediate evacuation to hospital for advanced treatment. Most cases of SIPE usually resolve within 24 h.

Conclusion

Being poolside or on the beach at an aquatic event is a pleasant working venue for any doctor. Working with the aquatic athlete provides an opportunity for the team doctor to develop a well-rounded skill set with experience in the management of acute trauma, artistic body image issues, overuse injuries, environmental medicine, and medical issues such as asthma. Being proactive in the implementation of preventive programs is equally important for the aquatic team doctor, as is having the breadth of skills to effectively manage aquatic health issues as they occur. Although the health risks to the aquatic athlete are lower than in many other sports, the team doctor should be aware of and be prepared for the physical and psychological health issues that are commonly seen in the aquatic disciplines. In all aquatic sports, it is essential that the team doctor develop a close understanding of the water rescue facilities and FoP medical treatment provided by the competition venue.

Bibliography

Bergeron, M.F., Bahr, R., Bartsch, P. *et al.* (2012) International Olympic Committee Consensus Statement on thermoregulatory and altitude challenges for the high-level athlete. *British Journal of Sports Medicine*, **46**, 770–779.

Stager, J. & Tanner, D. (2005) *Handbooks of Sports Medicine and Science: Swimming*, 2nd edn. Blackwell Science Ltd. ISBN:0-632-05914-1.

McDonagh, D. (2011) *FIMS Sports Medicine Manual, Event Planning and Emergency Care.* LWW; ISBN-10: 1582558736, ISBN-13: 978-1582558738.

Mountjoy, M., Junge, A., Alonso, J.M. *et al.* (2010) Sports injuries & illnesses in the 2009 FINA World Aquatic Championships. *British Journal of Sports Medicine*, **44**, 522–557.

Mountjoy, M. (2008) Injury & illness in synchronized swimming. Sixteenth FINA World Sports Medicine Congress. *Journal of Sport Science*, **26**, 1–3.

Mountjoy M. (2012) Sports medicine: illness and general health. In: S. Riewald, S. Rodeo (eds.) *The Science of Swimming Faster. Human Kinetics, Champaign*, McGraw-Hill, ISBN 9781559340366. [in publication].

Mountjoy, M. & Gerrard, D. (2011) Preserving and promoting health in the aquatic athlete. In: Seifert, L., Chollet, D. & Mujika, I. (eds), *The World Book of Swimming: from Science to Performance*. Nova Science Publishers, Hauppauge, New York. ISBN:978-1-61668-202-6.

Mountjoy, M. (2009) Injuries and medical issues in the synchronized Olympic sports. *Current Sports Medicine Reports*, **8**, 255–261.

Mountjoy, M., Alonso, J.M., Bergeron, M.F. *et al.* (2012) Hyperthermic-related challenges in aquatics, athletics, football, tennis and triathlon. *British Journal of Sports Medicine*, **46**, 800–804.

22 Emergency Care of the Adolescent Athlete

Lisa M. Vopat[1] *and Lyle J. Micheli*[2,3]

[1]*Children's Hospital, Harvard University, Boston, MA, USA*
[2]*Division of Sports Medicine, Boston Children's Hospital, Boston, MA, USA*
[3]*Orthopaedic Surgery, Harvard Medical School, Boston, MA, USA*

Article 42 of the Olympic Charter states:

> *There may be no age limit for competitors in the Olympic Games, other than as prescribed in the competition rules of an IF, as approved by the IOC Executive Board*

Most International Federations require competitors to be 18 years of age but some, notably gymnastics, have an age limit of 16 (or turning 16 within the calendar year of competition). This chapter deals with the pediatric and adolescent athlete aged 12 years and older.

Introduction

More than 38 million children and adolescents participate in sports each year in the United States alone. Over two and a half million children aged 19 and under were seen in emergency departments for injuries related to sports and recreation. Sports injuries account for 8% of all emergency department visits by pediatric patients. While most pediatric sport-related injuries are considered minor, life-threatening illness and injury do occur. Forty percent of life-threatening injuries for children aged 6–18 years were sport related. Life-threatening sports injury can include skull fracture, cervical spine fracture, intracranial hemorrhage, traumatic pneumothorax, liver and splenic laceration, and commotio cordis among others. Nearly a quarter of cervical spine fractures in children occurred during athletics (7% in adults). One hundred and ninety nine sports-related deaths of young athletes occurred in the 4-year period from 2008 to 2011. Traumatic brain injuries and sudden cardiac arrest are believed to be the leading cause of death in young athletes.

The IOC Manual of Emergency Sports Medicine, First Edition. Edited by David McDonagh and David Zideman.
2015 International Olympic Committee. Published 2015 by John Wiley & Sons, Ltd.

Knowledge of the anatomic and physiologic differences in the assessment and management of the pediatric athlete is critical. Smaller body mass, proportionally larger head size, higher ratio of body surface area, and a more pliable skeleton are a few of these unique characteristics. These age-related differences produce different patterns of injury and do not allow extrapolation of some adult skills and algorithms to the pediatric patient. The pediatric athlete requires an altered approach for effective evaluation and treatment.

Primary Survey and Stabilization (See Chapter 3)

The primary survey is a quick initial assessment to identify any acute and immediate medical threat. A quick and accurate baseline assessment of the child's physiologic status will determine the need for immediate life-sustaining therapies such as airway protection, cervical spine immobilization, oxygenation, ventilation, and cardiovascular support. This process can take as little as 10 s by adhering to the following ABCDE sequence of assessment:

A: Airway with cervical spine protection
B: Breathing
C: Circulation
D: Disability and neurologic status
E: Environmental control and exposure

Asking the athlete his/her name and to describe what happened is the quickest way to initiate this assessment. An appropriate response demonstrates that he/she can speak clearly (no airway compromise or breathing difficulty) and he/she is alert enough to describe the event (no significant decrease in level of consciousness).

Airway Maintenance with Cervical Spine Protection

In pediatric medical and traumatic emergencies, maintaining the airway is the highest priority. These patients are far more likely to suffer problems in sustaining a patent airway, thereby compromising ventilation and oxygenation. Maintaining cervical spine inline immobilization is of upmost importance throughout all airway manipulations.

Airway occlusion can also occur due to the relatively large soft tissues of the oropharynx (tongue and tonsils) falling posteriorly to obstruct the more anterior pediatric larynx and vocal cords. A jaw thrust maneuver combined with bimanual inline cervical spine immobilization will pull these tissues forward to open the airway.

For athletes without protective equipment, inline cervical spine stabilization should be secured with a rigid pediatric cervical collar. Attention to sizing is key as an ill-fitting collar can cause excessive distraction, hyperextension, or flexion of the neck, resulting in a rise in intracranial pressure.

Breathing

Hypoxia is the most common cause of cardiac arrest in a child and is of significant concern especially in a head-injured athlete. If breathing is inadequate and equipment is available, bag-valve-mask ventilation should be initiated. Care should be taken to avoid overventilation. Excessive tidal volumes can lead to barotrauma, and hyperventilation can worsen ischemia and outcomes, especially in cases of traumatic brain injury.

Circulation

Evaluation of circulation includes assessment of pulse and perfusion while controlling any sign of hemorrhage. Low blood pressure is less useful for the identification of shock than in adults as young athletes have increased physiologic reserve, which allows for the maintenance of normal blood pressure even in the presence of shock. Ambient temperature can affect evaluation of perfusion by capillary refill as well as color and temperature of the skin, making these parameters unreliable in certain situations. Level of consciousness is an effective estimation of central perfusion except in cases of traumatic brain injury.

Disability and Neurologic Status

The pediatric brain is particularly susceptible to injury. During the primary survey, the goal is to assess the *general* level of injury until there is more time for an indepth evaluation. This is best accomplished by evaluating the level of consciousness using the AVPU mnemonic. Those athletes who are not fully alert and only respond to voice, pain stimuli, or not at all should be defined as being unresponsive – which in competing athletes is most likely to be due to trauma but may have other sinister causes (subarachnoid hemorrhage, cardiac dysrhythmias, hypoglycemia, etc.). This should be followed by the evaluation of pupil size and reactivity and gross assessment for movement and sensation in each extremity to identify a possible spinal cord injury. In cases of head injury, optimization of the "ABCs" is critical as hypoxia and hypercarbia are associated with a worse outcome.

The Glasgow Coma Scale (GCS) is a quick, objective, and reproducible method of defining a child's level of consciousness and neurologic status. A GCS score of 13–15 may indicate mild brain injury while scores lower than 12 may be due to serious brain injury and are predictive of worse outcome (See Chapter 3).

Exposure and Environmental Control

The final component of the primary survey includes undressing the patient to ensure a thorough assessment. The patient should then be covered with warm blankets to maintain a normal body temperature after the assessment. The increased metabolic rate, thin skin, and lack of subcutaneous tissue in the pediatric patient may contribute to heat loss. Blankets, heaters, and warm fluids may be necessary to preserve body heat. Privacy and confidentiality must be maintained during exposure, especially in the adolescent athlete.

Sudden Cardiac Arrest (See Chapter 4)

If a player collapses to the ground especially without contact, immediate recognition and treatment is critical to survival. Any athlete who collapses without contact and is found to be unresponsive should be assumed to have a potentially serious cardiac or cardiovascular condition and if not breathing, in cardiac arrest.

If unresponsive and breathing abnormally, cardiopulmonary resuscitation (CPR) must be initiated immediately while the automated external defibrillator (AED) is being acquired. Commence 30 chest compressions at the rate of 100 compressions per minute followed by two ventilations and repeat in 2-min cycles. Hands-only CPR is an acceptable alternative for the lay responder without ventilation training. Once an AED is available, the pads should be placed on the chest. The AED prompts should be followed and CPR continued. Rapid extrication from the Field of Play (FoP), not waiting for a return of spontaneous circulation, and direct transfer to hospital is essential.

Differences in Injury Pattern

Head Trauma

The pediatric brain is particularly susceptible to injury. Anatomic and physiologic differences are thought to contribute to this vulnerability, although the extent to which each difference contributes is not entirely clear. The larger head-to-body ratio results in a higher center of gravity and head momentum especially in the younger age groups. The head therefore is likely to be the leading force of impact regardless of where the force is applied to the body. It has also been suggested that less developed neck and shoulder musculature do not effectively dissipate the energy from the head impact to the rest of the body. Although there are significant gains in weight and mass during adolescence, there is also increased force and momentum without simultaneous gains in neck strength. An immature or incompletely myelinated brain is also more susceptible to shear forces resulting in neuronal injury.

The degree to which changes in cerebrovascular physiology influence vulnerability of the pediatric brain is not completely understood. Normal cerebral blood flow increases to twice that of adults by the age of 6–9 years and then progressively decreases. It is believed that children are more vulnerable to alterations in cerebral blood flow and autoregulation after brain injury. The mismatch of metabolic supply and demand may contribute to cerebral hypoxia and hypercarbia. After a moderate-to-severe injury has occurred, children are more likely to suffer from prolonged and diffuse cerebral edema compared to adults with traumatic brain injury.

These differences in structure, growth, and physiology account for variations in head injury pattern compared to adults. Skull fractures are more common in children but are less likely to be associated with epidural hematomas. Traumatic intracranial hemorrhage is rare but can include intracerebral, subdural, epidural, and subarachnoid hemorrhages. Subdural hemorrhages occur 5–10 times as often as epidural hemorrhages. In general, children have a larger subarachnoid space and cisterns that allow for better tolerance of expanding hemorrhagic mass lesions, but only to a point. Focal mass hemorrhages occur less often in children (15–20%) compared to adults (30–40%).

Concussion in the pediatric and adolescent athlete is very different to concussion in the adult athlete. The rate of concussion in high school athletes is higher than that of older athletes. Neurocognitive testing reveals that younger athletes have a longer recovery time compared to professional athletes. High school students take on average 10–14 days to return to their neurocognitive baseline compared with 5–7 days in college athletes and 3–5 days in professional athletes. High school students are also more likely to have persistent neurocognitive deficits despite becoming asymptomatic. Therefore, a more conservative approach to return to play for the child and adolescent athlete is recommended (See Chapter 11).

Cervical Spine

The pediatric cervical spine can be difficult to evaluate and presents a diagnostic challenge. The developing cervical spine has unfused synchondroses, incomplete ossification centers, and epiphyseal growth plates. Synchondroses can be visible until adolescence; secondary ossification centers can appear in childhood and fuse in the second or third decade, and the apophysis of the vertebral body can give the appearance of slight anterior vertebral wedging. All of these developmental findings can easily be confused with acute fractures. Children have increased ligamentous laxity and more vertebral mobility compared to adults. This can result in absent lordosis seen on lateral radiograph. This extreme laxity can also exaggerate the vertebral override, which in children is known as pseudosubluxation. Children can also have normal widening of the prevertebral space, which in an adult would otherwise signify hemorrhage or edema from underlying injury. The pediatric spinal column does not take on more adult characteristics until 8 years of age.

Depending on the size and age of the child, patterns of injury differ from the distribution of injuries seen in the adult population. Cervical spine fractures are less common in children than adults, but the incidence increases with age. Younger children with a higher head-to-body ratio have a higher fulcrum about which flexion and extension occurs (C1–C3 regions). Therefore, children younger than 8 years of age have higher cervical spine fractures, while those older than 12 have more lower cervical spine injuries with patterns similar to adults (C5–C6). Children ages 8–12 have a fulcrum at the C3–C5 levels reflective of their transitioning state. Children aged 8–16 have a greater incidence of neurologic deficit with cervical fracture (40%) compared to the younger ages (20%).

Since 2005, 7.9% of all new cases of spinal cord injury in the United States were related to sport, ranking the fourth most common cause of spinal cord injuries in the USA. While spinal cord injuries can occur in conjunction with cervical fracture or dislocation, the pediatric patient is uniquely at risk of Spinal Cord Injury With Out Radiographic Abnormality (SCIWORA). The flexibility and elasticity of the vertebral column is greater than that of the spinal cord, thus cord injury can occur without anatomic defects. Most cases of SCIWORA present with paresthesias, or some variation of motor or sensory neurologic deficits. A SCIWORA injury usually involves the upper cervical spine of children aged 9–11 due to these age-related anatomic differences. In sports-related cervical spine injuries, there is an overwhelmingly high rate of SCIWORA (50–75%) compared to other injuries and is most prominent in older children and adolescents (See Chapter 19).

Chest

The young athlete is at risk for a unique pattern of medical and traumatic thoracic emergencies based on age and anatomy. The chest wall of children is much more pliable and compliant than that of adults. As a result, the force from an impact may be directly transmitted to the underlying structures such as the heart or lungs without an associated chest wall injury. Pulmonary contusions are more likely than rib fractures and direct evidence of a chest injury such as a chest wall swelling or bruising may be absent. Sport-related traumatic pneumothorax (abnormal accumulation of air in the pleural space) is rare, especially in the absence of fractured ribs. A spontaneous pneumothorax is also rare but has been reported in various sports including weightlifting due to valsalva and scuba diving due to barotrauma. If a pneumothorax is present, the increased mobility of the mediastinal structures makes the child more susceptible to a tension pneumothorax, which is immediately life threatening if not recognized and treated. A tension pneumothorax results in shifting of the mediastinal structures away from the side of the pneumothorax with resultant decrease of blood returning to the heart, leading to a cardiac arrest.

The compliant chest wall of children and adolescents also puts them at risk for commotio cordis from blunt chest trauma. This syndrome is typically triggered from a blow to the chest resulting in a rhythm disturbance, rapid cardiovascular collapse, and in most cases sudden death. This occurs in the absence of structural damage and any underlying cardiovascular issues. This condition predominantly affects young adolescents with 75% of cases occurring in children under the age of 18. Young men participating in organized sports such as baseball, football, hockey, and lacrosse are at highest risk. Survival rates have improved in the last four decades from 10% in 1970 to 58% in 2012. This improved survival can be attributed to the initiation of prompt CPR and early use of an AED. While the use of sport-specific chest protectors are recommended to decrease the incidence of commotio cordis, the effectiveness of such protective equipment in preventing sudden cardiac arrest is debatable. Similarly, use of a softer (safety) baseball has been used in Japan for children under14 years of age, with an anecdotal decreased rate of commotio cordis in the country.

The adolescent athlete is also at risk from other rare causes of sudden cardiac arrest. Eighty-five percent of these cases are attributed to cardiac events while additional causes include heat illness, pulmonary disorders, and drug-induced system failure. Hypertrophic cardiomyopathy (HCM) is the most common cause of cardiac death in athletes under the age of 30. This inherited disorder results in the muscular enlargement of the left ventricle and the septum leading to dysfunction and various cardiac complications. Young athletes with HCM are at highest risk during strenuous exercise. Most are asymptomatic and are unaware of the problem before collapse. Screening and early identification through preparticipation in physical exams is the cornerstone of prevention (See Chapter 5). In the event of onfield collapse, immediate recognition, CPR, and use of an AED are critical to survival.

Abdomen

Sport-related abdominal injuries in children are rare, but if present can be serious and diagnosis is often delayed due to subtle presentation. The pediatric abdominal wall is thin and less muscular. Therefore, an external force is more readily transmitted to the internal organs, increasing the risk of internal injury in the absence of external findings. Collisions are the most common mechanism of injury in children aged 12 or over, while falls account for the most injuries in the younger (5–11-year-old) age group. Males are four times more likely than females to have an intraabdominal injury due to more forceful collisions. The most commonly injured organ in sports trauma is the spleen followed by renal and liver injuries. While hollow viscous injury (intestinal contusion or perforation) is infrequent, it tends to occur in the younger age group and is associated with multiple injuries due to the close proximity of other organs such as the pancreas, stomach, liver, and spleen. Owing to the child's smaller size, a single force will cover a greater surface and involve injury to more structures. The subtle presentation of abdominal injury warrants a high index of suspicion to ensure early diagnosis and treatment.

Musculoskeletal

Musculoskeletal injury is the most common type of sport-related injury among children. Sprains, strains, fractures, and contusions are the most common injury types, while dislocations are less common. Body parts most injured are the ankle and knee followed by the wrist, hand, and elbow. The developing pediatric musculoskeletal system is susceptible to a unique pattern of injury compared to that of an adult. This is a reflection of persistent growth, open growth plates, and elastic bones in the setting of year round training, repetitive activities, and overtraining.

Emergency Planning and Fieldside Preparedness

Proper sideline preparation with a rapid, well-designed, and rehearsed emergency plan can make the difference between an effective and an ineffective emergency response. Life-threatening and limb-threatening events are unpredictable and therefore easily hindered by heightened emotions and a chaotic atmosphere.

Preparedness begins with the development of an emergency action plan. This plan acts as a blueprint for handling emergencies and should be practical and flexible in order to adapt to any athletic situation. This written plan should detail a chain of command; the proper personnel needed to carry out the plan and ensure qualified personnel are present. Sports medicine doctors, trainers, officials, and coaches should be trained in how to use an AED, CPR, and first aid. Adult equipment can be used on all children 8 years and older. A clear mechanism of communication, transportation, and a predetermined emergency facility should be detailed in the plan. This plan should be frequently reviewed and rehearsed by all FoP medical responders to ensure seamless execution. Promotion of proper education, training, and preparation is critical to the emergency management of the pediatric athlete.

Conclusion

Life-threatening illness and injury of the pediatric athlete can occur during any physical activity and at any level of competition. Knowledge and recognition of the age-related anatomic and physiologic differences is critical to accurate assessment, resuscitation, and appropriate management. Athletes, coaches, officials, athletic trainers, and other sports medicine practitioners should be familiar with the ABCDE sequence of assessment to identify significant pediatric injury and initiate treatment. The pediatric population is susceptible to differences in injury pattern, which can alter triage, management, and consideration for return to play. Although life-threatening situations can be rare, a substantial proportion of life-threatening pediatric injury is sport related. Preparation is key; a well-planned and rehearsed emergency action plan should not be underestimated. Increased training and a knowledgeable and conservative approach to assessing and treating pediatric sports injury will optimize successful emergency management and promote safety in sports participation.

Bibliography

Safe Kids Worldwide (SKW) (2013) *Sports and Recreation Safety Fact Sheet.* SKW, Washington, DC. Accessed October 31, 2013. https://www.safekids.org/sites/default/files/documents/skw_sports_fact_sheet_oct_2013.pdf

Meehan, W.P. III & Mannix, R. (2013) A substantial proportion of life-threatening injuries are sport-related. *Pediatric Emergency Care*, **29**, 624–627.

Andersen, J.C., Courson, R.W., Kleiner, D.M. *et al.* (2002) *National Athletic Trainers' Association position statement: emergency planning in athletics*, Journal of Athletic Training **37**, 99–104.

Wolfson, A.B. (ed) (2010) Pediatric trauma. In: Harwood-Nuss' Clinical Practice of Emergency Medicine, 5 edn. Lippincott Williams & Wilkins, Philadelphia, pp. 1089–1117.

Maugans, T.A., Farley, C., Altaye, M. *et al.* (2012) Pediatric sports-related concussion produces cerebral blood flow alterations. Pediatrics, **129**, 28–37.

Gottschalk, A.W. & Andrisk, J.T. (2011) Epidemiology of sports injury in pediatric athletes. Sports Medicine and Arthroscopy Review, **19**, 2–6.

Soundappan, S.V., Holland, A.J. & Browne, G. (2005) Sports-related pneumothorax in children. Pediatric Emergency Care, **21**, 259–260.

Madden, C.C., Putukian, M., Young, C.C. & McCarty, E.C. (eds) (2010) The pediatric athlete. In: Netter's Sports Medicine. Saunders Elsevier, Philadelphia, pp. 55–64.

23 Emergency Medical Care in Paralympic Sports

Peter Van de Vliet[1] and Mike Wilkinson[2,3,4]

[1]*International Paralympic Committee, Bonn, Germany*
[2]*Department of Sports Medicine, University of British Colombia, Vancouver, Canada*
[3]*Sports Medicine and Human Performance, Vancouver Canucks, Vancouver, Canada*
[4]*FISA Medical Commission, Canada*

The Paralympic Athlete

Sport for an athlete with a disability has existed for more than 100 years. In the eighteenth and nineteenth centuries, new contributions proved that sport activities were very important for the rehabilitation of injured persons. Following World War II, traditional methods of rehabilitation could not meet the medical and psychological needs of the large numbers of injured soldiers and civilians. Professor Ludwig Guttmann introduced sport as a form of recreation and as an aid for remedial treatment and rehabilitation. The inspiration for incorporating sport in the rehabilitation program came from the patients themselves who had developed their own "active" programs. On July 28, 1948, the day of the Opening Ceremony of the Olympic Games in London, the Stoke Mandeville Games were founded and the first competition for athletes with spinal cord injury took place on the hospital grounds in Stoke Mandeville, just 35 miles outside London. Two British teams, comprised 14 former servicemen and 2 former servicewomen, competed in the archery event. At the following Games, Dr. Guttmann, declared his hope that the Games would become international and achieve "world fame as the disabled men and women's equivalent of the Olympic Games." In 1952, the event became "international" with the participation of exservicemen from The Netherlands and 8 years later, in 1960, the International Stoke Mandeville Games were staged for the first time in the same country, Italy, and city, Rome, as the Olympic Games. The first Paralympic Winter Games took place in Örnsköldsvik in Sweden in 1976.

From this early beginning, the Movement grew into a professional organization, now known as the International Paralympic Committee (IPC), which is the global governing body of the Paralympic Movement, as well as the organizer of the Paralympic Summer and Winter Games. Today, this event involves 4200 athletes competing in 20 summer sports and 600 athletes in 5 winter sports (see Table 23.1).

The IOC Manual of Emergency Sports Medicine, First Edition. Edited by David McDonagh and David Zideman.

	Impaired muscle power	Impaired range of motion	Limb deficiency	Leg length difference	Short Stature	Hypertonia	Ataxia	Athetosis	Visual impair-ment	Intellectual impairment
Archery	x	x	x	x		x	x	x		
Athletics	X	X	X	X	X	X	X	X	X	X
Boccia	X	X				X	X	X		
Canoe[a]	X	X	X	X		X	X	X		
Cycling	X	X	X	X		X	X	X	X	
Equestrian	X	X	X	X	X	X	X	X	X	
Football 5-a-side									X	
Football 7-a-side						X	X	X		
Goalball									X	
Judo									X	
Powerlifting	X	X	X	X	X	X	X	X		
Rowing	X	X	X			X	X	X		
Sailing	X	X	X	X	X	X	X	X	X	
Shooting	X	X	X			X	X	X		
Sitting volleyball	X	X	X	X		X	X	X		
Swimming	X	X	X	X	X	X	X	X	X	X
Table tennis	X	X	X	X	X	X	X	X		x
Triathlon[a]	X	X	X			X	X	X	X	
Wheelchair basketball	X	X	X	X		X	X	X		
Wheelchair fencing	X	X	X	X		X	X	X		
Wheelchair rugby	X	X	X			X	X	X		
Wheelchair tennis	X	X	X	X		X	X	X		
Alpine skiing	X	X	X	X		X	X	X	X	
Biathlon	X	X	X	X		X	X	X	X	
Cross-country Skiing	X	X	X	X		X	X	X	X	
Ice sledge hockey	X	X	X	X		X	X	X		
Snowboard	X	X	X	X		X	X	X		
Wheelchair curling	X	X	X			X	X	X		

[a] New sports included in the Rio 2016 Paralympic Games program.

Table 23.1 Impairment types eligible to compete in different Paralympic sports (further details on eligible impairments can be found in the IPC Policy on Eligible Impairments in the Paralympic Movement, IPC Handbook, Section 2, Chapter 3.13, www.paralympic.org/The-IPC/Handbook)

With participation in sport comes an associated risk of injury and despite the growing awareness and popularity of Paralympic sport there continues to be a relative paucity as to the understanding of injury patterns and risk factors for injury among these athletes. Such understanding however, is crucial for planning appropriate emergency medical care.

Although athletes with impairments can experience the same spectrum of medical conditions as their able-bodied counterparts, furthering the understanding through longitudinal and systematic investigation of injuries and illnesses in elite athletes is extremely helpful in this regard. The few studies that have been published comparing sport participation in both able-bodied and disabled individuals suggest that the latter do not have a significant greater overall risk of injury than their able-bodied counterparts, although the functional consequences of injury to an athlete with an underlying impairment can be considerably greater than for an able-bodied athlete. For example, a comparatively "routine" shoulder overuse injury that might be a mere "nuisance" for an able-bodied athlete, may compromise the ability of a C6-lesion tetraplegic athlete (athlete with high neck lesion, impacting the function of both lower and upper limbs) to remain independently mobile, to say nothing about dramatically interfering with their participation in sport.

The assessment of risk of injury in Paralympic sport is complicated by the different nature of impairments in the paralympic athlete. Athletes with different degrees of physical, visual, and/or intellectual impairment compete in the 28 Paralympic sports; some are unique to a particular impairment category (see Table 23.1). In this chapter, both injury and illness types as well as impairment-related medical care are addressed.

Injury and Illness in Paralympic Athletes

Up to the present time, the only available data on injury and illness are medical encounter data reported by the Organizing Committees (OCOG, Olympic Games Organizing Committee) as part of the transfer of knowledge to the next OCOGs. Vancouver 2010 was the first Games to systematically report on these medical encounters of Paralympic Games in the public domain. Whereas the initial aim of such reporting is to gain insight into the medical services as part of the planning for future Games, such data is very useful to identify areas of high needs. In the case of the Vancouver 2010 Paralympic Games, a majority of the medical encounters were musculoskeletal related and the findings also identified a high demand for dental, optical, imaging, and therapy services.

For the purpose of identifying the specific needs of emergency medical care, a more accurate or detailed reporting mechanism is required. This system includes data from the team doctors, typically "first-line" responders for many minor or nonacute medical incidents. Both the International Olympic Committee (IOC) and the IPC, respectively, have initiated such surveys during recent Games and with each successive Games, these surveys have become more detailed in identifying mechanisms of injury, and most recently, illness. The highest incidence (23.8%) was reported in the Vancouver in 2010 compared to 8.4% and 9.4% in Salt Lake City and Torino, respectively. This high incidence in Vancouver was probably due to the high compliance rate of injury reporting by team physicians, thus reflecting a more accurate reporting of medical incidents. Fortunately, the vast majority of medical encounters recorded were minor impact-related injuries, with only 14 of the 120 injuries recorded resulting in the athlete being unable to continue with training or to participate in competition.

1. Ice sledge hockey had the highest reported incidences (33.9%, 40 injuries/118 competitors). In 2010, only 1 lower limb fracture was recorded out of 40 encounters (2.5%), compared to 4 out of 12 (33%) in 2002. These 2002 findings led to the introduction of a regulation change on protective equipment and sledge height

and these efforts would seem to have been effective. Other injuries included muscle strains and ligament strains, fractures (three in total: phalanx, calcaneal, and rib), contusions, lacerations, and one glenohumeral dislocation. About 40% of the injuries could be categorized as less well defined (i.e., lower back pain, scapulothoracic dysfunction, impingement, and hypertonicity). The incidence proportion in alpine skiing was 21.1% (41/194), with 24 injuries (58%) occurring during training (15) or competition (9).
2. When analyzed by event, downhill produced most of the new acute injuries (4.1 injuries/100 race exposures), compared to Super Combined (1.2/100), Super-G (0.8/100) and Giant Slalom (0.6/100). Slalom events did not lead to any new acute injuries. Three acute injuries involved injury to the head that prevented further competition. Other injuries included neck and shoulder strain, chest contusion, and sprains to the metacarpophalangeal joint of the thumb (related to holding the sticks).
3. Among the athletes competing in cross-country skiing and biathlon, 18.6% (26/141) sought medical support for musculoskeletal problems. Similarly, in alpine skiing, injuries during training seemed to occur more when compared to competition (16 versus 10, respectively), with 2/3 of the injuries being related to overuse mechanisms. All acute injuries were related to falls and included concussion, lower limb contusion, and one case of pneumothorax.
4. Wheelchair curling can be considered a sport of minimal injury risk with medical encounters related to overuse/strain of the spine or upper limb; the majority accountable to pre-Games nonsport-related symptoms.

In summary, across winter sports, medical services should be prepared to deal with a wide diversity of injuries in terms of mechanism and location, having a minimal impact on the further continuation of competition, but with an increased number of injuries classified as overuse resulting from pre-Games activities.

Valuing the importance of this systematic and longitudinal data on prevention of injury and illness and the protection of athletes' health, the IPC conducted a web-based surveillance system during the London 2012 Paralympic Games. For the first time, illness was recorded as part of a surveillance system based on data indicating that up to 50% of the medical consultations in these settings were for illness in athletes.

1. In 2012, an injury rate of 12.1/1000 athlete-days with an incidence proportion of 11.6% was reported
2. The highest incidence rates for injury, per thousand athlete-days, were found in the following:
   a. Football 5-a-side (22.4)
   b. Goalball (19.5)
   c. Powerlifting (19.3)
   d. Wheelchair fencing (18.0)
   e. Wheelchair rugby (16.3)
   f. Athletics (15.8)
   g. Judo (15.5)

There was a predominance of injuries to the following:

1. Shoulder (17.7%)
2. Wrist and hand (11.4%)
3. Elbow (8.8%)
4. Knee (7.9%)

Acute injuries accounted for 51% of all injuries and were predominantly found in the following:

1. Boccia
2. Track cycling
3. Road cycling

The London 2012 conclusions revealed a higher incidence of injuries in athletes with visual impairment that will, in the future, require specific attention to the vulnerability of these athletes to specific environmental risk factors.

The 2012 incidence rate of illness was 12.8/1000 athlete-days with an incidence proportion of 10.2%. The sports with the highest incidence rates, per thousand athlete-days, were the following:

1. Equestrian (20.7)
2. Powerlifting (15.8)
3. Athletics (15.4)
4. Table tennis (15.2).

The highest system rates were reported for respiratory (27.4%), skin (18.3%), and gastrointestinal problems (14.5%). Of particular interest is the higher incidence for genitourinary problems (8.5%) compared to similar information in able-bodied athletes. This is primarily due to athletes with spinal cord injuries being vulnerable to urinary tract problems.

The clinical relevance of such data in planning emergency medical care is important. For a 10-day multisport event, these figures would suggest 12–13 injuries per 100 participating athletes, about half of which will be new onset acute injuries and will primarily be injuries of the upper limb region. An additional 10–11 athletes will seek medical treatment for illness related discomfort, most commonly of a respiratory nature.

Emergency medical care should not only focus on incidents that happen on the Field of Play (FoP) or during training, but they should also be prepared to care for the rare but significant number of noncompetition-related medical interventions. It is also important to not only plan for Paralympic-specific emergency conditions, but also to include medical incident scenarios found in able-bodied events.

Impairment-Specific Considerations of Medical Care

Athlete impairment types are known to affect injury characteristics and advances in the use of assistive propulsion and protective devices as allowed by the sport-technical rules (orthotic or prosthetic devices, wheelchairs, throwing chairs, sit-skis, sledges, use of goggles, etc.) have brought an additional component of medical care, which must be included when planning emergency medical services in Paralympic sports. Familiarization with the different types of equipment is essential as is the rapid, safe extrication and transport of the athlete from the FoP. Certain pieces of equipment, for example, sit-skis and sail boats, may require very specific extrication tools that will need to be procured before the event as part of the sport specific FoP medical equipment.

In the lead up to the Event, all medical personnel must train and practice using the equipment that will be present at the event. A good process that was used with great success at the 2010 Paralympic Games included the following steps:

1. Theoretical walkthrough and discussion of a particular medical event
2. Focused medical stabilization and extrication exercises
3. Full FoP emergency scenario practices

At the 2010 Games, these full scenario exercises were run daily with each FoP team at the venue with the FoP equipment provided. With each repetition, the efficiency improved so that when actual events occurred, there was a well-rehearsed response with no compromise to the medical care provided.

Awareness of the risks of common medical problems experienced by Paralympic athletes is essential to prevent serious sequela from unfortunate conditions and it is important for care staff to identify in advance the possible medical problems that athletes might face. Issues include the following:

1. The extent of muscle and joint involvement
2. Muscle tone and coordination
3. Sensory loss
4. Heat/cold intolerance
5. Susceptibility to fractures
6. Dangers of exacerbation or the likelihood of progression of disease symptoms

These are all important considerations in anticipation of sports participation.

A key aspect that needs to be appreciated when dealing with Paralympic athletes is how an otherwise minor injury affects the athlete as a whole:

1. A spinal-cord-injured athlete who develops a shoulder injury may lose some of his/her independence through the inability to perform activities of daily living, such as getting in and out of bed or general mobility if he/she uses a self-propelled wheelchair
2. A small abrasion or ulcer at the site of a prosthetic leg may prevent the athlete from wearing his/her prosthesis and in the same way limit daily mobility

It can be seen that a seemingly simple injury could have serious implications for the broader and longer term wellbeing of the athlete. FoP medical staff should be familiar with and trained in the diverse nature of impairment associated with Paralympic sports (see Table 23.1). International Sport Federations recommend that Emergency Medical Care is complemented with rehabilitation expertise and experience when planning the operational management of an event. At the London 2012 Paralympic Games, 82 of the 160 delegations did not bring their own Medical Officer and relied on the medical services of the Organizing Committee. Many medical volunteers will not be familiar with Paralympic sports and consequently specific Paralympic training must be included as part of the role-specific training. It should emphasize the important interface of the athlete with his/her equipment and sport and include potential Paralympic-specific issues:

1. Athletes are particularly at risk from accidental scrapes, cuts, bruises, blisters, and floor and wheel burns as a result of incidental contact with a wheelchair, prosthesis, or the ground after a fall
2. Occasionally, friction burns occur due to an inappropriate fitting of the device (wheelchair too wide, prosthesis to small); particular attention should be given to problems that can occur when the skin is wet (e.g., swimming, rowing, and sailing)
3. Soft-tissue injuries (abrasions, contusions, strains, and sprains) often occur as a result of repetitive stress on joints and muscles
4. Attention should be given to shoulder rotator cuff and carpal tunnel syndrome in wheelchair users
5. In addition to soft-tissue problems, degeneration of bony surface coverings (cartilage), tears in the fibrous tissue surrounding the joint, and loss of bone circulation may occur over time
6. Extensor forces imposed by weight-bearing and continuous overhead activity decreases the circulation to the shoulder in wheelchair users and hip in lower limb amputees

Although fractures are not a common problem and occur in few Paralympic sports (e.g., alpine ski), bones in paralyzed athletes are often osteoporotic and may fracture from minor injuries. As many athletes lack the sensation that accompanies a bone fracture, any evidence of an abnormal body position, swelling, redness, bruising, or grinding sensations should be stabilized or splinted and referred for further examination and imaging. Falls, as a consequence of reduced balance, also increase the chance of fractures and may have been the result of the following:

1. The loss of sensation (e.g., incomplete lesions)
2. Coordination problems (e.g., cerebral palsy (CP) athletes)
3. Loss of proprioception (e.g., prosthesis running)
4. Unforeseen obstacles (e.g., visual impaired athletes)

Specific Paralympic Medical Concerns

1. Systematically inspect insensitive skin
2. Be attentive to dehydration
3. Be attentive to bladder problems
4. Persistent redness, hardening of the skin, or a raised area are the first signs of a pressure sore and the area should immediately be relieved from all pressure caused by sitting, wearing restrictive clothes, or prosthesis fitting
5. Check for impaired circulation
6. Check for the ability to perspire below the site of the lesion. This is commonly seen in athletes with high spinal lesions and is not exclusive to extreme cold or hot environments
7. Opening and closing ceremonies, which incur long periods of waiting and sitting in combination with insufficient hydration

Autonomic Dysreflexia

Autonomic dysreflexia is a reflex syndrome that is unique to individuals with spinal cord injury at above T6 spinal level. This reflex can occur spontaneously resulting in a sympathetic discharge, which elevates the arterial blood pressure and associated cardiovascular responses. It is a medical emergency as it is a cause of very high blood pressure and can result in stroke. The stimulus usually occurs in an area without sensation and triggers a series of reflexes resulting in the following:

1. Abnormally high blood pressure
2. Sweating
3. Goose bumps
4. Flushing of the face and neck
5. Significant headache

Athletes with spinal cord injuries who compete in wheelchair sports can voluntarily induce autonomic dysreflexia prior to, or during the event, in order to enhance their performance. Research has demonstrated that this practice, which is commonly referred to as "boosting" in athletic circles, improves middle distance wheelchair racing performance by approximately 10% in elite athletes with quadriplegia.

Treatment:
Autonomic dysreflexia is a medical emergency

1. The situation is triggered by a stimulus from a full bladder or bowel obstruction
2. Immediately empty the bladder or evacuate the bowels
3. Sit the athlete up to reduce blood pressure

It is estimated that 20% of athletes vulnerable to autonomic dysreflexia have used the mechanism to voluntary enhance performance.

Conclusion

The diversity of Paralympic sports requires emergency medical services to be tailored to the needs and demands of each particular sport. The following criteria should be considered:

1. The athletes (impairment groups and wheelchair users versus standing athletes with a diversity of impairment profiles)
2. The adaptive equipment to be used
3. The venue (outdoor versus indoor and water environment)
4. The environmental conditions (winter versus summer, altitude, and air quality)

The considerations all potentially have an even greater impact on the athlete's health in Paralympic sports than is seen in able-bodied sport and they need to be addressed throughout the planning and running of medical services for Paralympic events. The more integrated these services and protocols are to the entire event and planning process, the greater the likelihood of excellent athlete care.

Bibliography

Derman, W., Schwellnus, M., Jordaan, E. *et al.* (2013) Illness and injury in athletes during the competition period at the London 2012 Paralympic Games – development and implementation of a web-based surveillance system (web-IISS) for team medical staff. *British Journal of Sports Medicine*, **47**, 420–425.

McDonagh, D. (2012) *FIMS Sports Medicine Manual Event Planning and Emergency Care*. Lippincott Williams & Wilkins, Philadelphia.

Taunton, J., Wilkinson, M., Celebrini, R. *et al.* (2012) Paralympic medical services for the 2010 Paralympic Winter Games. *Clinical Journal of Sports Medicine*, **22**, 10–20.

Webborn, A.D.J. (2010) Paralympic sports. In: Caine, D.J., Harmer, P.A. & Schiff, M.A. (eds), *Epidemiology of injury in Olympic Sports*. The Encyclopaedia of Sports Medicine, Oxford, Wiley-Blackwell, pp. 475–488.

Willick, S., Webborn, N., Emery, C. *et al.* (2013) The epidemiology of injuries at the London 2012 Paralympic Games. *British Journal of Sports Medicine*, **47**, 426–432.

24 Cold Injuries

Ken Zafren[1,2,3], *Gordon Giesbrecht*[4] *and David McDonagh*[5,6,7]

[1]*Emergency Programs, State of Alaska, Anchorage, AK, USA*
[2]*Division of Emergency Medicine, Stanford University Medical Center, Stanford, CA, USA*
[3]*Alaska Native Medical Center, Anchorage, AK, USA*
[4]*Kinesiology and Recreation Management, Departments of Anaesthesia and Emergency Medicine, University of Manitoba, Winnipeg, Canada*
[5]*Emeregency Deptartment, St. Olavs Hospital, Trondheim, Norway*
[6]*Faculty of Medicine, NTNU - National University of Science and Technology, Trondheim, Norway*
[7]*Medical Commission, AIBA - International Boxing Association, Lausanne, Switzerland.*

Cold injuries can be categorized as hypothermia, frostbite, and nonfreezing cold injuries. It is highly unlikely that a doctor will be required to treat any of these conditions within the confines of Olympic Sport competition. Even at the 1994 Olympic Winter Games in Lillehammer where temperatures dropped to –35 °C, no incidences of cold injuries were reported, even among spectators. Cold injuries are more likely to be seen in more extreme endurance events in harsher climates. Both FIS (Skiing) and IBU (Biathlon), the two IFs who have athletes competing outdoors in potentially extremely cold climates, have stringent regulations regarding acceptable climatic conditions for allowing competitions to take place.

Accidental hypothermia is defined as an unintentional drop of core temperature (T_{co}) from a normal value of ~37 °C to 35 °C or below. *Hypothermia* is classified as mild (T_{co}, 35–32 °C), moderate (32–28 °C), or severe (<28 °C). These categories are useful for guiding treatment, but there is great variability among individuals in the response to hypothermia. Hypothermia can occur in outdoor endurance sports such as cycling, long-distance running, sailing, and open-water swimming. Hypothermia can usually be prevented by the use of adequate dry clothing. Athletes who are exercising in extreme cold should avoid overheating, which causes excessive sweating. The most practical method of regulating clothing in endurance sports is to dress in layers, removing some layers just prior to periods of high exertion.

Frostbite is a risk whenever skin is directly or indirectly exposed to cold temperatures, especially in windy conditions, as are *nonfreezing cold injuries* (NFCIs).

A healthcare provider is therefore unlikely to ever see a severe cold injury after an organized ski event and is not likely to be required to enter the Field of Play (FoP) to treat a cold injury. The most likely cold weather scenarios are that of finding a cold collapsed athlete lying in snow or floating in water, an athlete retiring from an event due to extreme cold or an athlete contacting the ED post-event due to symptoms of

The IOC Manual of Emergency Sports Medicine, First Edition. Edited by David McDonagh and David Zideman.
2015 International Olympic Committee. Published 2015 by John Wiley & Sons, Ltd.

cold injury. This chapter therefore varies from the standard approach in this manual and discusses these various scenarios.

The Collapsed Cold Athlete

An athlete who has collapsed and been left lying in snow or floating in the water may develop hypothermia. An athlete will not remain lying in snow unless suffering from injury or illness, total exhaustion, or severe hypothermia. In water events, the dangers are compounded by the possibility of immersion. Any situation in which a patient collapses is potentially serious and the possible causes are many. The situation may then be further compounded if the patient becomes hypothermic. In an organized sports event, severe hypothermia is most likely the result of having been lying on the cold ground rather than the cause of collapse.

Primary Survey in a Cold Athlete

Rapidly evaluate the patient following the ABCDE mnemonic.

Inspection: The patient may be pale and there may be local skin coloration changes. There may be ice on the hair or beard and frozen secretions around the mouth and nose. If an athlete is found in a cold environment, they may be alert or have altered consciousness. Severe hypothermia is associated with a marked decrease in the level of consciousness and the patient may score a P or U on the alert, verbal stimuli response, painful stimuli response, or unresponsive (AVPU) Scale. The patient may be motionless but with no shivering. The absence of shivering should not delude the ED into believing that the patient is only slightly cold – in a patient with shallow respirations and with a normal or low RR, weak and probably slow pulse, with a GCS of 14 or less; the most important clinical finding is that the patient looks to be cold, complains of being cold and is cold on palpation. The presence of shivering would indicate that the patient is cold or suffering from mild or moderate hypothermia. With moderate hypothermia, there may be a decreased level of consciousness with slurred speech and unsteady gait, but the patient may still be shivering vigorously.

With mild hypothermia, the patient is usually alert, will feel cold, and will usually be shivering vigorously although not all alert, shivering patients are hypothermic.

Airway: The airway is most likely normal unless there has been an injury.

Breathing: May be absent or superficial in the severely hypothermic patient. The respiratory rate may be elevated with milder forms of hypothermia.

Circulation: There may be a weak or absent pulse. The capillary refill time (CRT) may be prolonged due to peripheral vasoconstriction.

Disability: An AVPU evaluation must be performed early in the patient assessment.

Palpation: Place an ungloved hand on the thorax under the patient's clothing. If the skin feels warm, the patient is not likely to be hypothermic. If the skin is cold, then the patient probably is hypothermic. If the patient is obtunded, cold and not shivering, then the patient is probably severely hypothermic.

Exposure/Environment: Try not to expose a hypothermic patient in a very cold environment unless essential. If exposure is necessary, cover the patient immediately after evaluation. If a cold injury is suspected, particularly frostbite, then the feet should also be exposed and examined in a sheltered area. Promptly protect from further heat loss and transport as quickly as possible to a warm environment for further evaluation and treatment. Evaluate and treat a patient with an altered level of consciousness for immediate life-threatening injuries or other conditions. Hypothermia and local cold injuries are almost never immediately life-threatening conditions.

Management:

1. *Prevent further heat loss*: Remove the patient from cold exposure. Protect from the wind. Insulate the patient from the ground. Cover as much of the patient as possible with a vapor barrier (plastic, bubble wrap, etc.) to decrease evaporative heat loss from wet clothing and to decrease convective heat loss due to the wind. Eventually, wet clothing will need to be removed and replaced with dry insulation; this should not be done until a sheltered area can be reached. At that time, the vapor barrier should be placed between the patient and the insulation in order to keep the insulation dry and effective.

2. *Apply heat*: If available, apply heat to the upper torso (specifically the chest, axillae, and back). This can be accomplished in the field using large chemical or electric heat packs or blankets or the Norwegian Charcoal Heatpac. The Hypothermia Prevention and Management Kit (HPMK), developed by the United States military is an excellent method of preventing heat loss. It consists of a blanket with four large chemical heat packs and a vapor barrier. The HPMK is easy to use and is widely available commercially. These methods do not increase the core temperature of a shivering patient faster than shivering alone, but active warming is still advantageous due to decreased energy requirements and increased thermal comfort resulting from decreased shivering. In a nonshivering patient, exogenous heat is necessary to increase core temperature because the patient's metabolic heat production will decrease from normothermic levels of ~100 W to as low as 50 W or even less.
3. Move the patient to a warm environment as soon as possible.

Remove wet clothing only after the patient is in a warm environment.

Prehospital Treatment for a Cold But Nonhypothermic Patient or for a Mildly Hypothermic Patient

If it is to take more than 30 min to arrive at a medical facility, attempt to rewarm the conscious co-operative patient by administering food or fluids that contain carbohydrates, including sugars, as patients will have significant energy requirements to support shivering which is the most effective method for increasing heat production. Carbohydrate content is more important than the heat in a hot drink. Do not allow a patient to eat or drink unless the patient is conscious and alert and can swallow and protect the airway.

Exercise, such as walking, will produce heat and may be helpful. However, exercise increases afterdrop, which is a continued decrease in core temperature after cold exposure that occurs before rewarming measures become effective. Increased afterdrop and peripheral vasodilation caused by exercise have the potential to cause cardiovascular collapse or ventricular fibrillation (VF). Exercise should only be allowed if the patient is conscious and alert, dry, has had calorie replacement and has been stable for at least 30 min. Continuous monitoring of vital signs is therefore essential. Prevent further heat loss and keep the patient in a warm place.

Do not put a cold patient in a shower or bath. This increases afterdrop and may cause cardiovascular collapse or VF.

Prehospital Treatment of a Patient With Moderate or Severe Hypothermia

Manage a patient with moderate-to-severe hypothermia with extreme care and keep the patient in a horizontal position. Prevent further heat loss and apply heat to the upper torso as described earlier. Transport the patient by stretcher to an ambulance or athlete medical room. If available, use forced-air warming with a heating blanket applied to the chest. Forced-air warming is effective at raising core temperature.

Proper management of these patients includes continuous vital sign monitoring and also includes the following list of what NOT to do:

1. Do not get the patient to move or exercise, as patients are prone to developing VF even after minor physical activity. Even placing a patient in a vertical position may induce severe cardiovascular stress
2. Do not give the patient food or oral fluids
3. Do not put the patient in a shower or bath

Rapid transfer to an appropriate medical facility is advised.

CPR and Severely Hypothermic Patients

Hypothermia is one of the (4Hs) reversible causes of cardiac arrest (see Chapter 4).

A severely hypothermic patient may be in a state of "suspended animation" or in a "metabolic icebox" (that is although cardiorespiratory activity is greatly diminished, the reduced metabolic needs of the cold body are still being met). Severely hypothermic patients have been known to survive neurologically intact for long periods of time even if they are in asystole. If the patient is not breathing, and the airway appears to be patent, initiate CPR and transport the patient immediately to a hospital with critical care capabilities.

Resuscitation should be initiated in the accidental hypothermic patient using the same procedures as for normal resuscitation (See Chapter 4). Commence resuscitation at 30 compressions to two ventilations using high-quality CPR and transfer immediately to hospital; do not try and rewarm in the field, as this will prolong the arrest/resuscitation phase without any specific outcome. VF may be resistant to defibrillation below 30 °C and some authorities have suggested that it be withheld after the first attempt until the core temperature has been rewarmed to at least 30 °C. Adrenaline Repeated adrenaline dosage should also be withheld at low temperatures as drug metabolism is slowed. Resuscitation should continue until the athlete reaches hospital and core rewarming has been attempted, usually by extracorporeal circulation at a rate of 8–12 °C per hour. Hyperthermia must be avoided at all costs.

Therapeutic temperature management (TTM) is now the recommended management of a postcardiac arrest patient who has achieved return of spontaneous circulation (ROSC). In most facilities, patients are actively cooled to a core temperature of between 32 and 34 °C and maintained at this level for approximately 24 h. This cooling reduces cerebral metabolic rate for oxygen by 6% for each 1 °C reduction and production of harmful neurotransmitters (glutamate and dopamine). Recent studies have questioned the ideal temperature and have suggested that a target core temperature of 36 °C produces outcomes equivalent to the lower range and local protocols reflecting the latest advice should be followed. Studies to determine optimal temperature management are ongoing. Therapeutically induced hypothermia should not be confused with accidental hypothermia.

Frostbite

Frostbite is the freezing of tissue usually seen in the face (especially the nose and ears), hands, and feet. Damage to frostbitten tissue is caused by ice crystal formation in tissues, by resulting changes in electrolyte concentration within cells and by the destruction of capillaries required for oxygen exchange with the tissue. Damage occurs during the freezing process and during reperfusion. Tissue temperatures must be well below freezing for frostbite to occur. Frostbite does not usually occur at air temperatures above −7 °C. Contact frostbite can occur rapidly due to direct contact with very cold objects that have high thermal conductivity (e.g., metal). Note that tissue cannot become frostbitten when immersed in cold water, but may freeze after removal and exposure to very cold air.

The onset and severity of frostbite is affected by air temperature, wind speed, duration of exposure, amount of exposed area, insulation, blood flow, and predisposing conditions such as the following:

1. Poor or inadequate insulation from the cold or wind
2. Impaired circulation from tight clothing, including gloves, mittens, or footwear
3. Fatigue
4. Injuries
5. Dehydration
6. Hypothermia

Frostbite is classified as superficial or deep. It is often difficult to distinguish clinically between the two categories, even after frostbite has been thawed. The older classification, first through fourth degree, is not useful clinically.

Superficial frostbite affects the dermis and shallow subcutaneous layers of the skin. It is characterized by white- or gray-colored patches. The affected skin feels firm, but not hard. The skin initially turns red and, once frostbitten, is not painful. No tissue loss will occur if superficial frostbite is treated with rapid rewarming.

Deep frostbite affects the dermal and subdermal layers. It may involve an entire digit or other body part. The affected skin is white or gray and feels hard and cold. A pulse cannot be felt in the deeply frostbitten tissue and skin will not rebound when pressed. Tissue loss will result even with rapid rewarming.

Frostbite prevention requires covering and insulation of all exposed skin, including the face, during very cold temperatures. Hands and feet should be protected by adequate insulation. Mittens, including "lobster-claw" mittens are better than gloves. Handwear and footwear should not be too tight. A common error is to wear too many pairs of socks or socks that are too thick, resulting in constriction of the feet, which decreases blood flow and increases risk of freezing. It should be noted that frostbitten areas are at higher risk of future frostbite because of damage to capillaries and nerves that may subsequently result in decreased circulation (and therefore delivery of heat) to the area.

Clinical Findings/Management Frostbite

White or gray skin is an early sign of frostbite. Numbness of the hands or feet are symptoms of imminent frostbite or nonfreezing cold injury. Healthcare providers should carefully monitor athletes for signs or symptoms of frostbite. In some sports, it is also important for athletes to keep an eye on each other, looking for early signs and symptoms of frostbite. Athletes should remember never to accept numbness. This is a sign that skin receptors and afferent nerves are cold enough that they are not functioning properly. If they cool further, they will cease functioning and the athlete may incorrectly assume that no feeling means the situation has improved. In fact, the tissue is at risk of freezing. Skin numbness is a warning that the athlete should do something to prevent frostbite, either by increasing insulation, active warming, or seeking shelter from the cold exposure.

Management:

Potentially life or limb-threatening conditions, including hypothermia, must be evaluated and treated prior to the treatment of frostbite.

Any athlete with possible frostbite should immediately be removed from the FoP and brought into a warm area. The definitive treatment for frostbite is thawing the frostbitten area in warm water (37–39 °C). Frostbite of the face or ears can be gently rewarmed with a warm washcloth. If a thermometer is not available to measure water temperature, a healthcare provider should be able to leave his/her hand in the water without discomfort; this should prevent burning the patient's skin. If warm water is not available, frozen tissue may be thawed by pressing it against the warm skin of a colleague or medical provider (e.g., the chest or axilla).

Do not do the following:

1. Rub the frozen part
2. Apply ice or snow
3. Attempt to thaw the frostbitten part in cold water
4. Attempt to thaw the frostbitten part with high temperatures such as those generated by stoves, fires, engine exhaust, and heating pads; these might result in burn injury to an area where thermal sensors are not functioning to warn the patient of impending burning

Tissue, which has been frozen, thawed, and refrozen is severely damaged and will likely be lost. The decision to thaw frostbitten tissue in the field commits the healthcare provider to a course of action that may involve pain control, maintaining warm water baths at a constant temperature and protecting the tissue from further injury during later transport. If a frostbitten foot is rewarmed in the field, the patient should not walk on it. If just toes are frostbitten, the patient may still be able to walk after they are rewarmed, but only if there is no chance of refreezing.

Transport

If transport time is short (less than 2 h), the risks posed by improper rewarming or refreezing outweighs the risks of delaying treatment for deep frostbite.

If transport time is prolonged (more than 2 h), frostbite will often thaw spontaneously. In the field, it is more important to treat or prevent hypothermia than to rewarm frostbite rapidly in warm water. This does not mean that a frostbitten extremity should be kept cold to prevent spontaneous rewarming. Anticipate that frostbitten areas will rewarm as a consequence of keeping the patient warm and protect these areas from refreezing at all costs.

In most cases, the patient should be transported as soon as possible. When frostbite is mild, is not complicated by other injuries, and there are resources available to care for the patient without transport, it may be appropriate not to transport the patient to a medical facility. This should only be done in consultation with a doctor knowledgeable in the treatment of frostbite.

Determine whether frostbitten tissue will be rewarmed in a medical facility. If so, transport the patient while protecting the tissue from further injury by wrapping it with a bulky dressing and insulation.

Frostbitten tissue should be handled gently before, during, and after rewarming.

Stabilizing for Transport

When moving a patient with frostbite by helicopter, care must be taken to protect the patient from additional exposure to cold due to the increased wind chill caused by rotor wash.

Assess and treat the patient for hypothermia and other injuries, if present.

Assess frostbitten areas carefully. Loss of sensation may cause the patient to be unaware of soft tissue injuries.

Most patients with frostbite will be volume-depleted. Administer intravenous or intraosseous boluses of warmed normal saline for volume replacement.

Remove jewelry and clothing from affected areas.

If there is frostbite distal to a fracture, attempt to align to ensure maximal circulation. Splint the fracture in a manner that does not compromise distal circulation. A patient with frostbitten feet may walk prior to rewarming if necessary for evacuation or rescue. Once frostbitten feet are rewarmed, the patient probably will not be able to walk.

Rewarming

If the decision is made to rewarm a frostbitten extremity in the prehospital environment, prepare a warm water bath in a container large enough to accommodate the frostbitten tissues without touching the sides or bottom of the container. The temperature of the water bath should be in the range 37–39 °C (the caregiver should be able to leave a hand in the water without thermal discomfort). This temperature range is lower than that recommended by many older guidelines. Using water at or just above normal body core temperature limits pain without significantly slowing rewarming. A source of additional warm water must be available to keep the bath at the proper temperature. Cold tissue will rapidly cool the surrounding water. Water should be maintained at approximately 37–39 °C and gently circulated around the frostbitten tissue until the whole frostbitten part becomes flushed (pink colored). This process usually takes about 15–30 min.

Ideally, a temperature-controlled whirlpool bath should be used for rewarming.

Administer analgesics and anxiolytics as needed. Pain after rewarming usually indicates that tissue has been successfully rewarmed.

After rewarming, let the frostbitten tissues dry in warm air. Do not towel dry or rub the injured area in any way.

After rewarming, tissues with deep frostbite may develop blisters or appear cyanotic. Large blisters are usually filled with clear or cloudy fluid and may be tensely distended. These may be drained by sterile needle aspiration if necessary for dressing the wound or for transport. Small, hemorrhagic blisters should not be drained.

Pad between affected digits and bandage affected tissues loosely with a soft, sterile dressing. Do not put pressure on the affected parts.

Rewarmed extremities should be kept at a level above the heart, if possible.

Protect the rewarmed area from refreezing and other trauma during transport. A frame around the frostbitten area can be constructed to prevent blankets from pressing directly on the injured area.

Patients who clearly have only superficial frostbite can be treated as outpatients if they have no other medical problems such as hypothermia that require admission. They must have appropriate resources and appropriate follow-up must be arranged. All other patients with frostbite should be admitted to a hospital unit that has experience in caring for patients with frostbite. Inappropriate amputations are commonly performed by doctors inexperienced in caring for frostbite patients. Normally, a line of demarcation separates living tissue from mummified tissue that will not survive. However, the line of demarcation on the surface hides live tissue that usually extends well past the line of demarcation.

Nonfreezing Cold Injuries (NFCI)

These injuries include trench foot, immersion foot, and pernio (chilblains).

Trench foot and immersion foot are identical injuries that are caused by prolonged exposure to cold wet conditions that do not cause actual freezing of tissue. Usually, the feet are affected, but hands are also susceptible to NFCI. Trench foot is caused by exposure to cold wet conditions on land and immersion foot is caused by exposure to cold water. These injuries are often associated with immobility and usually require days to develop fully. Early injury may develop in a few hours, however, especially with repeated exposures. Combined injury with frostbite and nonfreezing cold injury may occur.

Pernio consists of localized nodular lesions in susceptible patients. Pernio is caused by exposure to cold with less moisture than the amount necessary to cause trench foot or immersion injury. An unusual form of pernio, equestrian pernio, may affect the lateral thighs of riders. Pernio from brief cold exposure during river crossings has also been described.

Prevention of nonfreezing cold injury is best accomplished by the use of appropriate handwear and footwear, keeping feet and hands dry and avoiding constriction. Feet should be inspected daily for signs of injury. Athletes who are susceptible to pernio may need to pay special attention to keeping hands and feet warm and dry.

Initial assessment of NFCI: In the first stage of trench foot or immersion foot during cold exposure, injured tissue will usually be completely anesthetic. The extremities are initially bright red but later turn pale or white. There is no pain or swelling unless attempts are made to rewarm the affected part. The second stage (prehyperemic) begins immediately after removal from cold exposure and usually lasts a few hours, although occasionally it can persist for several days. The extremities turn a mottled pale blue, but pigmented skin can obscure the color change. The affected parts remain cold and numb. Swelling may take place. Long-range sequela may include chronic severe pain and decreased circulation with increased risk for further cold injury.

Pernio takes several hours to develop and will seldom be diagnosed in the field.

Management of NFCI

Potentially life-threatening conditions, including hypothermia, must be evaluated and treated prior to treatment of NFCI. The patient should be brought to a warm environment as soon as possible.

There is no standard initial treatment regimen for trench foot or immersion foot. Injured parts should be elevated and warmed as soon as possible. Unlike frostbite, rewarming should not be rapid as the goal is to relieve discomfort rather than to thaw frozen tissue. If it is clear that the injury does not involve freezing, standard treatment is slow rewarming in air. Under no circumstances should nonfreezing cold injuries be exposed to snow or ice. Mixed frostbite and NFCI injuries require rapid rewarming for the frostbite injury (in 37–39 °C water) if the frostbite has not already thawed.

Pernio should be treated by drying and gentle massage. Active rewarming is contraindicated.

Bibliography

Giesbrecht, G.G. (2000) Cold stress, near drowning and accidental hypothermia: a review. *Aviation, Space, and Environmental Medicine*, **71**, 733–752.

Giesbrecht, G.G. & Wilkerson, J.A. (2006) *Hypothermia, Frostbite and Other Cold Injuries: Prevention, Survival Rescue and Treatment*. Mountaineers Books, Seattle, WA.

Imray, C. & Castellani, J. (2012) Nonfreezing cold-induced injuries. In: Auerbach, P.S. (ed), *Wilderness Medicine*, 6th edn. Elsevier, Mosby, Philadelphia, PA.

Luks, M. *et al.* (2010) Wilderness Medical Society consensus guidelines for the prevention and treatment of hypothermia. *Wilderness & Environmental Medicine*, **21**, 146–155.

McIntosh, S.E. *et al.* (2011) Wilderness Medical Society practice guidelines for the prevention and treatment of frostbite. *Wilderness & Environmental Medicine*, **22**, 156–166.

Department of Health and Social Services. Division of Public Health. Section of Community Health and EMD. *State of Alaska Cold Injury Guidelines* (2014). www.hypothermia.org/hypothermia_Ed_pdf/Alaska-Cold-Injuries.pdf.

25 Severe Dehydration and Exertional Heat Illness

Eunice M. Singletary

Department of Emergency Medicine, University of Virginia, Charlottesville, VA, USA

Introduction

Athletes are typically accustomed to prophylactic hydration prior to sporting events and thus serious dehydration is not a common medical illness encountered on the Field of Play (FoP). Environmental conditions however, especially over the course of several days and in the face of endurance competitions, can alter mechanisms of heat dissipation during thermal stress and contribute to dehydration, electrolyte imbalance, and exertional heat-related illnesses. The primary consequence of dehydration and minor exertional heat illness is impaired exercise performance. Exertional heat stroke (EHS) is a life-threatening illness with end-organ damage (most commonly involving the central nervous system (CNS)) that can lead to cardiac dysrhythmias, rhabdomyolysis, fluid and electrolyte disturbances, acute kidney injury, hepatic failure, coagulopathy, and death. Exercise-associated hyponatremia (EAH) is defined as a serum or plasma sodium level below the normal reference range of 135 mEq/L during or up to 24 h post-prolonged physical exertion or endurance events. It is the result of overhydration (i.e., ingestion of >1500 mL/h) and persistent secretion of arginine vasopressin (antidiuretic hormone), with subsequent impaired urinary water excretion. When symptomatic, EAH may result in collapse, significant mental status changes, seizures, and/or coma due to cerebral edema and less commonly, noncardiogenic pulmonary edema and death. Signs and symptoms of EAH can overlap with heat illness or dehydration, making diagnosis and proper field treatment difficult without point of care (POC) testing.

This chapter addresses the prehospital emergency diagnosis and treatment of several potentially life-threatening conditions seen in the sporting environment, including the following:

1. Severe dehydration
2. EAH
3. Exercise-associated (heat) muscle cramps (EAMC)
4. Heat syncope
5. Exertional heat exhaustion (EHE)
6. EHS

Fieldside Observation and Observations on Approaching the Athlete

Prior to competition, the team doctor should be aware of environmental conditions, which may place the athlete at risk of dehydration or heat illness and have adequate

The IOC Manual of Emergency Sports Medicine, First Edition. Edited by David McDonagh and David Zideman.
2015 International Olympic Committee. Published 2015 by John Wiley & Sons, Ltd.

supplies and equipment to care for heat illness. High ambient temperatures, combined with high humidity or a high "wet bulb globe temperature" (WBGT) reading will limit the ability of an athlete to effectively cool via evaporation of sweat. When high WBGT readings occur for several consecutive days of competition, this places further stress on an athlete's thermoregulation and ability to stay adequately hydrated.

1. Has the athlete had adequate time to acclimatize to the environmental conditions?
2. Establish if the athlete has collapsed without any preceding or associated trauma. A lack of trauma prior to collapse suggests a medical etiology such as dehydration, heat illness, cardiac dysrhythmias, or hypoglycemia
3. Did the athlete appear to have difficulty with coordination, or were they confused prior to collapse? An athlete, who develops mental status changes while exercising under conditions of high ambient temperature and without preceding trauma, should be presumed to have EHS until proven otherwise. Syncope and collapse are common symptoms of severe dehydration as well as EHS, but without significant mental status changes
4. Look to see if the patient is motionless or exhibiting seizure-like activity. Seizure-like activity may be the result of a preexisting seizure disorder, but it may also be associated with heat stroke or EAH

Primary Survey Severe Dehydration or Heat Illness

Begin with a quick survey of the scene and determine if the patient is conscious. If the patient has collapsed but is conscious, note if they are able to speak or seem confused or disoriented:

1. Is there obvious pilo-erection?
2. Does the patient appear to be in shock with cool, diaphoretic skin?
3. Is the patient hyperventilating?

Obtain a focused history, asking if the patient recalls what happened and what symptoms preceded the event:

1. Was the patient feeling lightheaded, dizzy, short of breath, or experiencing any pain prior to collapse?
2. Does the patient have a headache, nausea, chills, tingling sensations, or muscle cramps?
3. Were prophylactic hydration regimens followed prior to the event?
4. Has body weight been monitored and if so is there a record of weight gain or loss?
5. Does the patient have any medical condition or take any prescription medication that might predispose them to dehydration or heat illness?

If the patient has collapsed and is not conscious, begin the primary survey with the ABCDE mnemonic. Initiate cardiopulmonary resuscitation immediately if the patient is pulseless or apneic. Severe dehydration and exertional heat illness may be associated with hypotension, tachycardia, and tachypnea, but cardiac arrest suggests an alternative etiology.

Skin, mucous membranes, and body temperature Note if the skin is profusely diaphoretic or relatively dry. Moist cool skin is commonly seen with EHS and dehydration:

1. Are the eyes sunken?
2. Is there decreased turgor of the skin?

Core body temperature is a critical vital sign needed to differentiate between heat illness, dehydration, and EAH. As soon as practical, probably in the athlete medical room, obtain a core temperature using a rectal thermometer capable of reading extremely high temperatures. EHE is accompanied by the following:

1. Warm or hot skin
2. Signs of dehydration

3. A body temperature between 38.5 and 40 °C
4. Piloerection is a common finding with heat exhaustion

EHS is associated with a core temperature >40 °C. When hyperpyrexia is accompanied by mental status changes in the absence of head trauma, heat stroke is the likely culprit.

Blood Pressure and Pulse

Severe dehydration and heat stroke are associated with hypotension, which may result in loss of peripheral pulses and delayed capillary refill. Tachycardia is common with both dehydration and heat-related illness.

Lungs and musculoskeletal system If auscultation is possible, lungs are typically clear with heat illness despite tachypnea. Pulmonary edema and respiratory distress may suggest EAH. Muscle cramps, spasm, and tetany are occasional findings with heat illness.

Neurological With heat stroke/hyperthermia, neurological manifestations in the form of mental status changes are the sine qua none and distinguish this disorder from other forms of heat illness. Mental status changes in the face of normal or mildly elevated core temperature suggests EAH.

FoP Management Dehydration, Exercise-Associated Hyponatremia and Heat-Related Illness

Athletes with a heat-related illness or dehydration and who are alert and without mental status changes should be moved to a shaded area or a cool indoor rest area and allowed to rest while rehydrating. Oral rehydration is recommended with cold water or an electrolyte replacement fluid, with a goal of an intake of 1–2 L over an hour. However, it may require 24–36 h to fully rehydrate. If the athlete is unable to tolerate oral hydration (due to vomiting or progression of symptoms), intravenous hydration with normal saline or D5 normal saline will be necessary along with evaluation for end-organ damage. If the athlete has suspected heat injury, they should be observed in a fully equipped medical facility for progression of the illness.

EHS is a medical emergency and requires immediate treatment by rapid lowering of the core body temperature.

Initial resuscitative efforts and stabilization must be accompanied by rapid cooling. Shade the patient from sun or quickly move him/her to a shaded area. The most effective means of cooling is by cold water immersion up to the patient's shoulders. This can be accomplished using an inflatable pool or bath filled with ice water. If cold water immersion is not an option, use bed sheets soaked in ice water to cover the patient, including the head, and change or recool sheets every few minutes so that you are continuously applying cold sheets. The moist sheet will also enhance cooling by evaporation, which can be augmented by fans or fanning. Ice packs applied to the anterior neck, axillae, and groin are useful cooling adjuncts but are not effective alone. If ice is not available, use sheets wetted repeatedly with large volumes of tap water and fans to promote evaporative cooling.

FoP treatment of athletes with symptoms suggestive of EAH depends on the availability of POC testing for hyponatremia and the presence or absence of severe neurological or respiratory symptoms. It is also critical to differentiate between EAH and dehydration or heat illness, as the provision of isotonic or hypotonic fluids to someone with EAH can worsen hyponatremia resulting in disastrous consequences.

First, assess the volume status of the individual. If hypotension is present, intravenous fluids are indicated. In the face of suspected EAH with hypotension, hypotonic intravenous fluids should be avoided. Unfortunately, EAH can develop in the face of oliguria, making it extremely difficult to differentiate between EAH and dehydration. Fluid replacement is indicated for dehydration; fluid restriction in the face of dehydration may result in acute renal failure or cause further injury in the presence of rhabdomyolysis. Thus, the benefit of withholding fluids for suspected EAH versus the potential harm from withholding fluids for severe dehydration must always be considered.

1. *Where POC sodium measurement is not available*: If the blood pressure is stable in an individual with suspected mild symptoms of EAH and POC and sodium measurement is not available, treatment can be either fluid restriction or oral hypertonic solutions if tolerated, using (for example) three to four cubes of bouillon in 100 mL water, until the onset of urination. If the patient develops progressive neurological deterioration, a 100 mL bolus of 3% hypertonic saline should be considered if available and can be repeated twice at 10-min intervals while arranging transport to a medical facility.
   EAH can be difficult to recognize and if the FoP/athlete medical room treatment is unsuccessful, the patient should be transported immediately to advance care and the clinical suspicion of this diagnosis should be relayed to the Emergency Medical Service (EMS) and hospital personnel. If respiratory symptoms are present, administer oxygen at a rate of 2–4 L/min.
2. *POC sodium testing is available*: If POC testing for hyponatremia confirms the diagnosis of EAH, treatment is guided by the presence of absence of severe neurological or respiratory symptoms. In the absence of such symptoms, individuals with confirmed hyponatremia can be advised to limit fluid intake and to ingest salty snacks or hypertonic (~9%) saline solutions, such as three to four cubes of bouillon in 100 mL water, until urination resumes. If neurologic symptoms progress, treatment must be rapidly initiated with intravenous 3% hypertonic saline using 100 mL boluses delivered via a peripheral vein over 60 s. If cerebral symptoms do not improve, repeat treatment with hypertonic saline at 10-min intervals up for two further doses and prepare to transport the patient to an emergency medical facility for ongoing care.

   In the presence of symptoms of suspected severe EAH, if a POC sodium level is >/=135 mmol/L, consider alternative diagnoses such as hypoglycemia or heat stroke.

Specific Conditions

Severe dehydration:

Dehydration is by definition, a state of hypertonic hypovolemia brought about by a net loss of hypotonic body fluids. It is caused by sweat loss from exercise or heat stress, by inadequate fluid intake, or by osmotic diuresis from glycosuria. Gastrointestinal fluid losses are considered negligible except with diarrheal illness, which is a consideration during travel. Urine output varies as a mechanism for regulating water balance, averaging 1–2 L/day, so that net water gain equals water loss. In athletes, hydration guidelines are used to minimize water deficits but needs can vary with activity, body size, and the environment in which the athlete lives or exercises in. When net body water balance is disrupted by excessive fluid loss or inadequate intake, dehydration results. Physical exercise performance begins to degrade in temperate, warm, or hot environments once dehydration progresses to >2% body weight loss and may be the only sign or symptom of dehydration. As dehydration progresses, exercise performance degrades proportionally and additional signs and symptoms develop. With severe hypernatremic dehydration, thermoregulatory control is compromised and neurological symptoms may portend cerebral edema, intracranial hemorrhage, hemorrhagic infarcts, and permanent brain damage. Dehydration is a risk factor for the development of heat exhaustion and EHS. Symptoms of severe dehydration include headache, dizziness, fatigue, thirst, orthostasis, or syncope

Findings:
1. Diminished skin turgor, sunken eyes, evidence of diminished sweating, and dry oral mucous membranes
2. Elevated pulse rate, weak pulse quality, and delayed capillary refill
3. Blood pressure ranging from low normal to hypotension

When evaluating an athlete with signs and symptoms of dehydration, the triad of thirst, decreased body mass weight and/or increased concentration of urine, makes the diagnosis of dehydration likely.
Treatment:
1. Treatment begins with prevention using customized regimens for hydration of athletes
2. Once excessive dehydration develops (>2% body weight reduction from baseline body weight), athletes should drink ~1.5 L of fluid for each kilogram of body weight loss and when possible, this should occur over time and with sufficient electrolytes, rather than via large boluses to improve fluid retention
3. Salty snacks and beverages will promote a rapid and complete recovery by stimulating thirst and fluid retention
4. There is no advantage to using intravenous fluids for rehydration unless an athlete is unable to tolerate oral fluids
5. Severe dehydration (>7% body weight loss) with abnormal vital signs warrants intravenous fluid replacement with normal saline or D5NS. If a baseline body mass index is known, fluid loss can be estimated by bioimpedance measures or body weight, if available, but this may be difficult to obtain in the presence of orthostasis or hypotension. Urine osmolarity and specific gravity (SG) are other means to assess for hydration, with a euhydration SG level cutoff of <1.020 g/mL

Exercise-associated hyponatremia (EAH)

EAH is defined as a rapid reduction in serum or plasma sodium below the normal reference range of 135 mmol/L, during or up to 24 h after prolonged exercise. EAH may be asymptomatic in up to 50% of cases. Rates of symptomatic EAH vary widely with the duration of exercise and with different forms of exercise: approaching 38% in marathon and ultramarathon competitors. Mild symptoms include fatigue, weakness, nausea, vomiting, headache, dizziness, and oliguria. More severe symptoms include confusion, obtundation, coma, seizures, and respiratory distress. The pathogenesis of EAH is excessive fluid intake combined with impaired urinary water excretion due to persistent secretion of arginine vasopressin. In athletes, the primary risk factor is overhydration, which may be reflected by weight gain during exercise. Other possible contributing factors include excessive sodium loss from sweat, the inability to mobilize sodium stores, and atrial and brain natriuretic peptide elevations

Findings:
1. A normal to slightly elevated body temperature
2. Tachycardia and orthostasis
3. Varying degrees of mental status changes, hyperreflexia, seizures, and coma
4. Noncardiogenic pulmonary edema with tachypnea and hypoxia on pulse oximetry
5. Serum sodium levels if measurable by POC testing are <135 mmol/L

Treatment

1. If POC testing is not available:
   a. *Mild symptoms:*
      i. Fluid restrict or oral ingestion of salty snacks, hypertonic solutions such as three to four cubes of bouillon in 100 mL water until urination occurs
   b. *Progressive neurological symptoms or severe EAH*:
      i. Administer 3% hypertonic saline: 100 mL over 60 s via peripheral IV, repeating twice at 10-min intervals if no improvement
      ii. Transport by EMS to hospital. Communicate concern for possible severe EAH to medical staff
      iii. If hypertonic saline not available, establish saline lock and avoid hypotonic fluids
      iv. Administer oxygen at 2–3 L/min for symptoms of respiratory distress
   c. *If POC sodium testing available and hyponatremia confirmed*:
      i. Mild symptoms may be managed with fluid restriction or oral hypertonic saline/salty snacks until urination resumes
   d. *Progressive or severe symptoms*:
      i. Administer 3% hypertonic saline; 100 mL over 60 s via peripheral IV, repeating twice at 10-min intervals if no improvement
      ii. Transport to hospital. Communicate concern for possible severe EAH to medical staff
      iii. Administer oxygen at 2–3 L/min for symptoms of respiratory distress

Exercise-associated muscle cramps

Heat cramps are brief, intense muscle cramps in the arms, legs, or abdomen and are associated with dehydration, muscle fatigue, and electrolyte deficiencies, particularly when not acclimatized to heat. Profuse sweating with large quantities of sodium sweat losses may predispose to cramps

Findings:

1. Vital signs are normal or as expected with pain and strenuous exercise
2. Profuse diaphoresis may be present
3. Visible muscle spasm

Treatment:

1. Gentle stretching and physio massage of the affected muscle
2. Rest
3. Oral rehydration with electrolyte-containing fluids. Avoid salt tablets due to GI irritation

Heat syncope

Heat syncope or fainting is caused by blood pooling in the cutaneous or skeletal vasculature. It is more common in unacclimatized, dehydrated individuals following prolonged standing or after standing up quickly following lying or sitting down.

Findings: may be similar to those of dehydration:

1. Orthostatic changes with blood pressure and pulse
2. Body temperature is normal

Treatment:

1. Move the patient to a cool environment
2. Encourage oral hydration

Exertional heat exhaustion (EHE)

EHE is a mild-to-moderate heat illness associated with an inability to sustain cardiac output. It is frequently associated with dehydration and an elevation of core temperature between 38.5 °C and 40 °C. EHE can occur in relatively cool temperatures but is more common during exercise in temperatures >33 °C, with an air velocity <2 m/s, in those with a BMI >27 and in the presence of dehydration. As for EHS, EHE is more common in conditions of high humidity where evaporative cooling from sweating is impeded. EHE can progress to a more severe form of heat injury with end-organ damage. Symptoms include headache, nausea, fatigue and poor exercise performance, dizziness, and vomiting. Exercise training in heat for 7–9 days has been shown to improve acclimatization and reduce the risk of developing EHE

Findings:

1. The athlete with EHE may or may not have collapsed
2. *Skin*: Diaphoresis, pilo-erection, ashen color, and possible tenting
3. Hypotension: Elevated heart rate and respiratory rate
4. Core temperature ranging from 38.5 to 40 °C
5. A normal mental status examination, lack of neurological findings, and core temperature </=40 °C helps distinguish severe EHE from EHS

Treatment:

1. Remove the patient to a shaded cool area and maintain in a recumbent or supine position until blood pressure and orthostasis resolve
2. Remove or loosen restrictive or excessive clothing
3. Administer oral fluids with a ≤6% carbohydrate electrolyte solution with a goal of 1–2 L in the first hour. If oral fluids are not tolerated, administer normal saline intravenously
4. Initiate effective cooling measures with evaporative techniques or icepacks
5. Monitor mental status, core temperature, body weight, and urine SG. Once symptoms improve and are clinically stable, the athlete may be released with a friend or family to continue rest and hydration
6. Do not allow the athlete to return to exercise on the same day. For milder forms of EHE, the athlete may return to exercise in 24–48 h

Exertional heat stroke (EHS)

EHS is a medical emergency defined as follows:

1. Hyperthermia (core body temperature >40 °C) at the time of collapse
2. Multiorgan failure, most commonly involving the CNS

   Strenuous exercise in a hot and humid environment (especially with WBGT above 28 °C), lack of acclimatization to heat, and poor physical fitness are considered the main risk factors. However, highly trained and acclimatized athletes can develop EHS during high-intensity exercise if heat production exceeds heat dissipation. EHS may occur in the absence of significant dehydration.

Risk factors for EHS include the following:

1. Obesity
2. Lack of heat acclimatization
3. Cumulative effect of multiple days of heat exposure
4. Dehydration
5. Previous history of EHS
6. Sleep deprivation
7. Sweat gland dysfunction
8. Sunburn
9. Viral illness
10. Diarrhea
11. Medications with anticholinergic effects that may inhibit sweating

Signs and symptoms are initially subtle and include irrational or unusual behavior, inappropriate comments, clumsiness or stumbling, irritability, or headache. Symptoms can progress to confusion, hyperventilation, vomiting, seizures, collapse, or loss of consciousness. A change of performance or personality should trigger an evaluation for EHS.

Findings:
1. Core body temperature >40 °C
2. Systolic BP <100 mmHg, tachycardia, and tachypnea
3. A shock appearance with cool, diaphoretic skin
4. Varying degrees of CNS dysfunction from confusion to obtundation, seizures, or coma

Treatment:

The recognition of EHS is paramount to survival.
1. Maintain an open airway
2. Initiate immediate whole body cooling to <39 °C. In the absence of other life-threatening complications, cooling should be completed on site if possible, prior to transportation to advanced medical care
3. Cool
   a. Best accomplished with whole body cold-water immersion
   b. If not available, use ice water-soaked towels or sheets applied to the head, trunk, and extremities and rapidly replace towels
   c. Misting or covering the patient with water-soaked sheets and fanning is useful but most effective when relative humidity is low and evaporative cooling occurs
4. Establish a large bore IV access and begin rehydration with normal saline
5. Antipyretics are ineffective and not recommended
6. Transport to hospital; if the athlete's mental status returns to normal on scene with cooling measures, do not allow them to return to competition. A gradual return to training may be allowable 1 week following discharge from medical care

Bibliography

American College of Sports Medicine, Sawka, M.N., Burke, L.M. *et al.* (2007) American College of Sports Medicine position stand. Exercise and fluid replacement. *Medicine & Science in Sports & Exercise*, **39** (**2**), 377–390.

Armstrong, L.E., Casa, D.J., Millard-Stafford, M., Moran, D., Pyne, S.W. & Roberts, W.O. (2007) American College of Sports Medicine position stand: exertional heat illness during training and competition. *Medicine & Science in Sports & Exercise*, **39** (**3**), 556–572.

Brad L. Bennett, Tamara Hew-Butler, Martin D. Hoffman, Ian R. Rogers, Mitchell H. Rosner (2013). Wilderness Medical Society Practice Guidelines for treatment of exercise-associated hyponatremia. *Wilderness & Environmental Medicine* **24**, 3, 228–240, DOI: 10.1016/j.wem.2013.01.011.

26 Hypo- and Hyperglycemia

Kathryn E. Ackerman[1,2,3,4] *and David McDonagh*[5,6,7]

[1]*USA Rowing, Boston, MA, USA*
[2]*Female Athlete Program, Division of Sports Medicine, Boston Children's Hospital, Boston, MA, USA*
[3]*Sports Endocrine Research Lab, Neuroendocrine Unit, Massachusetts General Hospital, Boston, MA, USA*
[4]*Harvard Medical School, Boston, MA, USA*
[5]*Emeregency Deptartment, St. Olavs Hospital, Trondheim, Norway*
[6]*Faculty of Medicine, NTNU - National University of Science and Technology, Trondheim, Norway*
[7]*Medical Commission, AIBA - International Boxing Association, Lausanne, Switzerland.*

Diabetes mellitus (DM) is a chronic endocrine disorder characterized by hyperglycemia due to either decreased insulin secretion, decreased insulin action, or both. While many athletes with DM are well controlled, changes in physical activity combined with alterations in DM treatment and/or diet may cause unexpected hypoglycemia. Prolonged hyperglycemia is less commonly seen in a competing athlete with DM; however, transient hyperglycemia is often seen in sprinting and very high-intensity bouts of exercise.

Type 1 DM accounts for 10–15% of all cases of diabetes. It is characterized by the destruction of beta cells, leading to deficient insulin production but normal insulin sensitivity. Type 2 DM accounts for the vast majority of the other 85–90% of cases and is characterized by variable abnormalities in insulin secretion and insulin sensitivity. Both types of diabetes, in the uncontrolled state, will have increased hepatic glucose output and decreased glucose uptake in muscle and adipose tissue. However, in general, only patients with type 1 DM are at risk of severe lipolysis leading to diabetic ketoacidosis (DKA).

Various secondary causes of DM have been recognized and new categories of DM are being added as we learn more about genetic and environmental predisposing factors. But for the team doctor considering treatment modalities, it is most important to know if the athlete's disease is more similar to type 1 or type 2. Also knowing the athlete's general, diabetes control is important in anticipating their response to athletic activity and medical treatment. Thus, in this chapter, variations of DM will only be referred to under the global categories of "type 1" and "type 2."

Hypoglycemia

There are many factors that may play a role in the development of hypoglycemia during exercise. These include exercise intensity and duration, blood glucose concentrations before initiating exercise, the time relation of exercise to meals, basal/bolus

The IOC Manual of Emergency Sports Medicine, First Edition. Edited by David McDonagh and David Zideman.

insulin doses, an individual's physical fitness level, the athlete's insulin sensitivity, and the adequacy of the athlete's counterregulatory responses to exercise.

In the nondiabetic population, insulin levels decrease during exercise, however, in those with insulin-dependent diabetes insulin levels do not decrease with activity. Increased insulin impairs hepatic glucose production and can induce hypoglycemia 30–60 min after exercise begins. This is particularly the case with prolonged aerobic activity. Counterregulatory hormones (e.g., glucagon, catecholamines, growth hormone, and glucocorticoids) may be impaired in patients with neuropathy or frequent hypoglycemic episodes. In addition, exercise improves insulin sensitivity in skeletal muscle, leading to postexercise, late-onset hypoglycemia, often at night when the athlete is sleeping. In fact, in patients with type 1 DM, exercise increases the risk of severe hypoglycemia up to 31 h after cessation of activity. This is a potentially dangerous scenario.

Clinical Findings Severe Hypoglycemia

Conduct a primary survey including the basic neurologic assessment known by the mnemonic AVPU (alert, verbal stimuli response, painful stimuli response, or unresponsive). The patient may be unresponsive or may react slowly to verbal or pain stimuli.

Findings: Initially, milder symptoms will present. If the blood glucose level continues to fall, neuroglycopenic symptoms may be observed and include fatigue, blurry vision, impaired cognition, loss of coordination, aggression, confusion, seizures, and loss of consciousness.

Management: Check blood glucose. If patient is unconscious and/or unable to ingest carbohydrates and blood glucose is low:

Alternative 1: Dextrose: Administer 25 mL of 50% dextrose solution IV. Recheck blood sugar approximately 10 min after the dextrose bolus. When the patient has regained consciousness, administer supplemental carbohydrates orally.

Alternative 2: Glucagon: Administer a glucagon injection using, for example, a glucagon emergency kit (requires mixing prepacked powder and dilution fluid). Inject the mixture (1 mL) either IM or SC. This gives 1 mg of glucagon. Normal response time is about 10 min. As with dextrose, administer supplemental carbohydrates orally once the patient has regained consciousness. Recheck blood sugar 10 min after administering glucagon.

Alternative 3: If the athlete does not respond to either glucagon or 50% dextrose, rapidly transfer to a medical facility. Administer another dose of either 1 mg glucagon IM/SC or 50 mL 50% dextrose IV. If the athlete regains consciousness and is able to swallow, have the athlete eat complex carbohydrates (e.g., bagel, crackers).

The patient should be monitored at the event or medical facility and should not be discharged until he/she has normal blood sugar levels and is clinically normal. Same day return to play is not recommended. Fortunately, most well-trained athletes with DM are aware of their disease and know how to manage it.

There are variations in practice in the management of hypoglycemia with some authorities recommending the use of 20% Dextrose infusions instead of the higher 50% Dextrose solution. Local and national guidelines should be followed.

Mild hypoglycemic reactions are more likely when an insulin-dependent athlete is fasting or participating in endurance events.

Clinical Findings Mild Hypoglycemia

Symptoms: There is variation in the blood glucose level at which hypoglycemia occurs in different people as well as variability in different individuals' hypoglycemia symptoms. Early autonomic symptoms include sweating, tachycardia, palpitations, hunger, nervousness, trembling, headache, and dizziness. In general, signs and symptoms of hypoglycemia often occur when blood glucose drops below 70 mg/dL

(3.9 mmol/L). It can be challenging to differentiate between the exhaustion from vigorous exercise and early hypoglycemic symptoms.

Management:

Scenario 1

Symptomatic hypoglycemia in an alert patient with blood glucose levels between 50 and 70 mg/dL (2.8 and 3.9 mmol/L).

Administer 15 g of fast-acting solid (e.g., glucose tablets and honey) or liquid carbohydrates (e.g., juice and sugar-rich drink). Recheck blood sugar after 15 min and if still low, administer another 15 g of fast-acting carbohydrates and add 15 g of complex carbohydrates (e.g., bagels and crackers).

Recheck blood glucose after another 15 min. If glucose is in the normal range, the athlete is NOT on a long-acting glucose-lowering medication and is feeling better, monitor for 15–30 min and then consider allowing return to play. If the athlete is on a long-acting glucose-lowering drug, continue to monitor and do not allow return to play until after peak of medication has passed.

Scenario 2

Symptomatic hypoglycemia in an alert patient with blood glucose levels ≤50 mg/dL (2.8 mmol/L).

The athlete will usually have some form of neuroglycopenia symptoms. Administer 25–30 g of fast-acting solid or liquid carbohydrates.

Recheck blood glucose after another 15 min. If glucose is still low, readminister another 15 g of fast-acting carbohydrates and add 15 g of complex carbohydrates. Keep checking blood glucose and adding carbohydrates until normal blood glucose levels have been achieved. Do not allow same day return to play.

Hyperglycemia

Exercise may cause hyperglycemia in patients with DM. In athletes who are underinsulinized and/or have poor baseline control, exercise (particularly high-intensity, anaerobic exercise) leads to increases in blood glucose levels and may eventually lead to DKA. High-intensity exercise is associated with increases in catecholamines, free fatty acids, and ketones, all of which decrease muscle glucose utilization and increase blood glucose. In the well-controlled athlete, these changes may be transient (decreasing in 30–60 min), but poor insulin balance along with stress regarding sports performance may increase counterregulatory hormones and perpetuate the hyperglycemia.

Clinical Findings Hyperglycemia

Symptoms do not usually present until glucose levels are over 200 mg/dL (11 mmol/L).

As with hypoglycemia, some symptoms present early, allowing the athlete to adjust to activity, dietary intake, or medication.

Early symptoms include frequent urination, increased thirst, blurred vision, headache, and fatigue.

If hyperglycemia goes untreated, DKA may develop. Findings may include the following:

Nausea, vomiting, dry mouth, dyspnea, weakness, confusion, coma, abdominal pain, and classically a sweat fruit-smelling breath.

Management:

Type 1 DM:

1. 250–300 mg/dL (13.9–16.7 mmol/L): Check for urinary ketones, and if positive, do not allow exercise. If negative, ok to perform physical activity.
2. >300 mg/dL (16.7 mmol/L): Check for ketones, and if negative, may exercise with extreme caution.

Type 2 DM:

1. ≤350 mg/dL (19.5 mmol/L): May exercise.
2. >350 mg/dL (19.5 mmol/L): Do not allow to exercise. Hydrate and adjust the insulin/dietary regimen.

An athlete who experiences a change in mental status that does not improve within 15 min of treatment should be taken immediately to hospital.

Insulin Pumps

Athletes using insulin pumps receive insulin through a continuous subcutaneous infusion. They may have basal insulin settings that are consistent throughout the day (e.g., 1.0 unit/h for 24 h) or vary (e.g., 0.5 unit/h from midnight to 6 am, 1.2 unit/h from 6 am to 12 pm, 1.0 unit/h from 12 pm to 5 pm, 1.4 unit/h from 5 pm to midnight, etc.). In addition, pump users have bolus insulin doses administered prior to meals. Insulin pump settings may be adjusted prior to activity based on trial and error similarly to injectable insulin guidelines (See Table 26.1).

Activity	Exercise duration	Peaking insulin adjustment
Low, moderate, or high intensity	<30 min	No adjustment
Low intensity	30 to >60 min	Decrease by 5%
Moderate intensity	30–60 min	Decrease by 10%
	>60 min	Decrease by 20%
High intensity	30–60 min	Decrease by 20%
	>60 min	Decrease by 30%

Table 26.1 Injectable insulin adjustment guidelines (individual needs vary!)

Depending on the activity and athlete preference, pump users may discontinue the pump during sport and switch to injectable insulin. If the pump is removed before physical activity, hyperglycemia is more of a risk and a long-acting injectable insulin should be used appropriately. If the pump is continued during activity, pump malfunction or detachment (e.g., from contact or sweat) may lead to hyperglycemia, overinsulinization, and subsequent hypoglycemia. Pump athletes who experience hyper- or hypoglycemia should always have their pumps examined at the beginning of the athlete assessment.

Continuous Glucose Monitors

Continuous glucose monitoring (CGM) systems use a small sensor inserted under the skin to check glucose levels in tissue fluids. The sensor may stay in place for several days to a week and then must be replaced. A transmitter sends information about glucose levels to a wireless monitor. Because currently available CGM devices are not as accurate and reliable as standard blood glucose meters, they need to be recalibrated frequently against conventional glucose meters.

Advice to Athletes with DM Prior to an Event

Each athlete with DM should have a care plan for training as well as for matches/games/races.

Fasting glucose should be checked. The preexercise meal should be ingested 1–3 h before the activity, should consist of low glycemic index foods, and should include protein to ensure continuous, but not too rapid, glucose absorption. Immediately prior to the activity, the athlete should check blood sugar again, with an ideal goal of 120–180 mg/dL (6.7–10 mmol/L). The athlete should continue to monitor their blood glucose throughout the sporting activity, supplement with carbohydrate when needed, and continue to hydrate and reassess every 30–60 min depending on their baseline control and exercise level.

Often as athletes become more experienced with their glucose control and training habits, these intervals may lengthen. Elite athletes often get to an awareness of their personal responses to exercise such that they know when to consume extra carbohydrates or check a blood sugar based on exercise duration and/or symptoms. Those using insulin should inject in areas away from exercising muscles approximately 1 h before activity, as exercise, massage, and heat can increase the rate of absorption. If possible, the athlete should try to anticipate the intensity and duration of activity to better adjust insulin dosing and carbohydrate intake.

Bibliography

Albright, A., Franz, M., Hornsby, G. *et al.* (2000) American College of Sports Medicine position stand. Exercise and type 2 diabetes. *Medicine & Science in Sports & Exercise*, **32** (7), 1345–1360.

Colberg, S.R. *et al.* (1997) American College of Sports Medicine and American Diabetes Association joint position statement. Diabetes mellitus and exercise. *Medicine & Science in Sports & Exercise*, **29** (**12**), i–vi.

Beazer, R.S. (2007) *Joplin's Diabetes Desk Book – A Guide for Primary Care Providers*, 2nd edn. Joplin Diabetes Center, Boston.

Chu, L., Hamilton, J. & Riddell, M.C. (2011) Clinical management of the physically active patient with type 1 diabetes. *Physician and Sportsmedicine*, **39** (**2**), 64–77.

http://www.diabetes.org

http://www.insulindependence.org

Inzucchi, S.E. (2007) *Diabetes Facts and Guidelines*. Yale Diabetes Center/Takeda, New Haven.

Jimenez, C.C., Corcoran, M.H., Crawley, J.T. *et al.* (2007) National athletic trainers' association position statement: management of the athlete with type 1 diabetes mellitus. *Journal of Athletic Training*, **42** (**4**), 536–545.

Modigliani, G., Iazzetta, N., Corigliano, M. & Strollo, F. (2006) Blood glucose changes in diabetic children and adolescents engaged in most common sports activities. *Acta Biomedicine*, **77** (**Suppl 1**), 26–33.

Sigal, R.J., Kenny, G.P., Wasserman, D.H., Castaneda-Sceppa, C. & White, R.D. (2006) Physical activity/exercise and type 2 diabetes: a consensus statement from the American Diabetes Association. *Diabetes Care*, **29** (**6**), 1433–1438.

27 Wound Care

David McDonagh[1,2,3] *and Sally Whitmore*[4]

[1]*Emeregency Deptartment, St. Olavs Hospital, Trondheim, Norway*
[2]*Faculty of Medicine, NTNU - National University of Science and Technology, Trondheim, Norway*
[3]*Medical Commission, AIBA - International Boxing Association, Lausanne, Switzerland.*
[4]*District Nursing, UK*

Wounds are common in sports and can present as bruises, abrasions and burns, lacerations, punctures, blisters, or a combination of all these. Athletes tend to regard minor wounds as part of normal "wear and tear" and not much more than a minor irritation. However, seemingly minor wounds can, if left untreated/poorly treated, lead to serious infection and longer periods away from active sport.

FoP or Fieldside Management

Follow the ABCDE mnemonic approach (see Chapter 3) remembering that potentially catastrophic life-threatening hemorrhage must be controlled before the airway and breathing assessment. If a team of healthcare professionals are present, then one member should deal with the catastrophic hemorrhage immediately, while the other members assess the airway, breathing, and circulation. Each medical team must have access to a range of appropriate dressings, pressure dressings, hemostatic dressings, and possibly tourniquets if there is a danger of severe hemorrhage (see Chapter 6). Each member of the FoP medical team must be familiar with the use and application of all dressings (and tourniquet if included).

Clean the wound with bottled water and make a rapid assessment of how extensive the wound is. In some sports (if the International Federation (IF) permits), small cuts can be rinsed, cleaned, and covered with a nonadhesive dressing and finally a circular pressure bandage to stop minor venous seepage. Suturing or definitive wound care can wait until after the event, particularly if at a major competition. This may not be possible in other sports as removal from the FoP will result in disqualification of the athlete. However, if further wound evaluation or treatment is necessary, it is advised to remove the athlete to the athlete medical room for definitive treatment. Evaluate all wounds for underlying structural damage before deciding on further treatment and define if the wound is clean, clean contaminated, or contaminated/infected.

When evaluating wounds one must consider the following:

1. Is there significant bleeding?
2. Is the bleeding arterial or venous?

The IOC Manual of Emergency Sports Medicine, First Edition. Edited by David McDonagh and David Zideman.

3. If arterial bleeding continues despite continuous manual pressure, consider the need for arterial ligature. If ligature is possible and the doctor has the necessary skills, then remove the athlete to the medical room for suturing. If ligature is not possible, then the athlete should be removed to hospital for surgical treatment.
4. Once bleeding has been controlled, evaluate wound dimensions, for example, depth (superficial, partial, full thickness), length, width, and so on.
5. Note the anatomical position of the wound and relation to fixed anatomical landmarks, supraclavicular, midclavicular line, distance from the umbilicus, and so on.
6. Examine underlying or nearby structures for function before considering wound closure.
7. Examine carefully for foreign bodies, a good case history is imperative.
8. Note the time of injury and take a good case history, then classify the wound as follows:
   a. Clean (unlikely in a sporting environment) – Clean contaminated: a wound involving normal but colonized tissue.
   b. Contaminated: a wound containing foreign or infected material
   c. Infected: a wound with pus present.

This is an wound classification is important as clean wounds should be closed immediately, clean contaminated can usually be closed, whereas contaminated and infected wounds should be left open, treated with oral antibiotics and left to heal by secondary intention. Most sporting wounds can be classified as clean contaminated, though some may be defined as being contaminated.

When clean and clean contaminated wounds are more than 6–8 h old (opinions vary on this time factor), many recommend that the wound be cleaned, left open, and then closed by delayed primary closure after 48 h. Per oral antibiotics are often used.

1. Can the cut be treated with tape, strips, and wound glue or is suturing required?
2. Consider removing the athlete to the medical room for wound closure. Should the wound be closed using tape and glue or by suture? (see below).
3. Should the athlete be referred to hospital? Can the athlete return to play?

Wound Location

Wound location has significance in relation to the likelihood of there being complications and thus the need for monitoring and possibly hospitalization. Never close the wound if there is a suspicion of a muscle, ligament, major nerve, or capsule injury. If in doubt, cover the wound with a wet saline bandage and transfer the patient to hospital for further evaluation.

Evaluate the wound length, depth and location, the presence of bleeding, and the proximity of important structures (tear ducts, facial nerve, etc.). It is important to examine for underlying fractures; if these are present, then arterial bleeding should be stopped, if possible, by gentle compression. Arterial bleeding from a scalp wound may represent an underlying cranial fracture, so evaluate the patient's neurological status.

Wounds should be cleaned with saline and covered with a damp saline dressing. If on the Field of Play, clean the skin and irrigate the wound with saline while protecting the patient's eyes. Gross removal of foreign bodies is recommended, followed by gentle compression with a saline bandage. Once the athlete is taken to the medical athlete room, further evaluation and treatment can be conducted. The doctor must be aware of their own own surgical competency, particularly when dealing with hand or facial suturing, as there are several facial areas that require precise surgical technique, particularly with lacerations affecting the vermillion, the nostrils, eyebrows, and lacrimal duct.

If the decision is to suture, then the wound inspection and cleansing must be repeated. Debridement may be necessary, but if so, consider referring to a specialist clinic. Similarly, if there are damaged underlying structures, refer the athlete for specialist care.

If all is well and the choice is made to close the wound, close with simple monofilament 4/0 or 5/0 nonabsorbable sutures. If competent, then attempt to use intradermal or subdermal sutures as these often enhance the cosmetic result. Reinforce the sutured wound with several skin tapes, preferably at a 90° angle to the wound. For facial wounds, recommend that sutures be removed after 5 days, followed by supportive skin tape for a further 7 days; this reduces scarring and patients may avoid the "zipper" scar. A total of 12 days is usually sufficient before removing sutures from the upper extremity, whereas 14 days is often required for wounds to the torso, lower extremities, and over large joints. If there is suspicion of wound contamination, then prophylactic antibiotics may be recommended.

Larger lacerations and particularly those associated with tissue loss should be referred to a specialist unit. Attempt to stop bleeding, clean and irrigate the wound, remove all foreign material, and either cover the wound with a sterile saline bandage or gently pack the wound with sterile saline dressings.

Reassessment of Wounds and Dressing Changes

It is recommended that most wounds requiring treatment be reexamined after 24 h to allow for review of the wound, the integrity of the dressing(s), and any signs of infection. The exact extent of this reexamination and the requirement for dressing changes is a matter of professional judgment of the medical staff.

Specific Wounds/Injuries

Lacerations of the mouth, tongue, and lips (see Chapter 15). These lesions are best treated in a medical room. Most buccal lacerations should be sutured; however, some smaller lacerations can be left alone. After the event, the athlete should be advised to rinse the mouth frequently and to try a liquid diet for a few days, thus avoiding food particle entrapment. Cuts to the tongue may also need to be sutured, particularly if the wound is deep or there is significant bleeding.

If the lip needs to be sutured, then inject local anesthesia with adrenaline into the wound on each side and avoid piercing the lip again, as this often causes more bleeding. Waiting 5 min to allow the swelling from the injection to disappear facilitates correct realignment. Rinse the wound thoroughly. If possible, place the sutures on the buccal aspect of the lip and/or place a subcutaneous absorbable suture in the body of the lip, thus potentially allowing the front of the lip to be taped and glued for better cosmesis.

If the cut goes through the labial vermillion, then careful apposition and proper anatomical realignment with respect to anatomical subunit borders is important. This can usually be achieved by placing the first suture through the vermillion on each side of the cut; the borders can be marked with a pen before suturing. Vermillion borders can, however, be difficult to assess due to lack of definition or swelling, so consider referral to a specialized surgical unit if precise cosmesis is an issue.

Lacerations around the eye (see Chapter14) Beware cuts around the eyes and nose. Cuts involving the eyelids should be referred to a specialist. Similarly, cuts medial to the eye may encroach upon the lacrimal apparatus, so these wounds should also be referred to specialist treatment.

Lacerations in the temporal region Lacerations that affect the superficial temporal artery may cause profuse bleeding. There are two possible treatment options; external compression (often the best choice) or ligation of the artery proximal to the bleed placing a deep broad suture (using 3.0 non-absorbable thread) through the skin, to the bone, under and around the artery, then out through the skin again and knot the suture. This closed suture, that is, performed without a skin incision, may help stop profuse bleeding but requires skill and experience. The patient should be referred for further observation.

Laceration of facial nerves Deep lacerations may sever the supraorbital, supraglottic, infraorbital, facial, or trigeminal nerves. The Emergency doctor must be aware of these nerve locations and test for sensory and motor function before suturing. If a nerve lesion is found, then it is advisable to compress the wound with a saline-soaked bandage and refer to hospital.

Lacerations over joints Wounds over a joint necessitate the need for proper clinical assessment before closure. Cuts over the knees and hands are not unusual and may result in muscle, tendon, ligament, or capsular dysfunction locally and distal to the wound. If intact and function is normal, evaluate the wound for bleeding and if none, close the wound after thorough cleaning and apply an elasticized stretch bandage to prevent swelling and bleeding postoperatively.

Scalp wounds Scalp wounds can cause profuse venous bleeding (see Chapter 10).

Clenched fist human bite wounds Bites by humans do occur and can be intentional or accidental, classically when another athlete's teeth puncture the skin of the hand causing a wound.

These wounds are seldom large and the main concern is that of infection after a puncture wound. It is rare to have structural damage to muscles, nerves, capsules, etc., as human teeth are not that sharp. The commonest site of injury is over the dorsal surface of the metacarpophalangeal (MCP) joints, the so-called clenched-fist injury when a clenched fist comes into contact with another individual's teeth causing a small wound of the dominant hand. Skin, capsule, and extensor tendon injuries, even fractures, may occur. Approximately 10–15% of human bite wounds become infected. Infections can spread along the extensor tendons and deep purulent infections, often presenting several centimeters away from the initial wound. These infected wounds often require hospitalization with intravenous antibiotics and not unusually, open surgery. Prophylactic antiobiotics are usually recommended. Many recommend that bite wounds be left open and closed by secondary healing.

Wound hygiene, ice, and compression Saline solution and tap water are the most commonly used wound cleansing agents. If unsure of how clean tap water is, then bottled water may be used. The aim of wound cleaning is to remove foreign bodies and dead tissue and also to maintain the healing environment. The use of ice packs on swollen and lacerated wounds may be beneficial in preventing further swelling, however, may not be optimal for lacerated wounds, remembering that the optimal temperature for tissue repair is body temperature. Macrophages do not function properly at lowered temperatures. Elasticized compression bandages can be used both before and after wound closure. Wound debridement is best conducted in a medical room or surgical unit.

Glue and tape versus suture As a general rule, if there is no bleeding, tape and glue are effective. If there is bleeding, suturing is usually necessary. Tape and glue are usually used for small (wound width of 3 mm or less), straight edged, and nonbleeding wounds. Wounds that are bleeding, deep, with jagged edges should usually be sutured. Glue and tape seldom work with arterial bleeds as the wound usually swells up and the tape loosens. The bleeding also affects the tape's adhesiveness.

Always test for function at and distal to the wound, clean the skin, and wait for the skin to dry before closing the wound. Apply a compression bandage and evaluate the athlete's ability to return to play. As a rule, athletes can return to play (depending on the sport) if there is no fracture, head injury, organ contusion, or muscle/ligament or joint injury.

There are several ways of using glue. Glue can be applied directly into the wound, followed by apposition of the skin edges, which are held in position by the ED's fingers or by the use of tape. Another method is to adapt the wound with tape at a 90° angle to the wound with an equal amount of tape on each side of the wound (to ensure equal traction and better cosmesis) and leaving space between the strips as with sutures. This allows the ED to follow the line of the cut and helps prevent buckling of the skin. Glue can then be used to adhere the tape to the skin.

Some glues irritate wound tissue and patients may experience a mild burning sensation. Occasionally, some colored glues may cause pigmentation of scar tissue in white skinned patients. Avoid getting glue into the eyes as the eyelids can be glued together! Once the glue has dried, cover the wound with a thin dressing and then apply an elasticized stretch bandage to compress the wound. This prevents further swelling and bursting of the closed wound. Avoid using many or very thick dressings as this will just soak up more blood and reduce the compression effect.

Remove devitalized skin flaps (epidermal) as these often become necrotic. If the skin flap includes dermis, then it usually survives, so flap removal is not recommended unless circulation is definitely compromised.

Consider the need for antibiotics and vaccines

Tetanus Vaccines

Tetanus is acquired when a wound is infected with the spores of the bacterium *Clostridium tetani* but can be prevented through immunization. The World Health Organization Position Paper states: "The exact timing of the booster doses should be flexible to take account of the most appropriate health service contacts in different countries," as vaccination regimes vary from country to country. If an athlete has followed the recommended vaccination program, then they should have approximately 10 years of protection after their last booster, though the need for vaccination after a wound is usually based on a definition of that wound being clean or contaminated.

Burns, Abrasions, and Blisters

First- and second-degree burns and abrasions can occur after falls on artificial surfaces (cycling, road races, tennis, field hockey, winter sliding sports, etc.) and roads (marathon runs) causing asphalt burns.

Clean the wound with sterile water/saline. For asphalt burns, scrubbing the wound may be necessary (this is painful – dripping local anesthetic onto the wound may help, and creams tend to have a slow onset). Use a sterile surgical hand and nail scrub brush and try to remove all discoloration from the skin – this prevents infection and discoloration of scars.

Remove foreign bodies, stones, grass, and so on. Cover the wound with a nonadherent contact dressing pad held in place with a simple compression bandage, or a manufactured nonadherent pad attached to an adherent bordered dressing.

Blisters can be emptied on the second day and dead skin removed using a pair of small scissors. Leave 2–3 mm of skin at the wound's edge. For athletes wishing to continue their sport, a Duoderm, Comfeel, Angel Skin pad can be applied. Make sure the pad covers the whole of the sore and at least 10 mm of healthy skin. On the basis of the currently available evidence, blisters should wherever possible be left intact to reduce the risk of infection, but if anatomical position necessitates intervention for functional purposes, aspiration appears to result in less pain than deroofing.

Third-degree burns are unusual in most sports, but can occur. Treatment is as mentioned earlier, but as most surgical centers recommend skin transplantation, and referral to the local burns/surgical unit is probably advised. Prophylactic antibiotics are recommended in some centers as infection increases the depth of tissue damage. It is not absolutely vital that surgery takes place immediately, so an athlete may wait a couple of days and thus travel home, before receiving a surgical evaluation.

Artificial Grass Burns

While artificial grass sports fields have several advantages, they also have some potential drawbacks. Obviously, there is a risk of abrasions/burns caused by sliding over these synthetic fibers but increased rates of methicillin-resistant *Staphylococcus aureus* (MRSA) infections have also been reported in these wounds.

Friction Blisters

These develop in areas of constant friction, most typically on the feet or hands. Moisture contributes to their development. There have been some conflicting studies about the use of antiperspirants to prevent friction blisters. If blisters are painful, a small incision to allow drainage, but leaving the roof intact, may help during competition. There may be predisposing inflammatory conditions such as allergic or contact dermatitis, urticaria, or exercise-induced angioedema. Prevention of blisters can be achieved by keeping the feet dry, choosing correctly fitting shoes, using a thicker pair of socks, removing foreign bodies from the shoe, but they can still occur despite these preventative procedures. Blisters can be treated as burn injuries described above and using sterile hydrocolloid bandages.

Bruises and Contusions

There are several scales for classifying bruises, but they remain rather esoteric and obviously open for individual interpretation by the ED. Follow the PRICES mnemonic (protect, rest, ice, compression, elevation, support).

Splinters

Splinters are a foreign body, and on occasion can be problematic to remove. In general terms, they can be removed with a pair of fine tweezers and the entry wound cleaned and left to heal by secondary intent. Subungual splinters and deep splinters may well require anesthetic and surgical incision, preferably in the athlete medical room. Older splinters should be referred to a specialist as should those affecting ligaments, tendons, joints, or nerves.

Which Dressing?

There is no such thing as "the perfect dressing," with compromises having to made in each aspect of wound care and management. Whether the intention is to assist healing via moist wound healing and healing by secondary intention or to provide primary closure by suturing, there are an array of products available. A new (April 2014) online resource from *Wound Care Today*: woundcare-today.com/categories-pyramid/wound-contact-layers may provide assistance in the choice of bandage or dressing.

Bibliography

Marr, J.S., Beck, A.M. & Lugo, J.A. Jr. (1979) An epidemiologic study of the human bite. *Public Health Reports*, **94** (**6**), 514–521.

28 The Role of the Paramedic on the Field of Play

Mike Nolan[1] and David Whitmore[2]

[1]*Emergency Services, County of Renfrew, ON, Canada*
[2]*London Ambulance Service NHS Trust, London, UK*

In preparation for deployment to a major sports event, the paramedic must ensure an intimate knowledge of all planning, logistical, and operational considerations related to their role. It is highly recommended that any paramedic looking to work at a major sports event should gain experience beforehand at smaller but similar events. Even the most experienced paramedic may well find dealing with a cardiac arrest, fractured pelvis, or a life-threatening asthma attack on the Field of Play (FoP) challenging. Confidence in the surroundings and the others in the FoP team will increase the likelihood of enjoying the whole experience. This chapter focuses on the following:

1. Tasks the paramedic has to perform, both before and during the event
2. The relationship between doctor and paramedic
3. The legal aspects of emergency intervention

Planning and Logistics

With large-scale sporting events, it is necessary for the paramedic to understand the care and transportation expectations related to key participants. Participant groups often have individualized plans associated with their care and destinations in times of crisis. It is important to understand the transportation plan and to be aware of the intended receiving hospital/facility entrance and any security requirements for paramedic access and egress while providing care.

In addition to plans individualized to the FoP, the paramedic must be knowledgeable of event plans such as hospital notification systems, communication infrastructure, mass casualty plans, mass fatality plan, syndromic surveillance plans, severe weather plan, suspicious package plan, evacuation procedures, and security zone planning. Paramedics are ideally suited to bridge the planning and operational gap between the health systems and the security systems at large sporting events. Paramedics routinely work within both the public safety and health care spheres. They share common language and purpose with both groups and commonly function in a liaison role within multidisciplinary command operations. An example of this relationship role is exemplified in the traditional command and control structure utilized to deliver a paramedic service, yet providing health care as its primary function.

The paramedic must have a working knowledge of the event telecommunications guidelines and plans including the following:

1. Local emergency numbers
2. Call handling plan

The IOC Manual of Emergency Sports Medicine, First Edition. Edited by David McDonagh and David Zideman.

3. Venue emergency call plan including first responders
4. Radio call signs and priority codes, encrypted radio communications
5. Encrypted cellular phone communications
6. Subdued communications protocols
7. The use of direct land lines
8. Interoperable radio communications with offsite resources
9. Inventory controls and auditing
10. Satellite phone use
11. Dedicated communications support to commanders/command centers

If paramedics are expected to provide transportation services, they must adapt their stretcher mounts to accommodate enhanced requirements of the various shapes and sizes of athletes. The large heavy athlete may require specialized lifting and transfer equipment for sport-related injuries. The paramedic must ensure that the necessary venue access accreditation documentation is in place for all vehicles and occupants. Close collaboration with security officials is essential to establish vehicle security sweep protocols so as not to delay emergency exit transfers, or a return to the venue. If using an emergency vehicle, the paramedic must understand the event traffic management plan and road closures, and create response, and transport routes for all possible destinations to and from each event location. The paramedic is responsible for ensuring the availability and proper care of their vehicle, equipment, and supplies at all times.

Clinical Practice

The paramedic works within a framework of self-regulated and/or regulated clinical practice dependent on jurisdiction. They provide care based on evidence-based practice through their licensure level standards, clinical guidelines, and/or standing orders from a doctor or medical committee, professional body, or regulatory body (or combinations thereof). It is recommended that individual paramedics establish both clinical and operational expectations with all members of the medical team, that is, the venue medical manager, doctor, physiotherapist, ski patrol, marine rescue, etc. in advance of deployment at an event. It is crucial that the paramedic and sports doctor have a common understanding of each other's roles and responsibilities prior to engaging in athlete care. There must be a full understanding of who will provide initial medical assessment, treatment and coordinate extrication of athletes from the FoP. This should be a fully integrated response and rehearsed regularly using the FoP team of the day. The FoP Medical Team will, in all probability, be part of a multidisciplinary healthcare professional team whose collective skill base is relevant to the sport and who have all been trained in FoP assessment, treatment, and extraction (see Chapter 3)

The paramedic may be required to make accurate, rapid assessments, based on their interpretation of the mechanism of injury, presenting signs, symptoms, and history of the patient as part of the FoP team approach. Treatment decisions are typically made autonomously pertaining to the presenting medical condition and will follow current best practice guidelines such as Basic and Advanced Resuscitation, prehospital trauma management, or local medical protocol dependent on the environment and the availability of resources.

In an interdisciplinary team setting, the paramedic will work collaboratively to contribute their areas of expertise while maximizing the contribution of allied health professionals such as doctors, nurses, and physiotherapists. Where interventions may be required beyond the predetermined scope of independent practice of the paramedic, medical consultation or additional orders may be sought from a doctor. The doctor/paramedic relationship must be preestablished through mutually agreed upon clinical guidelines, training requirements, quality assurance mechanisms, and clear lines of communication given the dynamic environment of a large sporting event.

Paramedic Provider Levels

In many jurisdictions, there are two levels of paramedic qualifications; these are "Paramedic" and "Advanced Care Paramedic" or similar terminology.

The paramedic can provide the following:

1. Emergency patient care
2. Assessment
3. Immobilization
4. Extrication
5. Oxygen therapy
6. Mechanical ventilation
7. Basic trauma life support
8. Cardiopulmonary resuscitation

The paramedic is also licensed to perform a number of controlled medical acts for individuals experiencing acute injury or illness.

The basic paramedic skill set includes the following:

Laryngeal mask airway with $E_TCO_{2\ monitoring}$
CPAP
Pulse oxymetry monitoring
Peripheral intravenous cannulation
12-lead ECG application and interpretation of ST elevation myocardial infarction
Defibrillation
Blood glucose testing
Administration of medications such as acetylsalicylic acid, antiemetics, antihistamines, adrenaline, nitroglycerine spray, salbutamol inhalation, glucagon, and glucose gel

The Advanced Care Paramedic skill set includes the following

1. Advanced airway management
2. Orotracheal and nasotracheal intubation
3. Laryngeal mask airways
4. Orogastric and nasogastric tubes
5. Suction
6. SpO2 monitoring
7. Side stream E_TCO_2 monitoring (capnography and capnometry)
8. Mechanical ventilation
9. CPAP
10. Laryngoscopy and removal of foreign body obstruction using Magill forceps
11. Intravenous therapy
12. 12-lead ECG interpretation
13. Cricothyrodotomy
14. Needle thoracostomy
15. Chest tube monitoring
16. Intraosseous and external jugular IV cannulation
17. Manual defibrillation, synchronized cardioversion, and external transcutaneous cardiac pacing
18. Treatment of cardiac emergencies

Administration of medications according to Advanced Cardiac Life Support (ACLS) guidelines: (according to local protocol)

Cardiac Drugs
1. Adenosine
2. Adrenaline
3. Acetylsalicylic acid (aspirin) (ASA)
4. Atropine
5. Dopamine
6. Furosemide
7. Nitroglycerine

Sedatives and Analgesia
1. Diazepam
2. Midazolam
3. Morphine
4. Naloxone

Other Drugs
1. Ondansetron (or similar)
2. Dimenhydrinate (or similar)
3. Diphenhydramine
4. Glucagon
5. Lidocaine
6. Salbutamol
7. Sodium bicarbonate

Additional medications may be added based on anticipated need (see Chapter 30).

Medicolegal Considerations for the Paramedic Provider It is imperative that an individual paramedic is fully aware of any legal implication of practicing in what might be a foreign country, or even within a different state or jurisdiction within their own country.

Practitioners must be aware of any medicines, skills, or devices, which may not be allowed to be used and which would also limit their practice, as the paramedic may be required to use procedures which fall outside their normal scope of practice.

It will be necessary to check with the event organizer at least 6 months before the event that the temporary registration conditions are compliant with the requirements to practice as a paramedic. The local Olympic Games Organizing Committee will have established a detailed list of medication, equipment, and skills and drilled the FoP extrication process. The paramedic must be familiar with these procedures and agree that they fall within the individual's level of clinical competence and skills.

Additional Information

Paramedic competencies include those adapted from Paramedic Association of Canada, National Occupational Competency Profile, 2011 (www.paramedic.ca/nocp accessed December 20, 2013).

Professional Responsibilities

Function as a professional.
Possess an understanding of the medicolegal aspects of the profession.
Recognize and comply with relevant provincial and federal legislation.
Function effectively in a team environment.
Make decisions effectively.
Manage scenes with actual or potential forensic implications.

Communication

Practice effective oral communication skills.
Practice effective written communication skills.
Practice effective nonverbal communication skills.
Practice effective interpersonal relations.

Health and Safety

Practice safe lifting and moving techniques.
Create and maintain a safe work environment.

Assessment and Diagnostics

Conduct triage in a multiple-patient incident.
Obtain patient history.
Conduct complete physical assessment demonstrating appropriate use of inspection, palpation, percussion, and auscultation.
Assess vital signs.
Utilize diagnostic tests.

Therapeutics

Maintain patency of upper airway and trachea.
Prepare oxygen delivery devices.
Deliver oxygen and administer manual ventilation.
Utilize ventilation equipment.
Implement measures to maintain hemodynamic stability.
Provide basic care for soft tissue injuries.
Immobilize actual and suspected fractures.
Administer medications.

Integration

Utilize differential diagnosis skills, decision-making skills, and psychomotor skills in providing care to patients.
Provide care to meet the needs of unique patient groups.
Conduct ongoing assessments and provide care.

Transportation

Prepare ambulance for service.
Drive ambulance or emergency response vehicle.
Transfer patient to air ambulance.
Transport patient in air ambulance.

Health Promotion and Public Safety

Participate in the management of a chemical, biological, radiological/nuclear, explosive (CBRNE) incident.

29 The Role of the Physiotherapist on the Field of Play

Mark Brown[1], Michael Kenihan[2] and Marie-Elaine Grant[3,4]

[1]Sports Medicine Australia, Oceania National Olympic Committee Medical Commission, Griffith University Centre of Musculoskeletal Research, Southport, QLD, Australia
[2]Sports Medicine Australia, Albert Park, Victoria, Australia
[3]IOC Medical Commission (Games Group)
[4]Institute of Sport and Health, University College Dublin, Dublin, Ireland

Introduction

The IOC Sport Medicine Manual (International Olympic Committee 2000), which provides an introduction to the 2006 and 2009 versions of the IOC Medical Code, defines the physiotherapist as part of the sports medicine team and considers that all members of the team have the same obligation toward the athlete's well-being and also further recognizes that physiotherapists often travel with athletes and sporting teams without doctors. The physiotherapist has several functions at major sporting events, in addition to treatment and prevention of injuries; physiotherapists should consider their role in relation to emergency situations. Should the physiotherapist be working as part of a larger medical team where team physicians are available: the doctor will lead the management of an emergency situation. However, in certain cases, a physiotherapist may be traveling with a team alone and may be covering a sporting event with no other team physicians or paramedics covering the event at the same time.

The aim of this chapter is to outline the role and responsibility of the physiotherapist in the event of a medical emergency at a sporting event or training session in different scenarios such as the following:

1. An emergency situation when traveling with a team of athletes either nationally or internationally
2. An emergency situation either nationally or internationally where the physiotherapist is covering the event alone and there is no doctor or paramedic available
3. An emergency situation either nationally or internationally where the physiotherapist is working with other emergency professionals:
   a. Where a doctor is available
   b. Where a paramedic is available

The IOC Manual of Emergency Sports Medicine, First Edition. Edited by David McDonagh and David Zideman.
2015 International Olympic Committee. Published 2015 by John Wiley & Sons, Ltd.

The further aims of this chapter are to identify the skills that a physiotherapist should have in order to be able to provide a seriously injured or ill athlete with appropriate immediate emergency care and also to discuss the legal and ethical restrictions that must also be taken into consideration.

The World Confederation of Physical Therapy (WCPT) states that: "Physical Therapy provides services to individuals and populations to develop, maintain, and restore maximum movement and functional ability throughout the lifespan." Hence, the role and scope of practice of the physiotherapist in an emergency situation is not often clearly defined.

Physiotherapists who have undertaken postgraduate education in sports physiotherapy and who also have extensive experience in this area are recognized in many countries and use the title "sports physiotherapists." Throughout this chapter, the term physiotherapist is inclusive of sports physiotherapists and physiotherapists. (i.e., physiotherapy professionals who may work in sport but who may not necessarily have additional postsports physiotherapy qualifications). Physiotherapists have a responsibility to provide effective emergency care to the best of their ability. The ability of the physiotherapist to know both what to do in the event of a medical emergency, and also importantly what not to do, may be critically important to potentially saving an athlete's life and/or preventing further harm that may otherwise be caused by mismanagement of catastrophic injuries or medical conditions.

An Emergency Situation When Traveling with a Team of Athletes Either Nationally or Internationally

In many countries, it is a standard requirement that sports physiotherapists undertake first aid training to improve their ability to provide Field of Play cover at sports events. However, there is a wide variance internationally as to both the laws and also the sporting organizations and competition rules that are in place, as well as differences in the training and accepted scope of practice of physiotherapists. These variations create both a widely divergent range of necessary skills and also procedural restrictions, which affect the type of role the physiotherapist may undertake during an onfield medical emergency; hence, there is a global variance.

Factors to be Considered

The level of training and responsibility of physiotherapists for emergency response also varies between different countries. For example, in countries where physiotherapy training is at a more advanced level and where physiotherapists operate as first-contact practitioners, it is strongly recommended as a minimum requirement that sports physiotherapists undertake an approved first aid course including cardiopulmonary resuscitation (CPR) and recertify in first aid every 2–3 years and in CPR annually. In addition, sports physiotherapists often undertake additional training in emergency care, the management of concussion, suspected spinal cord injuries and also, though less commonly, Advanced Life Support (ALS) and Advanced Cardiac Life Support (ACLS). In Ireland and the United Kingdom, a high level of accreditation by the Association of Physiotherapists in Sports Medicine requires completion of approved courses in both first aid and sports trauma with recertification every 2 years. In the United States, in order to achieve Physical Therapy Specialist Certification in Sports within the Sports Physical Therapy Section (SPTS) of the American Physical Therapy Association, applicants must hold current certification in CPR, and SPTS also offers Emergency Medical Responder Courses which includes training in other components of emergency care.

While in some countries, first aid and emergency care is not considered as part of the role of the physiotherapist, and training may not be mandatory for sports physiotherapists, emergency and first aid training is nonetheless usually provided as part of undergraduate physiotherapy training programs.

Legal and Ethical Considerations (Both Nationally and Internationally)

The extent of the role and actions the physiotherapist may undertake in an emergency situation may be affected by their legal and ethical restrictions as established by their country's or state registration laws, and/or the rules established by the relevant professional association. These may therefore be different when traveling internationally, or even between states or territories within the physiotherapist's own country. In addition to the differences in the legal restrictions that exist, there can often be additional variations between sporting organizations procedures and even within specific sports, which may in turn further vary between different jurisdictions or levels of competition.

Scope of practice physiotherapy statements developed by many national regulating and professional physiotherapy bodies describes the role of the physiotherapist.

In some cases, the requirements for training and certification that relate to the legality or ethical appropriateness of the provision of emergency care by physiotherapists, is established within government legislation, the International Sports Federation or the National Physiotherapy Bodies. In other countries, legislation is silent on the matter of the role of the physiotherapist in the provision of emergency or first aid services.

In many countries, physiotherapists have a primary contact practitioner status (or direct access), which means physiotherapists can attend an injured athlete directly without the need for a medical referral. However, various differences between different sporting organizations' rules must also be taken into consideration. These rules may include important considerations such as under which circumstances a physiotherapist can enter the Field of Play to attend an injured athlete, as well as what procedures must be followed in the event of an emergency or acute injury situation. Physiotherapists who travel with their teams internationally must also be familiar with and comply with the laws and procedures of operation in that particular country.

Many people would argue that despite the apparent legal restrictions which may affect the physiotherapist's scope of practice, a competent person has an overriding ethical duty of care to assist in an emergency to the best of their ability. In some countries, the term "first responder" is applied to the first person to attend to a medical emergency. In many cases, the "first responder" is a physiotherapist, though generally the term incorporates an assumption that the first responder has at least some basic medical training such as a first aid course and that utilizing such training is a component of the person's designated role.

In the United States, state laws generally do not prohibit registered physical therapists from providing sports coverage. However, in some states of the United States, physical therapists require a physician's referral before assessing and treating a patient, while others do not. It is therefore important to identify in advance as to whether the physiotherapist is providing emergency care as a registered physical therapist, qualified in first aid.

There are some legal and ethical limitations as to what skills a physiotherapist can appropriately acquire or utilize, even in an emergency situation; this varies internationally. In some countries, physiotherapists are permitted to initiate advanced cardiac and trauma life support skills in the management of an athlete. But even though a physiotherapist may be able to recognize signs and symptoms of a tension pneumothorax, they cannot undertake any decompression procedures such as the insertion of a chest drain or perform emergency tracheostomies.

The Role of the Physiotherapist in Different Emergency Scenarios

The importance of the need for the physiotherapist to be clear about their role during an acute intervention situation, is referred to within the Sports Physiotherapy Competencies and Standards developed by the International Federation of Sports Physical Therapy (IFSPT) in section 2A:8, which calls upon sports physiotherapists to "locate information relating to specific regulations regarding the location of ultimate responsibility for first response in the event of injury or illness, whenever this is appropriate."

An Emergency Situation Either Nationally or Internationally Where the Physiotherapist is Covering the Event Alone and There is No Doctor or Paramedic Available

While ideally, teams should be accompanied by a doctor, particularly at high-risk sports events, it is often the case that only the physiotherapist covers moderate-risk sports events and regular training sessions where most injuries are minor or moderate in severity and often accompanies the team while traveling. Therefore, physiotherapists may find that they are the most qualified medically trained persons at sports events or training sessions. This necessitates that the skill set and scope of practice of physiotherapists is not confined only to the assessment and management of neuromuscular or musculoskeletal disorders, but also to emergency care. In the event of a medical emergency or catastrophic injury, the physiotherapist must be prepared and be able to provide immediate suitable emergency care, at least until more qualified medical care is available. Therefore, the skill set of a physiotherapist in these circumstances should include current competence in the recognition and management of medical emergencies.

The physiotherapist must establish in advance what procedures will be in operation for that particular event, especially those to be followed until the paramedics and/or physician reach the injured or ill athlete. Cooperation with local ambulance or other emergency services may also require establishing in advance the location of the nearest hospital or emergency center, as well as the communication procedures. These may also vary greatly from country to country, as well as possibly within countries, depending on factors such as state-specific differences and the location of the sporting or training venue.

When covering an event without a doctor or paramedic, the reasonable expectation of the physiotherapist in the event of an emergency situation is to be able to respond and address the emergency with competencies specified by the International Federation of Sports Physical Therapists (Competency 2). Physiotherapists who provide sideline coverage should have sufficient knowledge and skills to provide an onfield setting initial first response management of the following:

1. Cardiac and respiratory emergencies in sport
2. Torso injuries with abnormal vital signs
3. Major trauma including major bleeding, shock, major fractures, facial, and dental trauma
4. Suspected spinal injury

5. Head injuries with loss of consciousness and concussion, including sideline testing for return to play decisions
6. Environmental injuries and other medical conditions in sport, such as asthma, epilepsy, and hypoglycemic events and musculoskeletal issues, such as joint dislocations etc.

Onfield Assessment and Management

It is of vital importance that the physiotherapist undertakes a systematic approach to both the evaluation and treatment given in an emergency situation.

The primary role of the physiotherapist in those life-threatening injuries is to offer the patient-appropriate treatment. In order to achieve this, an agreed system for categorizing the injury severity must be in place.

Working with Other Emergency Professionals

An important additional factor that needs to be considered while planning the role of the physiotherapist in emergency situations is whether other medically trained personnel will be present.

1. *An emergency situation at a national or international event where the physiotherapist is covering and a physician is available*: In this situation, the doctor leads and the physiotherapist is in a position to provide care as a member of the emergency medical team. The physiotherapist is seldom at a venue alone, particularly at a time of major competitions; there will usually be other physiotherapists and team physicians available.

Categories of sports or events that can be considered as presenting relatively high risk are those that have potential for serious or life-threatening injury. In these cases, when organizing events for high-risk sports, it is suggested that the range of medical professionals required to be present at the event must include physicians supported by a therapist or a nurse and an ambulance with its attendants (See Chapter 3). The number of such professional teams of healthcare providers, including team doctors, will depend on the numbers of athletes involved in the location. For these reasons at competition, it is unlikely that the physiotherapist will be the only member of the healthcare team providing FoP cover.

2. *An emergency situation at an event either nationally or internationally where a paramedic and the physiotherapist are the only members of the multidisciplinary team available*:

In certain situations, it is likely that the team physiotherapist will be the most medically qualified person present who can provide immediate assistance as both the lead first responder and secondly coordinate and lead other healthcare professionals present in providing a coordinated and effective response.

IFSPT (Competency 2) codifies the importance of both preplanning and establishing in advance appropriate communication "with all other medical and site personnel in order to identify and establish the different responsibilities and lines of communication in case of injury or illness." The physiotherapist should "efficiently coordinate care in the acute sports emergency situation, to establish local processes and procedures for potential transfer of injured or ill athletes to medical facilities, including appropriate communication with:

1. ambulance personnel,
2. emergency department personnel and sports physicians, and
3. site personnel and other professionals."

Along similar lines, the IOC Sports Medicine Manual (International Olympic Committee 2000) describes one of the responsibilities of the medical team as the requirement to "establish an appropriate protocol among all members of the medical team for the management of a life-threatening situation."

It is likely that highly skilled emergency Healthcare professionals will be present at major sporting events and in these situations the role of the physiotherapist after the planning phase and during an actual emergency may revert to that largely of a first responder, providing additional assistance to the physicians or paramedics. If other medical personnel are present, sports physiotherapists should communicate with the other health professionals to establish in advance what each person's role will be in the provision of acute care, including the lines of reporting and communication.

If a doctor or paramedic is present and the physiotherapist is the in the role of first responder, the physiotherapist needs to be able to succinctly convey information about the cause of the problem, the signs and symptoms observed by them on initial examination of the athlete. They should also describe what treatment has been provided and also to convey any other medical information that has been previously identified. Appropriate records must also be documented.

At events when no doctor is available but paramedics are in attendance or may be called to attend, the team physiotherapist must establish in advance what procedures will be in operation for that particular event.

Regardless of whether other more highly trained emergency health professionals are in attendance, the duty of care of the physiotherapist to the athletes in his/her care is in no way abrogated and the physiotherapist must ensure that he/she is aware at all times of his/her athlete's condition and location.

Current and Future Emergency Management Skills and Training for Sports Physiotherapists

The IOC Medical manual section 6.2 states that: "Health care providers who care for athletes should have the necessary education, training and experience in sports medicine, and keep their knowledge up to date."

While there is variation between countries as to what legal and ethical constraints exist on the physiotherapist's scope of practice, the increased "globalization" of sport and sports medicine has highlighted both the inconsistencies that are in place and also the possible benefits associated with establishing consistent or at least minimum standards for physiotherapists who work with sports teams and athletes, including those who relate to the provision of emergency care and first aid. The most notable example of an attempt to establish consistent minimum standards for sports physiotherapists is the Sports Physiotherapy Competencies and Standards developed by the IFSPT. IFSPT Competency 2 – Acute Intervention specifically describes the role and required skills of the sports physiotherapist in emergency and acute situations: "Sports physiotherapists respond appropriately to acute injury or illness in both training and competition contexts, using prior communication with other professionals to identify and establish roles and responsibilities." This competency statement further describes the need for the physiotherapist to form: "rapid clinical judgements regarding the need for further intervention (i.e., triage) and appropriate referral" and also provide "basic life support and CPR" and "Stabilization and transport". The supporting list of competency statements provides guidance on several components of the specific skills and practices and the physiotherapist should have to effectively provide care in an emergency or acute situation.

It is reasonable to expect that all physiotherapists who work in sport should have as a minimum training and certification in the provision of CPR including the use of an automated external defibrillator (AED).

In many countries, Sports Emergency Medical Response courses for allied health professionals such as physiotherapists and other tertiary trained therapists have been developed. These courses use a case-based approach to address the emergency response competencies such as those specified by the International Federation of Sports Physical Therapists (Competency 2) and provide physiotherapists with the knowledge and skills to preserve life and reduce further harm until more qualified medical personnel arrive.

Crisis Management Procedures

Section 9.2 of the IOC Medical Code states: "In case of a serious incident occurring during training or competition, there should be procedures to provide the necessary support to those injured by evacuating them to the competent medical services when needed. The athletes, coaches, and persons associated with the sports activity should be informed of those procedures and receive the necessary training for their implementation."

Medical Screening and Emergency Care

The physiotherapist should also be aware of any preexisting medical conditions or risk factors the athletes in their care may have, so as to both be able to more rapidly respond in the event of an acute situation. Communication by the physiotherapist with the team doctor is therefore important so as to be aware of any identified risk factors that may be present in athletes for whom they are providing care.

Emergency Response Planning and the Physiotherapist

IFSPT Competency 2E.4 describes the role of the physiotherapist in participating in a multidisciplinary approach to planning, coordination, and intervention strategies to expedite a rapid and appropriate response in the event of a medical emergency or acute situation.

Emergency management planning has many components in addition to some of those outlined earlier. Additional components of the medical emergency plan that the physiotherapist should consider among other things include the following:

1. Ensure that appropriate equipment is available and in safe working order
2. Conduct an initial venue assessment coordination with local services

In Summary

While medical emergencies are infrequent in most sports, a comprehensive knowledge and training of emergency management skills combined with preplanning and team-based practice of the procedures that are to be utilized in a medical emergency provides the greatest likelihood that the physiotherapist can respond effectively if a crisis situation does occur.

Bibliography

Australian Resuscitation Council (2010) *Guideline 8 Cardiopulmonary resuscitation*. www.resus.org.au [retrieved on 11 October 2013]

Australian Resuscitation Council (2012) *Guideline 2 Managing an emergency*. www.resus.org.au [retrieved on 11 October 2013]

Chan, K., Micheli, L., Smith, A. *et al.* (eds) (2006) *F.I.M.S. Team Physician Manual*, 2nd edn. ISBN:962-356-029-X.

International Olympic Committee (2000) *Sport medicine manual*. www.olympic.org [retrieved 19 September 2011]

International Olympic Committee (2009b) *Olympic movement medical code*. www.olympic.org [retrieved on 11 October 2013]

Karges, J.R., Cross, P.S., Hauer, P.L. *et al.* (2013) Effectiveness of the emergency response course in improving student physical therapists' and licensed physical therapists' decision making related to acute sports injuries and medical conditions. *International Journal of Sports Physical Therapy*, **8** (**3**), 277–289.

McDonagh, D. (ed) (2012) *FIMS Sports Medicine Manual: Event Planning and Emergency Care*. ISBN:978-1-58255-873-8. Wolters Kluwer Health/Lippincott Williams & Wilkins, 2011

Smith, D. (2012) Are all Physical Therapists qualified to provide sideline coverage of athletic events? *International Journal of Sports Physical Therapy*, **7** (**1**), 120–123.

Sports Medicine Australia (xxxx) *Medical emergency planning*. www.sma.org.au/wp-content/uploads/2014/07/MedicalEmergencyPlanningGuideforClubs.pdf [retrieved on 17 November 2013]

Sports Medicine Australia (2012) *Sports Medicine for Sports Trainers*, 10th edn. Elsevier. ISBN:9780729541541.

World Confederation of Physical Therapy 2014 *Policy statement: description of physical therapy*. www.wcpt.org/policy/ps-descriptionPT

30 Emergency Medications and Equipment at the Fieldside

Mark Faulkner[1]*, Fionna P. Moore*[2,3] *and David Zideman*[2,4,5]

[1]*Major Trauma and Legal Services, London Ambulance Service NHS Trust, London, UK*
[2]*London Ambulance Service NHS Trust, London, UK*
[3]*Emergency Medicine, Imperial Healthcare NHS Trust, London, UK*
[4]*Anaesthesia, Imperial College Healthcare NHS Trust, London, UK*
[5]*Emergency Medical Services, London Organising Committee of the Olympic and Paralympic Games, London 2012, London UK*

The selection of medication and equipment available to the medical team for the trackside or Field of Play (FoP) will depend on a number of different variables:

1. The number of athletes
2. The age and fitness profile of the competitors
3. The duration of the event
4. The sport and likely pattern of injuries
5. The weather, altitude, and temperature

However, there are two broad categories; the equipment and drugs that need to be available as a basic minimum for any event, whatever the profile of the competitors and that which will reflect the more specialized equipment and drugs required as the result of a detailed risk assessment related to the specific event. At the London Olympics, London Organizing Committee for Olympic Games (LOCOG) Medical provided all the equipment and drugs required by the medical teams, standardized across all the FoP venues. By providing the equipment and drugs, LOCOG were able to specify the type and level of medical provision and they overcame the problems of individual preferences and omissions leading to gaps in medical care. In smaller events, this may not be possible and the level of medical provision should be agreed between the medical team and the event organizers prior to the event.

The selection of drugs and equipment needs to take into account weight, portability, and availability of backup arrangements. The selection of equipment and drugs needs to also allow for the experience, education, and training of the members of the team (Appendix 2). There is simply no point carrying an item of equipment if the team responding to an incident is not trained and familiar with its use.

The IOC Manual of Emergency Sports Medicine, First Edition. Edited by David McDonagh and David Zideman.

The Bag

There are a variety of medical carrying bags on the market and every responder is more than likely to have a personal preference. There are a number of key factors, which need to be considered when selecting bags to contain medical equipment:

1. *Weight*: If the emergency equipment weighs more than is manageable in a single bag, consider splitting the equipment between two bags and having first- and second-line of treatment equipment bags. Any member of the team should be able to comfortably carry a bag.
2. *Material*: Consider the material the bag is made from; is it suitably strong, can it be wiped clean of mud, body fluids, and is it waterproof?
3. *Method of carrying*: Should the bag be handheld or a rucksack? How will the bag be carried while removing a patient from the FoP?
4. *Different bags for different tasks*: It may be suitable to have several bags, each for a defined purpose – one for medication, one for airways, one for ABC, and so on. It may be appropriate to have these packed as units within a larger bag unit.
5. *Bag identification*: Color coding is useful for readily identifying types of equipment.
6. *Responding agencies*: Do bags need a different appearance to those of cooperating ambulance and paramedic/first aid agencies? It is easy for other groups to pick up the wrong bag before leaving scene if all the bags are identical.

In the London Olympics, three types of bag were provided:

1. A personal bag (green bum bag/fanny pack) – carried by all medical personnel containing basic simple equipment and drugs for immediate medical treatment and care
2. A medical bag (red rucksack) – containing emergency medical equipment and drugs (one per FoP team)
3. An advanced treatment bag (orange rucksack) – containing advanced emergency medical equipment and drugs (one per FoP)

Each rucksack was subdivided into compartments to facilitate the finding of individual items. The compartments – Diagnostic, Resuscitation, Breathing, IV, First Aid, and Extras – were mounted on Velcro and detachable from the rucksack. The FoP teams were required to check each compartment on a daily basis to ensure completeness of the equipment and to improve their knowledge of the position of individual items. Following inspection, each compartment and the rucksack was sealed with a snap seal.

The contents of the advanced trauma bag closely mirrored that of the medical bag but included the equipment and drugs required to undertake advanced airway and trauma care.

On the outside of the medical and advanced treatment bags was a separate sealed compartment which contained the medical drugs, stored in boxes, with a countdown check list of contents on the outside. Controlled drugs (e.g., morphine) were carried separately by individual FoP doctors, according to UK regulations. A lightweight portable oxygen cylinder was attached to the outside of the medical and trauma bags.

Whatever design of bag is chosen, all team members must be familiar with its contents and their location within the bag. For larger events, it may be necessary to have a duplicate bag to be able to respond to a second patient before rechecking and repacking the primary bag.

Each bag should have a contents list, which notes the location and number of the contents. This list can then be used for the basis of a challenge and response when restocking or checking the bag. Once checked, consider sealing the bag and dating it with the earliest expiry date; this saves considerable time when checking the bags. There should be an agreed process for how new items are added to the bag and for changes to the contents list.

Immobilization and Carrying

The event risk assessment should determine the need for the FoP team to enter the FoP and move a patient. For smaller events or for training venues, it may be the case that an ambulance will be called and the patient can be stabilized in situ by the event medical staff. This scenario would allow the event staff to utilize the ambulance's immobilization and carrying equipment.

It is recommended that the medical response team and the retrieval ambulance use similar equipment. This allows for swapping of equipment when an ambulance departs an arena with venue equipment, for example, when a patient is packaged on a scoop stretcher and then handed over to the ambulance. A similar policy is also useful for the ambulance service and the emergency department. Consider the use of single-use equipment, as a correctly applied splint will often remain in situ until operative fixation.

Stretcher or Trolley Bed

In the main, ambulance services utilize a trolley bed to move recumbent casualties. These can be wheeled and reduce the need to carry the patient over any distance. However, trolley bed stretchers can be unstable particularly over rough ground and are extremely difficult to wheel on grass or muddy ground.

The Spinal Board

The spinal or rescueboard has been a mainstay of prehospital care for many years. Its use is now regarded as suitable for extrication only. It provides a hard surface when carrying patients as well as providing a surface for spinal immobilization when used in conjunction with a hard collar, head blocks, and body straps. If recumbent, the patient will need to be log rolled, the board slid under the patient, and then the patient's position adjusted to the center of the board. This process may create considerable movement of the spine and other body structures, which may be an issue in the multi-traumatized patient with the potential to disrupt clot formation. The spinal board has some limitations, particularly when carrying a larger patient. All patients should be strapped to the board to enable safe transfer. Adapted spinal boards that float can be a useful adjunct when removing the patient from water.

The Scoop Stretcher

This device is used for both lifting patients and as a surface for spinal immobilization when used in conjunction with head blocks and a hard collar. The ability to split the stretcher and slide each half under the patient reduces the degrees of logrolling needed. More modern plastic scoops have reduced the negative effects of placing a cold metal structure under the patient. It should be noted that if the scoop is used as a carrying device, it might flex if carried over distances. The same is true for vacuum mattresses. The stretcher should ideally be placed within another nonflexible device (such as a basket stretcher) prior to carrying. The Faculty of Pre-Hospital Care of the Royal College of Surgeons Edinburgh has produced a useful consensus guideline on this subject (see Bibliography).

The Basket Stretcher

This device is an addition to the scoop stretcher and vacuum mattress in that the lifted patient can be placed within the basket stretcher to aid carrying and removal. It should be noted that unless a patient is placed on a scoop/vacuum mattress/carry sheet within the basket, it could be difficult to remove the patient from the basket stretcher.

Carry Sheet

The carry sheet is a simple to use device to aid lifting the patient who does not require spinal immobilization. Care needs to be taken to ensure the patient does not slip or slide from the carry sheet. A number of the military stretchers have adapted the carry sheet by adding securing straps and often have a tough base to facilitate the patient being dragged if required. This piece of kit can provide a rapid and useful way of moving patients particularly in mass participation events where they may need to rapidly extract numerous patients.

Semi-Rigid Cervical Collars

These form a part of the package of spinal immobilization. There are multiple brands and styles on the market. The adjustable telescopic collars, which allow the size to be altered, are of benefit as they reduce the number of sizes the team needs to carry. Collars should have an opening at the front to allow visualization of the trachea and carotid vessels. They should support the chin, occiput, and periauricular regions without compressing neck structures. In some small adults, the pediatric-sized collars may fit better than the adult-sized collars. A number of collars have small hooks that allow an oxygen mask to be easily attached with the collar.

Head Blocks

There are purpose-designed head blocks, which can be secured to both the scoop stretcher and spinal board. Although in the case of the scoop stretcher, some wide 7.5 cm elastic adhesive bandage is effective, and disposable head blocks provide a cheap alterative without the need for cleaning and the worry of product loss. A rolled blanket can be an effective emergency alternative.

Body Straps

Patients placed on scoops or spinal boards need to be effectively secured to the device. Body straps aid spinal immobilization and limit body movement while potentially allowing the patient to be tilted laterally in case of vomiting. Straps come in a number of styles including simple straps that are passed across the patient and single piece "spider straps." Straps can be difficult to clean and there are a number of single-use options on the market.

Vacuum Mattresses

Both the spinal board and scoop stretcher are hard surfaces and there is a risk of developing tissue ischemia when tissue is compressed between a dislocated fractured bone and the stretcher surface. There is a similar risk for spinal cord injury victims. Using a vacuum mattress may reduce this tissue pressure particularly where transit times to hospital are prolonged. Vacuum products are prone to puncture and leaking, so care must be exercised. It is important to check that correct adaptors and pumps are packed with the mattress/splints and that staff know how to lock and open valves.

Limb Splints (See Chapter 20)

There are numerous different types of limb splints on the market:

1. Light weight aluminum-lined foam splints provide a convenient way of immobilizing a number of different anatomical areas
2. Box or Loxley style splints provide a method of immobilizing a limb in an anatomical position. A range of sizes will often be needed. These are now also available in a single-use form

3. Vacuum splints provide a method of supporting a limb in an abnormal position and although prone to puncture, require a vacuum pump and adaptor to deflate. A range of sizes is often required
4. Inflatable splints have lost favor, as they limit space for the fracture to swell and can increase the risk of pressure ischemia
5. Traction splints are mainly designed for managing the fractured femur and there are many different styles and types. It is worth considering the ease of application, the ability to carry the splint; some are very bulky and it may be unclear if the splint can be used with concurrent fractures on the same limb or with a suspected pelvic injury. The "tent pole" style splints provide lightweight and convenient styles of traction splint. It is important that the proximal straps do not press upon the fractured area
6. Moldable splints: There are a number of ready-to-use splints available. Some are prehardened, others are applied in the style of a back slab plaster cast where lengths of material are cut to measure, dampened, and then applied to the patient before hardening after a few minutes. Operators need to be proficient in the application of a back slab.

Pelvic Splints (See Chapter 18)

These form a mainstay of treatment of the fractured pelvis, and there a number of styles on the market. Consideration needs to be given to the range of sizes needed: single cut to size or a range of sizes. Correct application of pelvic splints is necessary. It is also worth considering that with the growing use of interventional radiology in the management of hemorrhage from fractured pelvis, to consider splints where access to the groin is preserved or can be facilitated with the splint in situ.

Resuscitation (See Chapter 4)

Automatic External Defibrillator (AED)

Where the risk assessment identifies that the provision of Advanced Life Support is required, manual mode AEDs with cardiac rhythm display should be available. Consideration should be given to robustness and how weatherproof the device is. Devices will often be moved in and out of storage and will sit at the side of the FoP until needed, where they may be subject to inclement weather.

The AED pack should contain the following:

1. Adult defibrillation pads including a spare set in case of malfunction or a second cardiac arrest
2. Chest hair razors, for specific use with an AED, designed not to clog with hair
3. A small towel to dry a wet patient and aid application of the pads
4. A pair of trauma shears which can be used to remove clothing rapidly
5. Consideration should be given as to whether a spare battery is needed

Pocket Mask

This allows for the effective delivery of rescue breaths particularly if there is a sole responder.

Bag Valve Mask with Reservoir Bag

This provides a method of artificial ventilation but requires familiarity, skill, and practice to be able to use. A two-person technique is the optimal method in an emergency situation. A range of mask sizes should be carried as should anticrush oxygen tubing.

Other Masks

1. High-flow oxygen masks (reservoir bag) if oxygen is carried
2. Nebulizer mask if oxygen is carried

Airway Adjuncts

1. A full range of adult oral pharyngeal (OP) tubes (airways)
2. Size 6 and 7 nasal pharyngeal tubes (airways) with lubrication gel

Manual Suction Device

Ideally disposable

Advanced Airway Equipment

The event risk assessment should determine the need for advanced airway management facilities. The use of supraglottic airways has significantly enhanced emergency airway management in the prehospital environment though endotracheal intubation is still considered to be the best form of airway management. To master both techniques requires specialized training. The team must have a method of securing the airway during patient removal. Consider the following:

1. The range of endotracheal (ET) tubes that need to be carried. Most ambulance services avoid using half sizes
2. Methods of securing the ET tube (e.g. specifically designed tube holder)
3. *Laryngoscope*: Ensure that a range of blade types are available. The blade and handle must be compatible. There are a range of power sources and bulb types on the market, not all of which are interchangeable
4. A syringe for inflating the cuff
5. Catheter mount
6. Disposable intubation bougie
7. Magill forceps for removal of an upper airway obstruction
8. Where intubation is proposed, there must be a robust and evidential way of monitoring and documenting expired carbon dioxide levels ($ETCO_2$). This is imperative where intubation is undertaken
9. A clinical waste bag provides a useful surface for laying out equipment on a clean surface prior to use and for disposing of used equipment.

Depending on the risk assessment and the skills of the FoP team, it may be necessary to include an emergency surgical cricothyrotomy kit (scalpel, tracheal hook, and tracheostomy tube).

Dressings and Hemorrhage Control

A range of general dressings is recommended:

1. Pad and gauze bandages and dressings provide a simple method of hemorrhage control and come in a range of sizes
2. A pressure dressing or hemorrhage control dressing is a useful adjunct for controlling significant hemorrhage
3. Simple nonadherent absorbent wound pads: some products have nonadherent surfaces on both sides of the dressing which aids accurate placement in limited lighting
4. A range of plasters and adhesive dressings
5. Cohesive bandage (which is designed to stick to itself) is a useful way of securing dressings to the scalp and other difficult areas

6. A selection of bandages for securing dressings, supportive bandaging of joints
7. Blister (hydro colloid) dressings
8. Fabric, paper, and plastic tape are useful in securing dressings
9. Triangular bandages allow for the application of slings
10. Hemostatic dressings are recommended where there is a particular risk of hemorrhage. The FoP team needs to understand the style and constituents of the dressings and ensure that it can be easily packed into the wound. A number of these dressings also now contain an X-ray opaque strip so they can be detected on X-ray (See Chapter 6)
11. Where there is a particular risk of limb injury and hemorrhage, it is worth considering whether a specific arterial tourniquet should be added to the equipment. When used in a civilian context, these should be brightly colored to aid identification (See Chapter 6)
12. Where there is a risk of a penetrating injury, it is worth considering whether a chest seal with adherence dressing should be added to the equipment for use in a sucking chest wound

Ensure that all items of equipment are latex free as this considerably reduces the risk of an iatrogenic allergic reaction.

Drug Administration and Intravenous Access

1. A range of intravenous cannula should be included in the kit. It may be necessary to provide needle safer devices as this is mandated in some countries
2. A range of intravenous syringes
3. Intramuscular and subcutaneous needles. Again consider needle safer devices as there are now multiple syringes which the needle retracts into after use
4. A solution for cleaning venipuncture sites such as 2% chlorhexidine
5. Disposable venous tourniquets
6. Dressings for securing intravenous cannula
7. Spare syringe and cannula bungs
8. Blunt tip drawing up needles with filters
9. Three way taps or multiple port injection devices fitted with non-return valves.

Rapid and efficient venous access is important in an emergency situation. The Resuscitation Council (UK) currently recommends for the resuscitation situation that after two failed attempts at venous cannulations, there is a change to an intraosseous device. Small battery-driven electrical drills with a detachable needle are now available – the preferred insertion point being the anterior medial aspect of the tibia or the humeral head.

Medications

To be fully equipped, the FoP team must have a complete supply of emergency drugs. They should also carry a limited supply of some of simple commonly used medications. Most emergency drugs will be administered by the intravenous or intraosseous route or occasionally intramuscularly: tracheal drug administration has now been discontinued. Simple common medications are given orally or rectally.

Caution

Before administering a drug it is important for the prescribing doctor to be aware of relevant WADA regulations (see Chapter 31). However, it cannot be emphasized enough that the athlete's care and well-being *must* come before any consideration of antidoping regulations. This is most important in FoP emergency medicine where the timely and rapid administration of a life-saving drug may be critical; for example, injected adrenaline (epinephrine) is prohibited under WADA regulations (local administration, e.g., nasal, ophthalmologic or in coadministration with local anaesthetic agents is not prohibited on the 2014 Prohibited List). However, adrenaline is a primary drug in the treatment of cardiac arrest (1 mg intravenously) or in the treatment of acute anaphylaxis (0.5 mg by intramuscular injection). Any delay in giving this drug under these situations may delay recovery and could result in death.

Following the administration of a prohibited drug under emergency conditions, a retroactive TUE must be completed and submitted together with a full copy of the doctor's clinical notes as soon as possible after the patient has left the venue.

Emergency Drugs

Used in both cardiac arrest and anaphylaxis

1. Adrenaline (epinephrine)
   a. In cardiac arrest, administer 1 mg IV or intraosseous (IO). A total of 1 mg is 10 mL of 1 in 10,000 solution or 1 mL of 1 in 1000 solution. Repeat as per cardiac arrest algorithm (See Chapter 4)
   b. In anaphylaxis administer 0.5 mg IM (0.5 mL of 1 in 1000 solution). Repeat if the signs and symptoms of anaphylaxis return, or after 5 min if no improvement (See Chapter 7)
   c. Patients with a history of severe anaphylaxis may carry their own adrenaline in a self-injectable format (Epipen, Anapen). These devices usually provide 0.3 mg of intramuscular adrenaline and may need follow-up doses

N.B. Adrenaline IM, IV, SC, IO is prohibited on the WADA 2014 Prohibited List (see caution above).

Used with cardiac emergencies (see Chapters 4 and 5)

1. Amiodarone
   Used in refractory ventricular fibrillation and pulseless ventricular tachycardia as a bolus dose of 300 mg IV or IO. Administration may result in the cessation of the ventricular fibrillation or tachycardia but may cause a severe bradycardia. It should not be given concurrently with IV lidocaine.
2. Atropine
   Used in the treatment of severe bradycardia where there is evidence of severe adverse signs (cardiovascular shock, syncope, myocardial ischemia, and heart failure) in an IV dose of 0.5 mg, repeated as required to a maximum of 3 mg.
3. Adenosine
   For supraventricular tachycardia, administered in an initial rapid IV bolus dose of 6 mg over 2 s, followed by 12 mg after 1–2 min if required and a further dose of 12 mg after the same time interval. Administration must be under electrocardiogram (ECG) control and full clinical monitoring. Following a bolus dose, there may be a very brief period of asystole or severe bradycardia followed by a return of spontaneous circulation.

Used with allergy/asthma (see chapters 7 and 8)

1. Chlorpheniramine (chlorphenamine)
   This antihistamine can be given as a 10 mg IV or IM injection. It may be associated with drowsiness and affect motor skill performance. It is sometimes given orally, 4 mg, for symptomatic relief of pruritus or hay fever.
2. Salbutamol
   Prescribed for asthma or reversible airway obstruction, it is quickly administered by aerosol administration, 100–200 mcg (one to two puffs from a metered aerosol inhaler). Athletes who have clinically diagnosed asthma will usually carry their own (blue) inhaler. The use of a spacer device will aid the inhalation therapy by optimizing the inhalational dose and is the optimal method of delivery for mild/moderate attacks.

Alternatively, or for acute severe or life-threatened asthma it can be given as a nebulized solution, 5 mg repeated as required. Ipratropium (500 μg) can be added to the second nebulizer. If inhalation dosing is not reliable, salbutamol can be given as 50 mcg per mL by slow IV injection to a maximum dose of 250 mcg.
N.B. In the WADA 2014 List, salbutamol urine levels of more than 1000 ng/mL may be considered an adverse analytical finding (see WADA List).

3. Hydrocortisone
   Given in an IV dose of 100 mg or may be prescribed as 40–50 mg of oral prednisolone. These rarely have to be given on the FoP.

   N.B. Hydrocortisone administered IM, IV, rectally, or orally requires a TUE according to the 2014 WADA Prohibited List.

Analgesia

The provision of fast, effective, and appropriate analgesia is a critical function of the FoP medical team. These must be supplied by a range of analgesic drugs that will cover a wide range of scenarios.

Analgesia can be divided into simple and advanced.
1. Simple analgesia:
   a. Paracetamol
      A simple nonopioid analgesic with no antiinflammatory activity. It can be administered in a dose of 1 g every 4–6 h by mouth or by rectum and more recently an IV formulation has become available.
   b. Aspirin
      Probably not used as an analgesic but given in the early stages of cardiac chest pain in a dose of 160–325 g and chewed for its antiplatelet effects. Check for any history of allergy or gastrointestinal (GI) bleeding before administration.
   c. Diclofenac
      This nonsteroidal antiinflammatory analgesic is used for mild-to-moderate trauma-related musculoskeletal pain often in addition to the primary administration of paracetamol. The dose of 50 mg, 8 hourly (oral, rectal, IM, or IV) with a maximum daily dose of 150 mg must be adhered to, to avoid serious side effects.

2. Advanced analgesia:
   a. Tramadol
      Used for moderate-to-severe pain. This is a popular opioid analgesic as it has fewer of the true opioid side effects and can be carried and administered without all of the administrative complexities of a true opiate. The dose of 50–100mg can be administered by mouth, IV, or IM injection.
   b. Morphine
      The best known opiate analgesic, which can be administered in a dose of 1 mg/kg by IM injection or 0.1 mg/kg slow intravenous injection. If used by the intravenous route, administration should be titrated to effect, starting with 2.5–5 mg and adding 1–2.5 mg increments to achieve analgesia without the loss of consciousness or respiratory depression. Morphine can also be used in the early stages of ACS (see chapter 5). It is advised to consider giving an antiemetic following the administration of morphine.

      Athletes receiving morphine must be removed from the FoP and should be fully monitored.

      Morphine is considered a "Class A" controlled drug and is therefore subject to strict regulations as to how it is stored and who can carry and administer the drug. It is strongly advised that the advise of a pharmacist is sought on the supply and storage of morphine. However, considering its potency and effectiveness, it is well worth the effort to enable the FoP team access to morphine. Morphine is restricted in competition (2014 WADA Prohibited List).

c. Ketamine
Ketamine can be used in very low dosage as a very effective and fast acting analgesic. A dose of 0.1 mg/kg IV will provide intense rapid onset analgesia for 10–15 min, where there will be usually enough time to attach a traction splint or perform a fracture manipulation. The dose can be titrated and repeated as required. Ketamine is supplied in two formulations, 10 and 100 mg/mL. It is advised to use the drug as 10 mg/mL for FoP use.

Ketamine is used in higher doses, 2 mg/kg IV or 5 mg/kg IM for induction of anesthesia, but its use as an anesthetic is restricted to those healthcare professionals (HCPs) trained in the provision of anesthesia.

It is sometimes suggested that midazolam should be given prior to the administration of ketamine to reduce its side effects. This is not considered to be a major issue in low-dose ketamine.

Ketamine has been upgraded to a Class B substance under the UK Misuse of Drugs Act 1971. Guidance on the storage and administration should be sought to ensure local pharmaceutical regulation compliance.

Inhaled Analgesics

1. Entonox – this is a 50:50 mixture of oxygen and nitrous oxide that can be inhaled by the trauma casualty and provides rapid analgesia. However, its effects are somewhat unpredictable and unreliable. It should not be administered to casualties with a suspected pneumothorax or where there is intracranial air post head injury. Entonox is carried in cylinders and self-administered by the casualty through disposable tubing and a mouthpiece or facemask. It will separate out into its components at low ambient temperatures and is not recommended for use below 5°C
2. Methoxyflurane – this is an inhaled anesthetic agent commonly used in prehospital medicine in Australia. It was withdrawn from use in many countries because of its nephrotoxicity and is therefore not available outside Australasia

Sedatives/Antiepileptics

1. Diazepam
   This is the first-line therapy for convulsions or epilepsy administered per rectum in a dose of 10–20mg and repeated after 15 min if required. Alternatively it can be given IV, 1 mL (5 mg) per minute titrated to effect.
2. Midazolam
   This water-soluble benzodiazepine is widely used in preference to diazepam as it has a faster onset of action. It should be titrated to effect and should only be used by those trained in its use, as it will produce profound sedation that may require airway control. It is often used in epilepsy, as it can be administered by the buccal route.

Pharmacologic Antagonists

If morphine, diazepam, or midazolam is supplied in the medical kit, it is strongly recommended that the appropriate specific pharmacologic antagonists are also supplied. Patients who receive these antagonists must be carefully monitored and observed to ensure continuity of the pharmacologic reversal.

1. Naloxone – the specific antagonist for the respiratory depressions and sedative side effects of opiate analgesics in a titrated IV dose of 100–200 mcg. It has a relatively short duration of action compared with most opiates and may require a second dose after 20 min. It is not uncommon to split the initial dose and administer half IV and half IM
2. Flumazenil – the specific antagonist for the sedative effects of benzodiazepines in an IV dose of 200 mcg followed by a second dose of 100 mcg after 1 min if required

Antiemetics

As with analgesia, the prompt management of nausea and vomiting is an important function of the FoP team.

1. Cyclizine
   An antihistamine antiemetic with a common side effect of drowsiness. It can be administered as 50 mg orally, IV, or IM.
2. Metoclopramide
   Metoclopramide acts directly on the GI tract and although it is associated with less sedation than cyclizine, it can induce facial and skeletal dystonic reactions and oculogyric crises (treat with procyclidine). This is an effective antiemetic given in a dose of 10 mg orally or by IV or IM injection.
3. Ondansetron
   Ondanetron blocks 5HT receptors both centrally and in the GI tract. It can be administered in a dose of 4 mg by slow IV or IM injection.

Hypoglycemia Treatment

It is important to diagnose and treat hypoglycemia quickly and effectively (See Chapter 26). If the patient is conscious, then giving oral glucose, 10–20g, either as sugar, snack sweets, glucose drinks, or a commercially available product (Glucogel), will usually be sufficient. This should be followed up with carbohydrate-containing food to sustain recovery.

1. Glucagon
   A polypeptide hormone, 1 mg administered IV or IM to a hypoglycemic unconscious patient will raise blood sugar by mobilizing liver glycogen. It is often administered in insulin-induced hypoglycemia in insulin-dependent diabetics. Close monitoring of its effect must be undertaken and if there is no response within 10 min, then IV glucose should be given.
2. IV glucose
   Hypoglycemia – not responding to oral glucose or glucagon and should be treated with 50 ml of 20% glucose IV through a large vein. Alternatively, a larger volume of 10% solution can be used. Glucose 50% is recommended by some authorities but as it is difficult to administer and there is high risk of tissue injury from extravasation. Close monitoring of blood sugar levels must be undertaken during and after treatment.

Intravenous Fluids

There are a wide variety of intravenous fluids available. Emergency trauma resuscitation requires 250 mL boluses of saline to a systolic blood pressure of 90 mmHg and there is very little indication for dextrose-containing fluids directly on the FoP. In addition, it is important to consider the weight of carrying bags of fluids in the medical pack (See Chapter 6). It is recommended to restrict the emergency fluids to one 500 mL bag of 0.9% sodium chloride in the FoP medical pack as this has the widest therapeutic use.

The above-mentioned list of drugs is only a suggestion as to the basic drugs supplied and carried by the FoP medical team. The FoP team should ensure that they are fully up-to-date with the current pharmacy guidelines and WADA regulations for all drugs carried in their medical kit. They should be provided with access to the local/national pharmacopeia (the USP-NF, the British National Formulary, APF, Felleskatalogen, etc.) and the WADA List of prohibited substances: www.list.wada-ama.org. At an Olympic and Paralympic Games, the medical services publish specific formularies to be used during the Games.

If the FoP team has advanced airway or rapid sequence induction of anesthesia skills, then they may request further drugs to include anesthetic induction agents (etomidate, ketamine, and propofol), muscle relaxants (suxamethonium, pancuronium, and rocuronium), and alternative analgesics (fentanyl and remifentanyl) according to local practice and protocol.

FoP doctors must take full responsibility for the drugs they have been issued and carefully record all prescribed drugs together with the presenting signs and symptoms, the reason for prescribing/administration and the drugs effect. This record should accompany athletes should they be transferred to hospital and a copy kept by the venue doctor for possible drug exemption queries. Retroactive TUEs, together with the appropriate supporting medical notes, should be completed and submitted as soon as possible following the administration of a designated drug.

Bibliography

Faculty of Pre Hospital Care – Consensus statement on Patient Handling: http://www.fphc.co.uk/content/Portals/0/Documents/2013-12%20Consensus%20Handling%20v8.pdf

Faculty of Pre Hospital Care – Consensus statement on pre-hospital Spinal Immobilization: http://www.fphc.co.uk/content/Portals/0/Documents/2013-12%20Spinal%20Consensus%20COMPLETE.pdf

31 Emergency Medications and the WADA Prohibited List

Alan Vernec[1] and Eduardo de Rose[2]

[1] *World Anti-Doping Agency, Montreal, Quebec, Canada*
[2] *Brazilian Olympic Committee, Rio de Janeiro, Brazil*

Concern for the health of athletes and for fair play resulted in the creation of antidoping rules. International Federations initiated these rules, including the prohibition of specific substances, although many sports eventually followed the lead of the International Olympic Committee (IOC), which published the IOC Prohibited List for the first time in 1967. The World Anti-Doping Agency (WADA) was conceived in 1999 and by 2004 WADA had taken over the management of the Prohibited List. There are over 600 signatories to the World Anti-Doping Code, thus ensuring that the majority of sports worldwide accept the WADA Prohibited List. There are very few sports (e.g., American professional leagues) whose rules may differ slightly from those of the Code and thus do not abide by this List. It remains for the physician to verify the rules, which apply to their particular sport.

The first duty of any team doctor or healthcare professional treating athletes is to know what drugs are included on the current Prohibited List. A new List is published on the WADA website on January 1 of each year. It can also be found on many sport federation or National Anti-Doping Organization (NADO) websites. The List includes both prohibited substances and prohibited methods. The most recent version may be found on the WADA website: www.wada.ama.org.

The majority of the substances on the List are rarely prescribed by typical sport or emergency physicians. Examples include anabolic androgenic steroids, other anabolic agents such as clenbuterol, erythropoiesis-stimulating agents, blood or blood components, and human growth hormone or growth factors.

However, in an acute life-threatening situation, a physician may be obliged to administer potentially life-saving medications. *Many of these medications are on the WADA 2014 Prohibited List.* They include the following:

1. Adrenaline (epinephrine) – for serious allergic reaction or anaphylaxis
2. Hydrocortisone – for serious allergic reaction or anaphylaxis

The IOC Manual of Emergency Sports Medicine, First Edition. Edited by David McDonagh and David Zideman.

3. Salbutamol* or terbutaline – for an asthma attack or when there is a serious allergic reaction or anaphylactic reaction with a respiratory component
4. Insulin – for ketoacidosis, symptomatic hyperglycemia, may be indicated with hyperglycemia in the presence of a head injury – rapid action human insulin is commonly used
5. Diuretics – for emergency pulmonary edema
6. β-blockers† for symptomatic tachycardia

In emergency situations, the physician should focus on the appropriate treatment for the safe management of the athlete and not on whether the medication may or not be prohibited. Physicians may sometimes be anxious about breaching antidoping rules even when treating anaphylaxis, acute asthma, or delivering an emergency intravenous infusion. An athlete's health should never be put at risk by withholding or delaying necessary medications or treatments. The main goal is to preserve life and prevent further injury or illness. Once the life-threatening situation has been resolved, the athlete should not return to the Field of Play. An athlete in need of these emergency medications needs continued medical care in a carefully monitored environment and probably hospitalization.

A retroactive TUE should be applied for as soon as possible after the incident. The physician should record adequate notes of the medical situation, including all elements of the physical examination and any ancillary test results. The full documents should be sent to the appropriate antidoping authorities as soon as possible following the use of the prohibited substance or method. As the athlete has received a prohibited medication in an emergency situation, the onus is on the treating physician to inform the correct antidoping authorities about the necessary intervention and apply for a TUE.

It should be restated that the need for a TUE must be justified as per clause 4.1 of the WADA code and that a retroactive TUE could be refused with the possible consequence of an antidoping rule violation to the athlete. For example, an intramuscular or oral dose of glucocorticosteroids for fatigue is not something that would be accepted.

Fortunately, other important medications are not on the *2014 List of Prohibited Substances*. These medications are not a substitute but an adjunct to the above-mentioned prohibited medications. These common medications include the following:

1. H_2 antagonists – serious allergic/anaphylactic reaction with a gastric component
2. Nitroglycerine and salicylic acid – ischemic cardiac pain
3. Glucose – hypoglycemia
4. Diazepam – treatment of seizures
5. Amiodarone – for life-threatening dysrhythmias

Some medications are prohibited at all times, while others are prohibited only during the in-competition period. In-competition is typically defined as 12 h before a competition until the end of such competition. However, this period may be defined differently by the organization that has jurisdiction over an event. For example, the IOC considered the in-competition period as commencing at the opening of the Olympic village through to the end of the Games.

1. *Substances prohibited at all times* are listed in Sections S0–S5 and M1–M3 of the 2014 Prohibited List.

* Salbutamol is permitted in sport. However, levels must not exceed 1600 mcgs in urine collected over 24 h. These levels are very rarely exceeded with regular dosages, but if there is an asthma attack and the normal dosages are exceeded, a retroactive Therapeutic Use Exemption (*TUE*) should be requested.

† β-blockers are banned in certain sports.

2. *Substances prohibited in-competition* include those in the sections noted earlier as well as substances mentioned in Sections S6–S9; stimulants, narcotics, cannabinoids, and glucocorticosteroids

The categories are clearly spelled out in the Prohibited List.

Healthcare professionals should always verify that the prescribed medication is not prohibited, but be aware that not all prohibited substances are individually named on the List. Some sections, i.e., narcotics, are considered closed, whereby all substances named in that particular section are prohibited but those not mentioned would be permitted. Many of the sections, i.e., anabolic agents, peptide hormones, and stimulants, list a number of substances but add the important line: ... *and other substances with similar chemical structure or similar biological effect(s).*

The WADA Prohibited List is straightforward but if questions do arise, the physician should contact their NADO. A number of NADOs have very convenient online databases where generic or pharmaceutical formulations can be checked to see if they are prohibited and whether it is in-or out-of-competition (e.g., Global-DRO, which is used by the United Kingdom, Canada, and the United States, with Japan as a licensee). There is no single global online database as pharmaceutical formulations often differ throughout the world.

Another service offered by many NADOs is providing a short list of commonly prescribed drugs that are permitted, including the trade name of the product within their particular country. These often include antibiotics, nonsteroidal antiinflammatories, and importantly decongestants, which do not contain stimulants. These lists often exist as convenient pocket-sized cards and are usually intended for athletes but may be of reassurance to the prescribing physician.

Therapeutic Use Exemption

It is recognized that athletes may have legitimate medical conditions that require the use of prohibited substances. In these situations, athletes may request a TUE from their NADO or International Federation. A specific administrative process has been developed in order to obtain a TUE and this can be found as WADA's International Standard on Therapeutic Use Exemptions on WADA's website: www.wada-ama.org/ISTUE.

The fundamental principles that must be addressed before a TUE will be granted are as follows:

1. There would be significant impairment to the athlete's health without the use of the prohibited medication or substance.
2. The use of the substance or method will not result in an enhanced performance beyond a return to the athlete's normal state of health.
3. There is no reasonable permitted alternative medication or treatment.
4. The necessity for the use of an otherwise prohibited substance or method cannot be as a result of a previous unauthorized use of a prohibited substance or method.

Further advice on what is expected from a TUE application for different medical conditions may be found on the WADA website at: WADA TUE Physician Guidelines for Medical Conditions – www.wada-ama.org/MI.

As a general rule, TUEs should be requested as soon as possible. For substances prohibited in-competition, TUEs should be requested 30 days in advance of the upcoming competition. However, the reality is that some medical situations and treatments may arise precipitously. In this case, one can apply for a retroactive TUE as per section 4.3 of the ISTUE. Retroactive TUEs may be granted when during the following conditions:

1. Emergency treatment or treatment of an acute medical condition was necessary
2. Owing to exceptional circumstances, there was insufficient time or opportunity for the athlete to submit, or for the TUE committee to consider, an application for the TUE prior to sample collection

In the 2015 ISTUE, the general rules for retroactive TUEs will remain the same, but there will be further clauses added to cover situations for those athletes (usually lower than national level) who may not be required to submit TUEs in advance.

The use of intravenous infusion is a prohibited method that may be used during legitimate emergency situations. The List (M2.2) states that: *"intravenous infusions and/or injections of more than 50 mL per 6-hour period except for those legitimately received in the course of hospital admissions or clinical investigations are also prohibited"*. This means that on or near the Field of Play, in postrace tents or even in clinics, intravenous infusions are prohibited. Nevertheless, intravenous infusions may be given but one would need to document the medical situation and apply for a TUE. In these situations, the TUE would almost always be retroactive. More information on granting TUEs for intravenous infusions or injections may be found on the WADA website under the WADA TUE Physician Guidelines on Medical Conditions.

Strict Liability

Sport physicians who are entrusted with treating athletes subject to doping control must be diligent. There is a principle in antidoping referred to as strict liability which states that "each athlete is strictly liable for the substances found in his or her bodily specimen, and that an antidoping rule violation occurs whenever a prohibited substance (or its metabolites or markers) is found in bodily specimen, whether or not the athlete intentionally or unintentionally used a prohibited substance or was negligent or otherwise at fault." Although there are provisions in the Code where the athlete may in fact receive a reduced sanction if no significant fault is demonstrated, the burden of proof is on the athlete. The principle of strict liability has existed in sport for decades and has been upheld in the Court of Arbitration of Sport.

The athlete may be sanctioned even if the physician made an error, as the athlete has some responsibility in the process. While seemingly harsh, cheating athletes have on numerous occasions benefited from the performance-enhancing effects of a medication while finding a physician to take the blame with minimal consequence. In one recent example, an athlete tested positive for the use of anabolic steroids and in his defense he provided a statement from a physician who claimed that he was intending to inject a gluccocorticosteroid but gave an anabolic steroid by mistake. The case was reviewed and the athlete was sanctioned.

Supplements

Another area of significant concern for physicians and athletes is the use of supplements. The reason for concern is that anywhere from 5% to 15% of supplements have been shown in different studies to contain prohibited substances. Supplements may be inadvertently contaminated during a production process or may be deliberately spiked by the company. Athletes are advised to avoid supplements or take extreme caution to reduce the risks as the principle of strict liability applies.

Physicians may not be involved in the decision process on whether or not to use supplements, which may be covered by the team nutritionists or, hopefully not, the coach or trainer. However, the team physician is often considered to be the medical Team Leader and therefore has a duty of care to ensure that smart medical and correct antidoping practices are being followed. There are more than a few instances where supplement use within a team has gone astray with dire consequences for athletes and the team, all of which could have been avoided with strong physician leadership and accountability.

It is unfortunately not rare to hear of cases where athletes are being given supplements with stimulants on the sidelines or at half-time by trainers. These athletes usually end up being sanctioned. If a product is claiming to provide fantastic energy-boosting properties, it is either likely a fraud or actually may contain prohibited substances. Be aware and do not hesitate to intervene. Note there does not exist a permitted list of supplements, although some third-party companies exist which test products and claim to reduce, if not eliminate, the risk.

Possession of Prohibited Medication and Physician Responsibility

Physicians (as part of Athlete Support Personnel) should be aware of Code article 2.6.2 of the revised 2015 Code. It states that possession of any prohibited substance or method could result in a sanction, unless accompanied by a TUE for a specific athlete, who otherwise has an acceptable justification. *The comment to 2.6.2 states:* "Acceptable justification would include, for example, a team doctor carrying Prohibited Substances for dealing with acute and emergency situations."

Therefore, physicians working with teams or at an athletic event are advised to remove any substance that could not justifiably be present for the emergency treatment of athletes.

Furthermore, physicians are advised to label all prohibited substances in their medical kit in some manner, for example, with red stickers, to remind one that it is prohibited and should either not be given to athletes or if used, to subsequently request a TUE.

Physicians and athletes should be aware that the terms *prohibited* or *permitted* substances are antidoping terminology. Some substances may be permitted but are illegal in certain jurisdictions. One may have a TUE for a prohibited substance such as a narcotic or cannabis, but the athlete may be at risk from customs officials or local authorities despite the "authorization" by a TUE committee to use the medication. Traveling team physicians should also be aware of the rules concerning transporting medications. One may have to request permission from the relevant authorities before being allowed to carry medications or even practice in a country without a license.

Summary

The physician needs to know the basics of the prohibited list and should regularly check before prescribing or delivering medications. There is no shortage of information available on the internet. WADA has a comprehensive website and includes much information on Therapeutic Use Exemptions. Many International Federations have extensive information on antidoping, but generally the first point of contact should be the national (or regional) antidoping organization. They will know about national rules and any regional issues in relation to specific pharmaceutical formulations or supplement alerts. They will also know if and when a TUE should be redirected to an International Federation.

The Field of Play healthcare professional need not feel hampered by antidoping rules but must be aware of the present reality of elite sports where antidoping rules and regulations have become an inherent part of the game. The understanding of antidoping rules should be an integral aspect of the education of any healthcare professional working in or around the Field of Play.

32 Retrieval and Repatriation of Injured and Ill Athletes

Mark Brown[1] *and Glenn Brown*[2,3]

[1]*Sports Medicine Australia, Oceania National Olympic Committee Medical Commission, Griffith University Centre of Musculoskeletal Research, Southport, QLD, Australia*
[2]*Supreme Court of Queensland, Brisbane, Australia*
[3]*High Court of Australia, Kingston, ACT, Australia*

Introduction

Safe transport of injured or ill athletes always carries some challenges, but these may be further complicated when factors such as remote and/or international locations are added to the equation. In some cases, the nexus between the legal issues and insurance logistics can significantly impact how transport should be undertaken, therefore necessitating serious consideration as part of the medical decision in relation to the best available options.

There are many stages in the process between the onset of a serious injury or illness and the safe return of the affected athlete to either his/her home or a suitable medical facility for advanced care, with each stage requiring careful consideration of the medical and possibly legal factors involved.

For the purpose of this chapter, the term medical retrieval is used generically; though some practitioners and authors also use the terms medical repatriation or medical evacuation. Interestingly, while these terms are both extant, and often used interchangeably, a strict reading of the term suggests that medical repatriation should be used exclusively for medical retrievals involving a return to the person's place of origin or present citizenship, compared to transfer to another advanced medical care facility that may be suitable for ongoing medical management.

Preplanning

As is the case for all types of travel with athletes and teams, adherence to well-formulated and proven procedures that are understood by all relevant medical and support staff improves the likelihood of a successful outcome. In all cases, preplanning for the possibility of medical retrieval should include at least the following issues:

1. Consideration of the *medical skills* reasonably foreseeable to be necessary based on an assessment of the nature of the sport and the environment to be traveled

The IOC Manual of Emergency Sports Medicine, First Edition. Edited by David McDonagh and David Zideman.

to (environmental, social, legal, etc.), including those factors relevant to possible medical evacuation or repatriation
2. Consideration of what *equipment* may be most likely to be required to assist with safe transport and also whether such equipment is itself readily transportable or can alternatively be obtained at the destination locations
3. Investigation and recognizance of the *medical transport options* as well as the acute *medical facilities* available in the destinations to be traveled to, including obtaining contact details and information about access arrangements for them
4. Establishment of appropriate *travel insurance* that includes provision of suitable medical evacuation or repatriation services, including the possibility of transport by air ambulance
5. Development of *procedures* to be followed in the event that special transport arrangements are required for medical reasons, including communication procedures with the athlete's usual doctor, team management, the athlete's family, and so on

While the above-mentioned should not be considered an exhaustive list, it serves as a starting point for the steps necessary in the preplanning phase. Naturally, it should be tailored to suit the vicissitudes of the circumstances.

Team Medical Staff Skills

In the event of a serious injury or illness occurring to an athlete that requires medical retrieval and return travel, determining whether the team medical staff can safely transport the athlete, or whether additional assistance should be sought, remains a primary consideration.

This is especially relevant for teams traveling without a multidisciplinary medical team or doctor. In the case of teams where there is limited medical support, staff should consider both the practitioner type, as well as their specific expertise and level of training, for example, doctor, paramedic, or physiotherapist. For example, a physiotherapist may be eminently qualified to supervise the transport of an athlete with a musculoskeletal injury, and indeed may also possess a moderately high level of training in the provision of first aid, but may not be able to provide suitable care for a person requiring IV fluids or medications. The question therefore arises: is the team medical provider both professionally and legally able to provide the type of care required during the transport process, especially as medical registration acts and legal scope of practice varies from country to country? This is especially relevant for physiotherapists traveling in countries where physiotherapists cannot legally operate as primary contact practitioners.

While a doctor of any specialty may be able to provide improved care of athletes with medical conditions, in the event that more advanced care is required when transporting injured or ill athletes, specialist training in emergency medicine or anesthesia together with specific training in transport medicine is likely to be preferable. In some countries such as Australia, retrieval medicine exists as a distinct subspecialty of emergency medicine, anesthesia, and intensive care with specific training modules.

Statistics support the contention that medical escort staff for high-dependency patients should possess suitable training in advanced life support and also have sufficient experience and appropriate personal attributes to be able to maintain calm control during complicated and often also rapidly changing circumstances.

Equipment Requirements

It is essential that all sick and injured patients are retrieved or repatriated with appropriate monitoring. The movement of a patient between medical facilities should not compromise patient care or observation. Patients with serious illness or injury should be physiologically monitored during transfer. The minimal monitoring is electrocardiogram (ECG), pulse oximetry, and noninvasive blood pressure (and an expired carbon dioxide trace if the patient is sedated or ventilated). It is also very important that the patient's core body temperature is maintained and monitored throughout the transfer. This may require active methods of heating to overcome ambient conditions. Additional electric equipment that should be considered are infusion pumps (rather than gravity dependent IV infusions), suction device and a defibrillator.

Just as with the healthcare professional, personnel requirements described earlier, it is essential that all the relevant equipment for transport is available, that the team is trained in its use, and that all electrical equipment is compatible with and approved by the aeromedical service. There are many specific considerations relating to each piece of equipment that should be considered. For example, portable ventilators, ECG monitors, and other electronic equipment must be robust to withstand the rigors of travel, including changes in temperature and pressure, have sufficient battery life, not be easily compromised in their operation by road or turbulence vibration, have alarms that can be heard over aircraft or road noise, and have adjustable displays to be seen in bright sunlight.

Medical Transport Options

Transport for medical evacuation or repatriation can include ground and air-based transport options including road ambulances, helicopters, and fixed-wing aircraft all with varying levels of installed or transportable equipment.

Given that returning the athlete to his/her country usually involves air travel, determining whether a commercial airline or air ambulance is required, may also need to be made. If the level of care required does not necessitate an air ambulance, it still may be necessary to arrange extra seating space on a commercial airline to accommodate the medical needs of the athlete requiring transport, especially if additional medical equipment is required. As many athletes are very tall, this may present additional difficulties. Temperature variations during transport should also be considered to ensure that body thermoregulation is not overlooked; this may be further complicated with athletes with a disability such as spinal cord injury. The medical escort should be located in adjacent seating to facilitate easier ongoing monitoring of the athlete's condition.

Specific medical issues relating to the injured or ill athlete's condition also need to be considered when determining what sort of transport is most appropriate. However, there is variation in actual practice or management guidelines for some conditions. For example, a review of medical records of 32 patients with a pneumothorax who were transferred by commercial airlines identified that physicians recommend and follow markedly different management plans with variations in the number of days postdiagnosis, whether chest tubes were in situ or transfer delayed until removal and also whether a medical escort was in attendance or not.

Specialist Medical Evacuation and Repatriation Services

If the athlete's medical support personnel do not have the necessary medical skills or equipment to safely transfer the casualty, then coordination of the medical retrieval by the medical assistance provider nominated by the athlete's travel insurance may be required. Therefore, team medical personnel *must* have the contact details and relevant policy numbers of the athlete or team's travel insurance provider readily available to minimize delays. The commercial realities inherent in this process need to be accepted by the retrieval team and included in the planning stage.

The use of a medical assistance provider will almost invariably be necessary when transport by regular commercial means is not medically appropriate, either because of the severity of the condition or where there is a risk of crossinfection between passengers. When choosing travel insurance, it is therefore worth checking that their nominated medical assistance providers have ready access to appropriately trained medical staff to accompany the patient as well as suitable air ambulances that are equipped with suitable intensive care and other equipment.

Travel insurance companies may also be able to assist team medical staff with the provision of information about the local medical services available in a foreign country. For example, some travel insurance companies have developed global hospital rating systems that might be of benefit in determining whether local medical facilities are appropriately matched with the medical needs of the injured or ill athlete.

Insurance/Repatriation Processes

If an athlete's condition requires medical care beyond that which the team doctor is able to provide, early contact should be made with the travel insurance company to arrange transport by his/her nominated medical assistance organization.

The team doctor can expedite the transfer of care to the medical assistance organization by having available information such as the travel insurance policy number, as well as providing a summary of the athlete's current medical status, his/her location, and the contact details of the admitting physician if already admitted to a local facility. The medical assistance organization will then collate the available medical data and determine whether immediate transport to another location is appropriate, though usually emergency treatment will be initiated locally depending on the type and severity of the condition.

Decisions regarding the necessity for early or later transport to the athlete's home country may also depend on the level of care available in the event host country and also possibly the wishes of the injured athlete or his/her substitute decision maker.

There are complicated duty of care issues associated with the transfer of care of an injured or ill athlete to a third-party medical assistance organization. These issues should be discussed and considered in advance. Providers should ensure that they are protected by an appropriately and professionally drafted contract indemnifying the medical provider, in case of any injury or illness caused by the actions of third-party providers, acknowledging that it may be necessary to outsource such care and to list the possible reasons and circumstances in which outsourcing may be deemed necessary. Care should be taken to note that the list is inclusive, not exhaustive of all circumstances, lest force majeure-type situations arise.

Other Procedural Considerations

1. A full set of patient notes, X-rays, and scans should accompany the patient. These documents should be prepared and made available for the departure time and should be supplemented with ongoing records of appropriate clinical observations and monitoring findings. It is not unusual for travel insurance organizations to request a report of the transfer by the senior clinician accompanied by copies of these notes and observations
2. The athlete's family (or other nominated person or persons) should be informed of his/her condition and the medical and transport arrangements that have been made
3. Inform the receiving hospital/facility of the projected arrival time and update this frequently throughout the repatriation
4. It may be helpful to contact the athlete's local embassy or consulate for assistance

5. During an Olympic Games, the Organizing Committee for Olympic Games (OCOG) will always require information about the athlete's whereabouts!
6. Ensure that all the necessary travel documents of all injured athletes and accompanying medical staff are correct and in order to minimize delays at transport hubs

Bibliography

Dewhurst, A., Farrar, D., Walker, C., Mason, P., Beven, P. & Goldstone, J. (2001) Medical repatriation via fixed-wing ambulance: a review of patient characteristics and adverse events. Anaesthesia, 56 (9), 882–887.

Duchateau, F., Legrand, J., Verner, L. & Brady, W. (2013) Commercial aircraft repatriation of patients with pneumothorax. Air Medical Journal, 32 (4), 200–202.

Hearns, S. & Shirley, P. (2006) Retrieval medicine: a review and guide for UK practitioners. Part 2: clinical guidelines and evidence base. Emergency Medicine Journal, 23, 937–942.

Shirley, P. & Hearns, S. (2006) Retrieval medicine: a review and guide for UK practitioners. Part 1: safety in patient retrieval systems. Emergency Medicine Journal, 23, 943–947.

Appendix 1

International Olympic Committee Executive Board

Olympic Movement Medical Code
In force as from 1 October 2009

PREAMBLE

"Fundamental Principles of Olympism

1 *Olympism is a philosophy of life, exalting and combining in a balanced whole the qualities of body, will and mind. Blending sport with culture and education, Olympism seeks to create a way of life based on the joy of effort, the educational value of good example and respect for universal fundamental ethical principles.*
2 *The goal of Olympism is to place sport at the service of the harmonious development of man, with a view to promoting a peaceful society concerned with the preservation of human dignity."*

Olympic Charter, July 2007

1. The Olympic Movement, in accomplishing its mission, should encourage all stakeholders to take measures to ensure that sport is practised without danger to the health of the athletes and with respect for fair play and sports ethics. To that end, it encourages those measures necessary to protect the health of participants and to minimise the risks of physical injury and psychological harm. It also encourages measures that will protect athletes in their relationships with physicians and other health care providers.
2. This objective can be achieved mainly through an ongoing education based on the ethical values of sport and on each individual's responsibility in protecting his or her health and the health of others.
3. The present Code supports the basic rules regarding best medical practices in the domain of sport and the safeguarding of the rights and health of the athletes. It supports and encourages the adoption of specific measures to achieve those objectives. It complements and reinforces the World Anti-Doping Code as well as the general principles recognised in international codes of medical ethics.
4. The Olympic Movement Medical Code is directed toward the Olympic Games, championships of the International Federations and competitions to which the International Olympic Committee (IOC) grants its patronage or support, and to all sport practised within the context of the Olympic Movement, both during training and competition.

The IOC Manual of Emergency Sports Medicine, First Edition. Edited by David McDonagh and David Zideman.
2015 International Olympic Committee. Published 2015 by John Wiley & Sons, Ltd.

Chapter I: Relationships Between Athletes and Health Care Providers

1. General Principles

1.1. Athletes should enjoy the same fundamental rights as all patients in their relationships with physicians and health care providers, in particular, respect for:
  a. their human dignity;
  b. their physical and mental integrity
  c. the protection of their health and safety;
  d. their self-determination; and
  e. their privacy and confidentiality.

1.2. The relationship between athletes, their personal physician, the team physician and other health care providers should be protected and be subject to mutual respect. The health and the welfare of athletes prevail over the sole interest of competition and other economic, legal or political considerations.

2. Information

2. Athletes should be fully informed, in a clear and appropriate way, about their health status and their diagnosis; preventive measures; proposed medical interventions, together with the risks and benefits of each intervention; alternatives to proposed interventions, including the consequences of non-treatment for their health and for their return to sports practice; and the prognosis and progress of treatment and rehabilitation measures.

3. Consent

3.1. The voluntary and informed consent of the athletes should be required for any medical intervention.

3.2. Particular care should be taken to avoid pressures from the entourage (e.g., coach, management, family, etc.) and other athletes, so that athletes can make fully informed decisions, taking into account the risks associated with practising a sport with a diagnosed injury or disease.

3.3. Athletes may refuse or interrupt a medical intervention. The consequences of such a decision should be carefully explained to them.

3.4. Athletes are encouraged to designate a person who can act on their behalf in the event of incapacity. They may also define in writing the way they wish to be treated and give any other instruction they deem necessary.

3.5. With the exception of emergency situations, when athletes are unable to consent personally to a medical intervention, the authorisation of their legal representative or of the person designated by the athletes for this purpose should be required, after they have received the necessary information.

When the legal representative has to give authorisation, athletes, whether minors or adults, should nevertheless assent to the medical intervention to the fullest extent of their capacity.

3.6. Consent of the athletes is required for the collection, preservation, analysis and use of any biological sample.

4. Confidentiality and Privacy

4.1. All information about an athlete's health status, diagnosis, prognosis, treatment, rehabilitation measures and all other personal information should be kept confidential, even after the death of the athlete and all applicable legislation should be respected.

4.2. Confidential information should be disclosed only if the athlete gives explicit consent thereto, or if the law expressly provides for this. Consent may be presumed when, to the extent necessary for the athlete's treatment, information is disclosed to other health care providers directly involved in his or her health care.

4.3. All identifiable medical data on athletes should be protected. The protection of the data will normally be appropriate to the manner of their storage. Likewise, biological samples from which identifiable data can be derived should be protected from improper disclosure.

4.4. Athletes should have the right of access to, and a copy of, their complete medical record. Such access should normally exclude data concerning or provided by third parties.

4.5. Athletes should have the right to demand the rectification of any erroneous medical data in their files.

4.6. Intrusion into the private life of an athlete should be permissible only if necessary for diagnosis, treatment and care, with the consent of the athlete, or if it is legally required. Such intrusion is also permissible pursuant to the provisions of the World Anti-Doping Code.

4.7. Any medical intervention should respect privacy and be carried out in the presence of only those persons necessary for the intervention, unless the athlete expressly consents or requests otherwise.

5. Care and Treatment

5.1. Athletes should receive such health care as is appropriate to their needs, including preventive care, activities aimed at health promotion and rehabilitation measures. Services should be continuously available and accessible to all equitably, without discrimination and according to the financial, human and material resources available for such purpose.

5.2. Athletes should have a quality of care marked both by high technical standards and by the professional and respectful attitude of health care providers. This includes continuity of care, including cooperation between all health care providers and establishments involved in their diagnosis, treatment and care.

5.3. During training and competition abroad, athletes should receive the necessary health care, which if possible should be provided by their personal physician or the team physician. They should also receive appropriate emergency care prior to returning home.

5.4. Athletes should be able to choose and change their own physician, health care provider or health care establishment, provided that this is compatible with the functioning of the health care system. They should have the right to request a second medical opinion.

5.5. Athletes should be treated with dignity in relation to their diagnosis, treatment, care and rehabilitation, in accordance with their culture, tradition and values.

They should enjoy support from family, relatives and friends during the course of care and treatment, and to receive spiritual support and guidance.

5.6. Athletes should enjoy relief of their suffering according to the latest recognised medical knowledge. Treatments with an analgesic effect, which allow an athlete to practise a sport with an injury or illness, should be carried out only after careful consideration and consultation with the athlete and other health care providers. If there is a long-term risk to the athlete's health, such treatment should not be given.

Procedures that are solely for the purpose of masking pain or other protective symptoms in order to enable the athlete to practise a sport with an injury or illness should not be administered if, in the absence of such procedures, his or her participation would be medically inadvisable or impossible.

6. Health Care Providers

6.1. The same ethical principles that apply to the current practice of medicine should apply equally to sports medicine. The principal duties of physicians and other health care providers include:
a. making the health of the athletes a priority;
b. doing no harm.

6.2. Health care providers who care for athletes should have the necessary education, training and experience in sports medicine, and keep their knowledge up to date. They should understand the physical and emotional demands placed upon athletes during training and competition, as well as the commitment and necessary capacity to support the extraordinary physical and emotional endurance that sport requires.

6.3. Athletes' health care providers should act in accordance with the latest recognised medical knowledge and, when available, evidence-based medicine. They should refrain from performing any intervention that is not medically indicated, even at the request of the athletes, their entourage or another health care provider. Health care providers must also refuse to provide a false medical certificate concerning the fitness of an athlete to participate in training or competition.

6.4. When the health of athletes is at risk, health care providers should strongly discourage them from continuing training or competition and inform them of the risks.

In the case of serious danger to the athlete, or when there is a risk to third parties (players of the same team, opponents, family, the public, etc.), health care providers may also inform the competent persons or authorities, even against the will of the athletes, about their unfitness to participate in training or competition, subject to applicable legislation.

6.5. Health care providers should oppose any sports or physical activity that is not appropriate to the stage of growth, development, general condition of health, and level of training of children. They should act in the best interest of the health of children or adolescents, without regard to any other interests or pressures from the entourage (e.g., coach, management, family, etc.) or other athletes.

6.6. Health care providers should disclose when they are acting on behalf of third parties (e.g., club, federation, organiser, NOC, etc.). They should personally explain to the athletes the reasons for the examination and its outcome, as well as the nature of the information provided to third parties. In principle, the athlete's physician should also be informed.

6.7. When acting on behalf of third parties, health care providers should limit the transfer of information to what is essential. In principle, they may indicate only the athlete's fitness or unfitness to participate in training or competition. With the athlete's consent, the health care providers may provide other information concerning the athlete's participation in sport in a manner compatible with his or her health status.

6.8. At sports venues, it is the responsibility of the team or competition physician to determine whether an injured athlete may continue in or return to the competition. This decision should not be delegated to other professionals or personnel. In the absence of the competent physician, such professionals or personnel should adhere strictly to the instructions that he or she has provided. At all times, the overriding priority should be to safeguard the health and safety of athletes. The outcome of the competition should never influence such decisions.

6.9. When necessary, the team or competition physician should ensure that injured athletes have access to specialised care, by organising medical follow-up by recognised specialists.

Chapter II: Protection and Promotion of the Athlete's Health during Training and Competition

7. General Principles

7.1. No practice constituting any form of physical injury or psychological harm to athletes should be acceptable. Members of the Olympic Movement should ensure that the athletes' conditions of safety, well-being and medical care are favourable to their physical and mental equilibrium. They should adopt the necessary measures to achieve this end and to minimise the risk of injuries and illness. The participation of sports physicians is desirable in the drafting of such measures.

7.2. In each sports discipline, minimal safety requirements should be defined and applied with a view to protecting the health of the participants and the public during training and competition. Depending on the sport and the level of competition, specific rules should be adopted regarding sports venues, safe environmental conditions, sports equipment authorised or prohibited, and the training and competition programmes. The specific needs of each athlete category should be identified and respected.

7.3. For the benefit of all concerned, measures to safeguard the health of the athletes and to minimise the risks of physical injury and psychological harm should be publicised for the benefit all concerned.

7.4. Measures for the protection and the promotion of the athletes' health should be based on the latest recognised medical knowledge.

7.5. Research in sports medicine and sports sciences is encouraged and should be conducted in accordance with the recognised principles of research ethics, in particular the Declaration of Helsinki adopted by the World Medical Association (last revised in Seoul, 2008), and the applicable law. It must never be conducted in a manner which could harm an athlete's health or jeopardise his or her performance. The voluntary and informed consent of the athletes to participate in such research is essential.

7.6. Advances in sports medicine and sports science should not be withheld, and should be published and widely disseminated.

8. Fitness to Practise a Sport

8.1. Except when there are symptoms or a significant family medical history, the practice of sport for all does not require undergoing a fitness test. The recommendation for an athlete to undergo such a test is the responsibility of the personal physician.

8.2. For competitive sport, athletes may be required to present a medical certificate confirming that there are no apparent contraindications. The fitness test should be based on the latest recognised medical knowledge and performed by a specially trained physician.

8.3. A pre-participation medical test is recommended for high level athletes. It should be performed under the responsibility of a specially trained physician.

8.4. Any genetic test that attempts to gauge a particular capacity to practise a sport constitutes a medical evaluation to be performed under the responsibility of a specially trained physician.

9. Medical Support

9.1. In each sports discipline, appropriate guidelines should be established regarding the necessary medical support, depending on the nature of the sports activities and the level of competition.

These guidelines should address, but not be limited to, the following points:
- medical coverage of training and competition venues and how this is organised;
- necessary resources (supplies, premises, vehicles, etc.);
- procedures in case of emergencies;
- system of communication between the medical support services, the organisers and the competent health authorities

9.2. In case of a serious incident occurring during training or competition, there should be procedures to provide the necessary support to those injured, by evacuating them to the competent medical services when needed. The athletes, coaches and persons associated with the sports activity should be informed of those procedures and receive the necessary training for their implementation.

9.3. To reinforce safety in the practice of sports, a mechanism should be established to allow for data collection with regard to injuries sustained during training or competition. When identifiable, such data should be collected with the consent of those concerned, and be treated confidentially in accordance with the recognised ethical principles of research.

Chapter III: Adoption, Compliance and Monitoring

10. Adoption

10.1. The Code is intended to guide all members of the Olympic Movement, in particular the IOC, the International Sports Federations and the National Olympic Committees (hereafter the Signatories). Each Signatory adopts the Code according to its own procedural rules.

10.2. The Code is first adopted by the IOC. It is not mandatory, but desirable, that all members of the Olympic Movement adopt it.

10.3. A list of all Signatories will be made public by the IOC.

11. Compliance

11.1. The Signatories implement the applicable Code provisions through policies, statutes, rules or regulations according to their authority and within their respective spheres of responsibility. They undertake to make the principles and provisions of the Code widely known, by active and appropriate means. For that purpose, they collaborate closely with the relevant physicians' and health care providers' associations and the competent authorities.

11.2. The Signatories encourage the physicians and other health care providers caring for athletes within their spheres of responsibility to act in accordance with this Code.

11.3. Physicians and other health care providers remain bound to respect their own ethical and professional rules in addition to the applicable Code provisions. In the case of any discrepancy, the most favourable rule that protects the health, the rights and the interests of the athletes should prevail.

12. Monitoring

12.1. The IOC Medical Commission oversees the implementation of the Code and receives feedback relating to it. It is also responsible for monitoring changes in the field of ethics and best medical practice and for proposing adaptations to the Code.

12.2. The IOC Medical Commission may issue recommendations and models of best practice with a view to facilitating the implementation of the Code.

Chapter IV: Scope, Entry into Force and Amendments

13. Scope

13.1. The Code applies to all participants in the sports activities governed by each Signatory, in competition as well as out of competition.

13.2. The Signatories are free to grant wider protection to their athletes.

13.3. The Code applies without prejudice to the national and international ethical, legal and regulatory requirements that are more favourable to the protection of the health, rights and interests of the athletes.

14. Entry into Force

14.1. The Code enters into force for the IOC on 1 October 2009. It applies to all Olympic Games, beginning with the 2010 Vancouver Olympic Winter Games.

14.2. The Code may be adopted by the other members of the Olympic Movement after this date. Each Signatory determines when such adoption will take effect.

14.3. The Signatories may withdraw acceptance of the Code after providing the IOC with written notice of their intent to withdraw.

15. Amendments

15.1. Athletes, Signatories and other members of the Olympic Movement are invited to participate in improving and modifying the Code. They may propose amendments.

15.2. Upon the recommendation of its Medical Commission, the IOC initiates proposed amendments to the Code and ensures a consultative process, both to receive and respond to recommendations, and to facilitate review and feedback from athletes, Signatories and members of the Olympic Movement on proposed amendments.

15.3. After appropriate consultation, amendments to the Code are approved by the IOC Executive Board. Unless provided otherwise, they become effective three months after such approval.

15.4. Each Signatory must adopt the amendments approved by the IOC Executive Board within one year after notification of such amendments. Failing this, a Signatory may no longer claim that it complies with the Olympic Movement Medical Code.

Adopted by the IOC Executive Board in Lausanne on 16 June 2009.

Appendix 2

Sport-Specific Injury Profile and Equipment Guide

Below is a description of frequent accident types, injury patterns, essential skills, and equipment list as required by the various International Federations. For a definitive list, look up the federation website or of contact your national federation authorities.

All Fields of Play should have at least one dedicated cardiac defibrillator/automated external defibrillator (AED).

Winter Olympics Federations

Biathlon

Accident type	Falls
Injury profile	Extremity injuries
Essential skills required	Resuscitation General sports medical background
Essential equipment	Resuscitation equipment, bag-valve-mask with supplemental oxygen, intravenous (IV) access Neck, spine, limb immobilization units. Snow scooter/sled stretcher unit
Federation's qualification requirements?	Recommend certified sports medical doctors

Bobsleigh and Skeleton

Accident type	Sled crashes – high-velocity injuries Start area incidents
Injury profile	Head, neck, spinal injuries Friction burns on the back Contusions, sprains, fractures Ocular foreign bodies
Essential skills required	Resuscitation, safe helmet removal, extrication from a bobsled, skilled in neck, spine, extremity immobilization, wound care
Essential equipment	Resuscitation equipment, bag-valve-mask with supplemental oxygen, IV access Neck, spine, limb immobilization equipment
Federation's qualification requirements?	None – but rules state that doctor: "Should be competent in emergency medical procedures"

The IOC Manual of Emergency Sports Medicine, First Edition. Edited by David McDonagh and David Zideman.
2015 International Olympic Committee. Published 2015 by John Wiley & Sons, Ltd.

Curling

Accident type	Occasional fall on ice – but rare
Injury profile	Upper extremity, head injuries
Essential skills required	General medical skills
Essential equipment	None
Federation's qualification requirements?	None

Ice Hockey

Accident type	Injuries due to tackling, falls, blows from sticks or puck
Injury profile	Contusions, sprains, strains, cuts Fractures Head injuries, neck injuries
Essential skills required	Advanced trauma and cardiac skills, prehospital emergency medicine, sport medicine
Essential equipment	Resuscitation equipment, bag-valve-mask with supplemental oxygen, IV access Spine immobilization, splints, suture equipment, wound care
Federation's qualification requirements?	None – recommend experience in sports medicine and prehospital emergency care

Luge

Accident type	Sled crashes – high-velocity injuries Start area incidents
Injury profile	Head, neck, spinal injuries Friction burns to back, elbows Fractures of the foot, ankle Contusions, sprains
Essential skills required	Resuscitation, safe helmet removal, skilled in neck, spine, extremity immobilization, wound care
Essential equipment	Resuscitation equipment, bag-valve-mask with supplemental oxygen, IV access Spine immobilization, splints, suture equipment, wound care
Federation's qualification requirements?	None – doctor must be proficient in prehospital emergency medical procedures

Skating

Accident type	In ice dancing – falls from height; in all other disciplines potential for serious wounds from skates, also crashes
Injury profile	Cervical spine and spinal injuries, concussion Blade lacerations – major blood vessel lacerations Asthma exacerbations Contusions, sprains
Essential skills required	Good emergency skills – maintenance of airways, control hemorrhage, IV access, cervical and spinal immobilization, neurological assessment, management of concussion, safe removal of helmet, management of epistaxis, suture skills

Essential equipment	Airway (basic and advanced), spine/limb immobilization, IV access, wound care, suture equipment
Federation's qualification requirements?	Doctor must be skilled in prehospital trauma care, spinal immobilization, and advanced airway skills

Skiing

The FIS has several disciplines: alpine skiing, cross country skiing, skijumping, nordic combined, snowbord, freestyle skiing. Despite this variety of disciplines, injuries are often similar. Doctors must be skilled in prehospital trauma care.

Alpine Skiing

Accident type	Crashes – high-velocity injuries
Injury profile	Head, neck, spinal, thorax, abdominal, pelvic, limb injuries
Essential skills required	Maintenance of airways, control hemorrhage, IV access, cervical/spinal/limb immobilization on the slope, neurological assessment, safe removal of helmet, wound management
Essential equipment	Resuscitation equipment, bag-valve-mask with supplemental oxygen, IV access Neck, spine, limb immobilization, splints, suture equipment, wound care

Cross country skiing

Accident type	Falls, sprains, hypothermia, respiratory problems
Injury profile	Muscle injuries, joint injuries, joint strains
Essential skills required	General sports medical skills
Essential equipment	Resuscitation equipment, bag-valve-mask with supplemental oxygen, IV access Neck, spine, limb immobilization, splints, suture equipment, wound care

Skijumping

Accident type	Falls – high-velocity injuries
Injury profile	Head, neck, spinal, limb injuries Muscle/ligament/joint injuries
Essential skills required	Safe helmet removal; neck and spinal immobilization extremity immobilization, wound care, resuscitation competent in emergency medical procedures
Essential equipment	Resuscitation equipment, bag-valve-mask with supplemental oxygen, IV access Neck, spine, limb immobilization, splints, suture equipment, wound care

Nordic Combined

Accident type	As with skijumping and cross country

Freestyle and Snowboard

Accident type	Falls – high-velocity injuries
Injury profile	Head injuries, neck, spine injuries Muscle/ligament/joint injuries
Essential skills required	Safe helmet removal, neck and spinal immobilization, extremity immobilization, wound care, resuscitation, competent in emergency medical procedures
Essential equipment	Resuscitation equipment, bag-valve-mask with supplemental oxygen, IV access Neck, spine, limb immobilization, splints, suture equipment, wound care

Summer Olympics Federations

Aquatics

There are several aquatic sports: swimming, synchronized swimming, diving, water polo, and open water swimming. Aquatic sports are generally quite safe from a medical perspective. Obviously, there is a potential for drowning in all water sports.

Accident type	Swimming: overuse injuries Synchronized: traumatic injuries from acrobatic lifts Water polo: contact injuries Diving: traumatic injuries are rare Open water swim: immersion, hypothermia, bites
Injury profile	Arm, shoulder, knee injuries Head, neck, face, finger trauma
Essential skills required	Understanding of water rescue procedures FINA medical rules • Medical guidelines for FINA competitions • FINA sports medicine ethical rules in the FINA Rule Book
Essential equipment	See medical guidelines for FINA competition Special medical equipment required for open water swimming may be find in the "Open Water Swimming Manual"
Federation's qualification requirements?	The event doctor must be a "qualified medical officer" Water polo – requires dentist on FoP

Archery

There are several archery disciplines that basically involve shooting from different distances in different environments with various forms of equipment. The disciplines are outdoor archery, indoor archery, field archery, ski, 3D, run, flight, and clout archery.

Accident type	Heat related problems; hand/finger burns Penetrating shaft wounds
Injury profile	Heat-related problems, burns, wounds
Essential skills required	General medical skills Ability to treat musculoskeletal injuries Able to remove ticks, splinters
Essential equipment	Thermometer, IV infusion set and fluids, sphygmomanometer, wound care
Federation's qualification requirements?	None

Athletics

Athletics can be divided into four main areas: track, field, combined, and road events.

Accident type	Falls, sprains, strains Heat-related issues
Injury – illness profile	Joint sprains/dislocations/fractures Muscle/tendon injuries Concussion Heat-related illnesses Cardiac arrest Acute asthma Metabolic disorders
Essential skills required	Resuscitation. Spinal and extremity immobilization Competent in management of acute and chronic musculoskeletal injuries, heat-related illnesses Management of acute internal medical problems
Essential equipment	Resuscitation equipment, bag-valve-mask with supplemental oxygen, IV access Neck, spine, limb immobilization, splints, suture equipment, wound care Diagnostic equipment (electrocardiogram (ECG), glucose test, etc.)
Federation's qualification requirements?	None

Badminton

Accident type	Blows from racquet, shuttlecock Sprains, strains Abrasions
Injury profile	Eye injuries, lacerations (racquet) Muscle – shoulder, low back, hamstring, calf, Achilles injuries Knee and ankle sprains Wounds
Essential skills required	Accident and emergency medicine
Essential equipment	Resuscitation equipment, bag-valve-mask with supplemental oxygen, IV access Neck, spine, limb immobilization, splints, suture equipment, wound care Stretcher, wheelchair
Federation's qualification requirements?	Registered doctor with Diploma in Sports Medicine/ Emergency Medicine

Basketball

Accident type	Blows, falls with sprains, strains, concussion, dental injuries
Injury profile	Head injury – concussion, joint and muscle injuries
Essential skills required	None
Essential equipment	None
Federation's qualification requirements?	Orthopedic surgeons preferred Requires dentist on Field of Play (FoP)

Boxing

Accident type	Cuts, abrasions, blows to head, sprains
Injury profile	Facial cuts, nasal injuries, concussion, hand fractures, knee/ankle sprains
Essential skills required	Boxing experience Pre competition – determine if athlete is fit to box Safe removal of head-guard and mouthpiece Treat serious head, thorax, abdominal injuries Advanced First Aid skills and airway skills
Essential equipment	Resuscitation equipment, bag-valve-mask with supplemental oxygen, IV access Neck, spine, limb immobilization, splints, suture equipment, wound care Pre-bout medical examination equipment
Federation's qualification requirements?	Boxing experience Must be approved as a Ringsde Doctor

Canoeing

There are many disciplines in Canoeing and the accident types are quite diverse.

Accident type	Blows from poles, paddles, walls Immersion
Injury profile	Head injuries Any trauma/LOC could result in potential drowning Contusions, shoulder, upper extremity injuries
Essential skills required	Understanding of water rescue procedures Flatwater: First aid, appreciation of overuse injuries Slalom: General emergency medicine skills
Essential equipment	Resuscitation equipment, bag-valve-mask with supplemental oxygen, IV access Advanced First Aid equipment
Federation's qualification requirements?	None

Cycling

There are many disciplines including road, track, mountain bike, cyclo-cross, BMX trials.

Accident type	High-velocity injuries, falls, blows Burn wounds, splinters from the track
Injury profile	Head, neck, spinal injury Thoracic injury Extremity injuries – contusions, burns, sprains, fractures
Essential skills required	Safe helmet removal, competent with neck, spine, extremity immobilization, wound care, resuscitation
Essential equipment	Resuscitation equipment, bag-valve-mask with supplemental oxygen, IV access Neck, spine, limb immobilization, splints, suture equipment, wound care, splinter removal, burn care
Federation's qualification requirements?	Doctor experienced in sports medicine and/or emergency medicine or traumatology In mountain bike downhill (MTB) events (downhill), experience in mountain rescue

Equestrian Sports FEI

Recognized competition disciplines include dressage, combined driving, endurance riding, eventing, para-equestrian, reining, show jumping, and vaulting. Some disciplines require athletes to wear specialized protective equipment (approved helmets, back protectors, etc.).

Accident type	Falls, blows from fences or horses, injury from falling horse
Injury profile	Multitrauma with potential for head, spinal, thoracic, abdominal, pelvic, and extremity injuries
Essential skills required	Experience with equestrian sport Emergency trauma management, basic and advanced airway management, fluid resuscitation, fracture management, head injury evaluation
Essential equipment	Equestrian ambulance, resuscitation equipment, bag-valve-mask with supplemental oxygen, IV access Neck, spine, limb immobilization, splints, suture equipment, wound care
Federation's qualification requirements?	Equestrian prehospital trauma course recommended

Fencing

Three disciplines – Foil, Épée, and Sabre. Athletes wear protective head and body equipment. Accidents are infrequent, but there is always the (rare) possibility of a very serious injury.

Accident type	Life-threatening penetrating injuries with broken blade Falls, sprains, strains, superficial lacerations
Injury profile	Penetrating injuries to the head, neck, thorax, abdomen Ankle, foot, knee injuries, muscle strains, bruising
Essential skills required	Advanced Life Support Competent and experienced in dealing with acute and chronic sports injuries
Essential equipment	Resuscitation equipment, bag-valve-mask with supplemental oxygen, IV access Dedicated FoP ambulance present or maximum 10 min away. Appropriate first aid equipment, ice, bandages, dressings, stretcher, wheelchair
Federation's qualification requirements?	Medical doctor, paramedic, physiotherapist – Advanced Life Support is obligatory for all official FIE events

Field Hockey

Accident type	Athlete hit by ball or stick, collisions, turf burns/skin abrasions
Injury profile	Fractures, joint sprains, lacerations, dental injuries
Essential skills required	Spinal immobilization. Limb splint application
Essential equipment	Spinal immobilization. Limb splint application, wound care
Federation's qualification requirements?	None Usually orthopedists, physical rehabilitation specialists or Primary Care doctors (general practitioners)

Football

Accident type	Contact injury from tackles, contact with other players Falls, sprains, strains
Injury profile	Muscle strains and contusions, tendon injuries, muscle tears, head and neck injuries, limb fractures A total of 70% of injuries involve the lower limb (most common foot and ankle injuries, second are groin and thigh injuries) and 30% upper limb and back
Essential skills required by an Event Doctor	Management of head and neck injuries on field with correct removal of unconscious or head injured player from FoP. Immobilization of limbs after injuries. Resuscitation on FoP. Initial management of soft tissue injuries
Essential equipment	See FIFA manual
Federation's qualification requirements?	FIFA competitions require fully equipped emergency teams including trained doctors at all games. All FIFA requirements regarding staff and infrastructure are laid out in detail in the "Medical services at FIFA tournaments" document provided to the respective local organizing committee in preparation of the competition At national level, large disparity at present depending on the role and standard of sports medicine in the respective member association and the level of the competition. At present FIFA is aiming to establish requirements for team doctors to be trained in Football Medicine with all relevant related medical injuries, complaints, and illnesses to be covered

Gymnastics

The are many various gymnastic events – Floor Exercise and the Horse Vault Events for both Men and Women. For Men – the Horizontal Bar, Parallel Bars, Pommel Horse, Rings, and Individual All-Around and Team Artistic Gymnastics. Women's events include Asymmetric Bars, Balance Beam, Individual All-Around, and Team Artistic Gymnastics.

Accident type	Falls, tumble, contact with apparatus
Injury profile	Head, spinal, limb, hand and toe injuries, fractures, dislocations, muscle, ligament injuries
Essential skills required	Spinal immobilization, reduction of dislocations and fractures, splintage of fractures, wound care, resuscitation
Essential equipment	Resuscitation equipment, bag-valve-mask with supplemental oxygen, IV access Neck, spine, limb immobilization, splints, wound care
Federation's qualification requirements?	None

Handball

Accident type	Falls, contact with other athletes
Injury profile	Joint dislocation/sprains/fractures of shoulder, elbow, knee, ankle Concussion Facial injuries
Essential skills required	Resuscitation, spinal immobilization, wound care

Essential equipment	Resuscitation equipment, bag-valve-mask with supplemental oxygen, IV access Neck, spine, limb immobilization, splints, suture equipment, wound care
Federation's qualification requirements?	None Traumatologist, orthopedic surgeon or sports medicine specialists preferred

Judo

Accident type	Falls, sprains, strains, contact with other athlete
Injury profile	Joint dislocation/fracture to shoulder, elbow, knee, finger, toes Rib fractures Facial injuries – cuts around the eyes Strangulation – legal hold.
Essential skills required	Spine, extremity immobilization, wound care, resuscitation
Essential equipment	Resuscitation equipment, bag-valve-mask with supplemental oxygen, IV access Neck, spine, limb immobilization, splints, suture equipment, wound care. Dedicated ambulance for athletes
Federation's qualification requirements?	Must have experience in Judo

Modern Pentathlon

Combination of five disciplines: fencing, swimming, show jumping, running, and pistol shooting.

Accident type	Potential from an array of injuries (see fencing, equestrian sports, aquatic sports, etc.)
Injury profile	Multitrauma with potential for injury to all body parts
Essential skills required	Spine, extremity immobilization, wound care, resuscitation
Essential equipment	Resuscitation equipment, bag-valve-mask with supplemental oxygen, IV access Neck, spine, limb immobilization, splints, suture equipment, wound care
Federation's qualification requirements?	Equestrian experience advisable

Rowing

Accident type	In a regatta – collisions, dehydration
Injury profile	Head, upper extremity, back injuries
Essential skills required	See FISA rules Knowledge of water rescue procedures
Essential equipment	See FISA rules
Federation's qualification requirements?	None

Rugby 7's

Accident type	Falls, sprains, strains, contact with other athlete, goalposts Cuts
Injury profile	Concussion Neck and spinal injuries (especially cervical injuries) Sprains/luxations/fractures to knee, ankle, elbow, wrist, hand Muscle rupture contusions Lacerations – often to the face and head
Essential skills required	Competent sports trauma management, spinal immobilization, able to reduce luxations, acute fracture management. Concussion assessment, resuscitation
Essential equipment	Resuscitation equipment, bag-valve-mask with supplemental oxygen, IV access Neck, spine, limb immobilization, splints, suture equipment, wound care
Federation's qualification requirements?	Emergency medical skills

Sailing

Common to both men and women are the Laser One Person Dinghy, Windsurfers, 470 Two Person Dinghy, Keelboats as well as Men's Skiff, Finn and Tornado classes. Sailing does not have a Medical Committee. Safe rescue is paramount. The distance from land could require an emergency sea airlift by helicopter.

Shooting Sports

There are several different disciplines for men and women such as target, clay, international, Olympic Air, shotgun, and rim-fire.

Accident type	Repetitive stress type injuries usually musculoskeletal from holding a firing position. Eye injury from powder, particle, fragment blow-back; rare since the introduction of shooting safety glasses
Injury profile	Muscle strain. Eye foreign body
Essential skills required	Manipulative/manual medicine as most shooters are reluctant to take oral medications. General medical knowledge/practices for those rare unforeseen situations such as new onset seizure, cardiac arrest, heat injury, limb injury from fall
Essential equipment	General medical equipment. Physiotherapy, massage
Federation's qualification requirements?	None

Table Tennis

Accident type	Strains and sprains
Injury profile	Muscle – tendon – joint strains
Essential skills required	General medical skills
Essential equipment	General medical equipment. Physiotherapy, massage
Federation's qualification requirements?	No

Taekwondo

Accident type	Falls, contact with other athletes, sprains
Injury profile	Muscle/tendon/joint strains Head, neck, chest and back injuries
Essential skills required	Trauma and general medical skills
Essential equipment	Resuscitation equipment, bag-valve-mask with supplemental oxygen, IV access Neck, spine, limb immobilization, splints, suture equipment, wound care
Federation's qualification requirements?	None

Tennis

Accident type	Sprains and strains, falls, blows from ball or racket, contact with apparatus
Injury profile	Muscle/tendon/joint strains
Essential skills required	Resuscitation, IV access, limb immobilization, musculoskeletal examination
Essential equipment	Resuscitation equipment, bag-valve-mask with supplemental oxygen, IV access Neck, spine, limb immobilization, splints, suture equipment, wound care
Federation's qualification requirements?	None

Triathlon

Accident type	Falls, contact with roadside objects (see aquatic and cycling injuries)
Injury profile	Head injury, oculofacial trauma, barotraumas Shoulder, hip, wrist injuries, Low back pain Acute and overuse injuries Heat stroke
Essential skills required	Competent in acute and overuse injuries, heat incidents, wound care, resuscitation
Essential equipment	Resuscitation equipment, bag-valve-mask with supplemental oxygen, IV access Neck, spine, limb immobilization, splints, wound care Blankets and ice
Federation's qualification requirements?	None – two doctors must be present (+ 1 doctor per 200 athletes)

Volleyball

Accident type	Falls, contact with athletes or apparatus, sprains and strains
Injury profile	Ankle, knee, finger sprains, dislocations fractures Beach volleyball – dehydration, hyperthermia
Essential skills required	Resuscitation. Beach volleyball – rehydration and cooling
Essential equipment	Resuscitation equipment, bag-valve-mask with supplemental oxygen, IV access Neck, spine, limb immobilization, splints, wound care
Federation's qualification requirements?	Must have sports medical training and certification as provided by national authorities

Weightlifting

Accident type	Balance problems with muscle/joint injury or inability to control weight with weight falling down
Injury profile	Extremity, spinal injury Acute patellar tendon rupture Shoulder, elbow dislocation Syncope Palm and shin abrasions
Essential skills required	Knowledge of competition rules and spinal immobilization. Reduction of dislocations and fractures, limb immobilzation muscle injury care. Wound care, resuscitation
Essential equipment	Resuscitation equipment, bag-valve-mask with supplemental oxygen, IV access Neck, spine, limb immobilization, splints, wound care. Dedicated athlete ambulance
Federation's qualification requirements?	None

Wrestling

Accident type	Falls, contact with other athletes
Injury profile	Neck and spinal injuries (especially cervical injuries) Joint strains – knee, ankle, elbow, wrist Luxations of shoulder, elbow Epistaxis Contusions, abrasions
Essential skills required	Sports trauma management, spinal immobilization, ability to reduce luxations, knowledge of osteopathy, resuscitation
Essential equipment	Resuscitation equipment, bag-valve-mask with supplemental oxygen, IV access Neck, spine, limb immobilization, splints, suture equipment, wound care
Federation's qualification requirements?	Sports medicine specialist with emergency medical skills

Appendix 3

Healthcare Professional Skillbase

Field of Play (FoP)

1. The Field of Play retrieval team will consist of two parts:

   a. Immediate response (Team Leader):
      i. Doctor and/or paramedic or nurse
   b. Retrieval
      i. Up to four healthcare professionals who can package and retrieve an athlete from the FoP.

2. The skillbase should be developed on a "generic team" basis and will be common for most sports and venues. Some sports will require additional skills (e.g. equestrian) or supplementary specialist teams (mountain bike).
3. Teams must have an excellent knowledge and understanding of the FoP rules and regulations, especially in relation to their specific sport's FoP access and retrieval.
4. All team members must be capable of the following:

   a. Basic life support skills, including airway management
   b. Advanced life support team response
   c. Casualty handling
   d. Communication skills (radio and telephone)

5. Immediate response doctor:

   a. Diagnostic skills:
      i. Acute injury assessment and management
      ii. Sports trauma injuries
      iii. Medical events including hypo/hyperthermia

   b. Advanced life support skills:
      i. Advanced airway management
      ii. Advanced venous access
      iii. Drugs and defibrillation

   c. Trauma management
      i. Provision and maintenance of analgesia
      ii. Fracture and dislocation management and splintage
      iii. Diagnosis and management of spinal injuries
      iv. Cardiovascular stabilization skills

The IOC Manual of Emergency Sports Medicine, First Edition. Edited by David McDonagh and David Zideman.
2015 International Olympic Committee. Published 2015 by John Wiley & Sons, Ltd.

d. Command and control
   i. Team leadership
   ii. Team worker
   iii. Advanced communication skills
   iv. Understanding of multiagency working and lines of responsibility
   v. Understanding of medical command and control
   vi. Transportation procedures

6. Immediate response paramedic or nurse

   Although these may seem the same as for the immediate response doctor, they should be complimentary to the 'doctor' skillbase and appropriate to the healthcare profession.

   a. Diagnostic skills
      i. Acute illness assessment and management
      ii. Sports trauma injuries
      iii. Medical events including hypo/hyperthermia

   b. Advanced life support skills:
      i. Advanced airway management
      ii. Advanced venous access
      iii. Drugs and defibrillation

   c. Trauma management
      i. Provision and maintenance of analgesia
      ii. Fracture and dislocation management and splintage
      iii. Diagnosis and management of spinal injuries
      iv. Cardiovascular stabilization skills

   d. Command and control
      i. Team leadership
      ii. Team worker
      iii. Advanced communication skills
      iv. Understanding of multiagency working and lines of responsibility
      v. Understanding of medical command and control
      vi. Transportation procedures

7. FoP retrieval healthcare professionals

   a. Advanced life support skills:
      i. Advanced airway management
      ii. Advanced venous access
      iii. Drugs and defibrillation

   b. Trauma management
      i. Provision and maintenance of analgesia
      ii. Fracture and dislocation management and splintage
      iii. Management of spinal injuries
      iv. Cardiovascular stabilization skills
      v. Designated Team Leader
      vi. Good communication skills

   c. Command and control
      i. Team leadership (as appropriate)
      ii. Team worker (as appropriate)
      iii. Good communication skills
      iv. Understanding of multiagency working and lines of responsibility
      v. Understanding of medical command and control
      vi. Transportation procedures

   This team will have a variable composition of healthcare professionals and should support the immediate response team. They will be responsible for packaging and retrieval of casualties from the FoP to the Athlete Medical room.

8. FoP teams should work in close cooperation with the sports medical teams, team doctors, and the ambulance service to deliver first-class immediate medical care.

Appendix 4 Treatment Algorithms at a Glance

Adult Basic Life Support

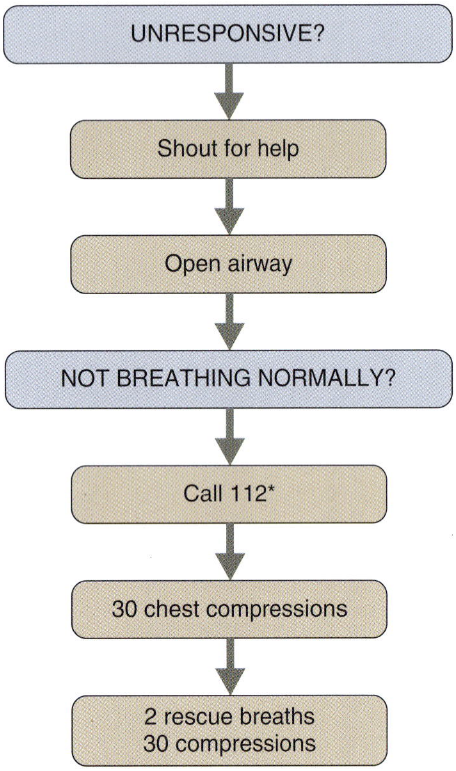

*or national emergency number

Source: Copyright European Resuscitation Council – www.erc.edu – 2014/012.

The IOC Manual of Emergency Sports Medicine, First Edition. Edited by David McDonagh and David Zideman.
2015 International Olympic Committee. Published 2015 by John Wiley & Sons, Ltd.

Adult Foreign Body Airway Obstruction Treatment Algorithm

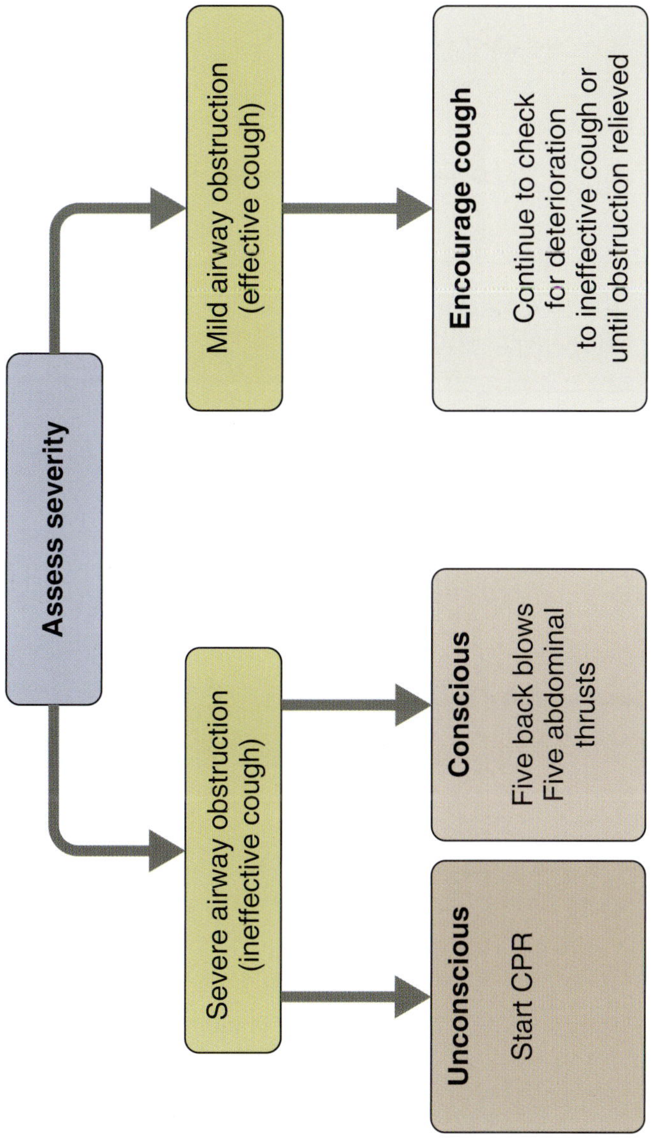

Source: Copyright European Resuscitation Council – www.erc.edu – 2014/012.

Automated External Defibrillation Algorithm

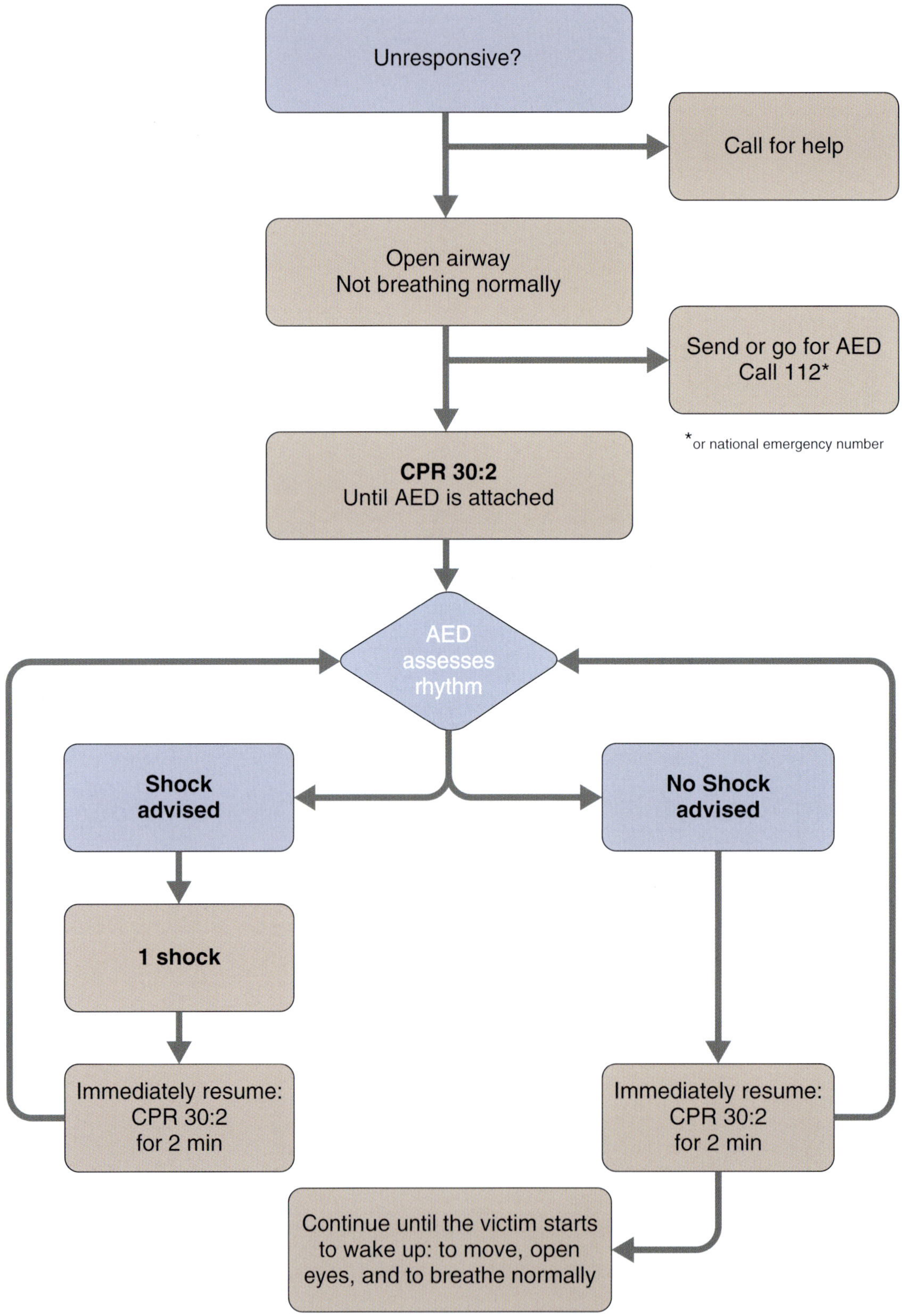

Source: Copyright European Resuscitation Council – www.erc.edu – 2014/012.

Advanced Life Support

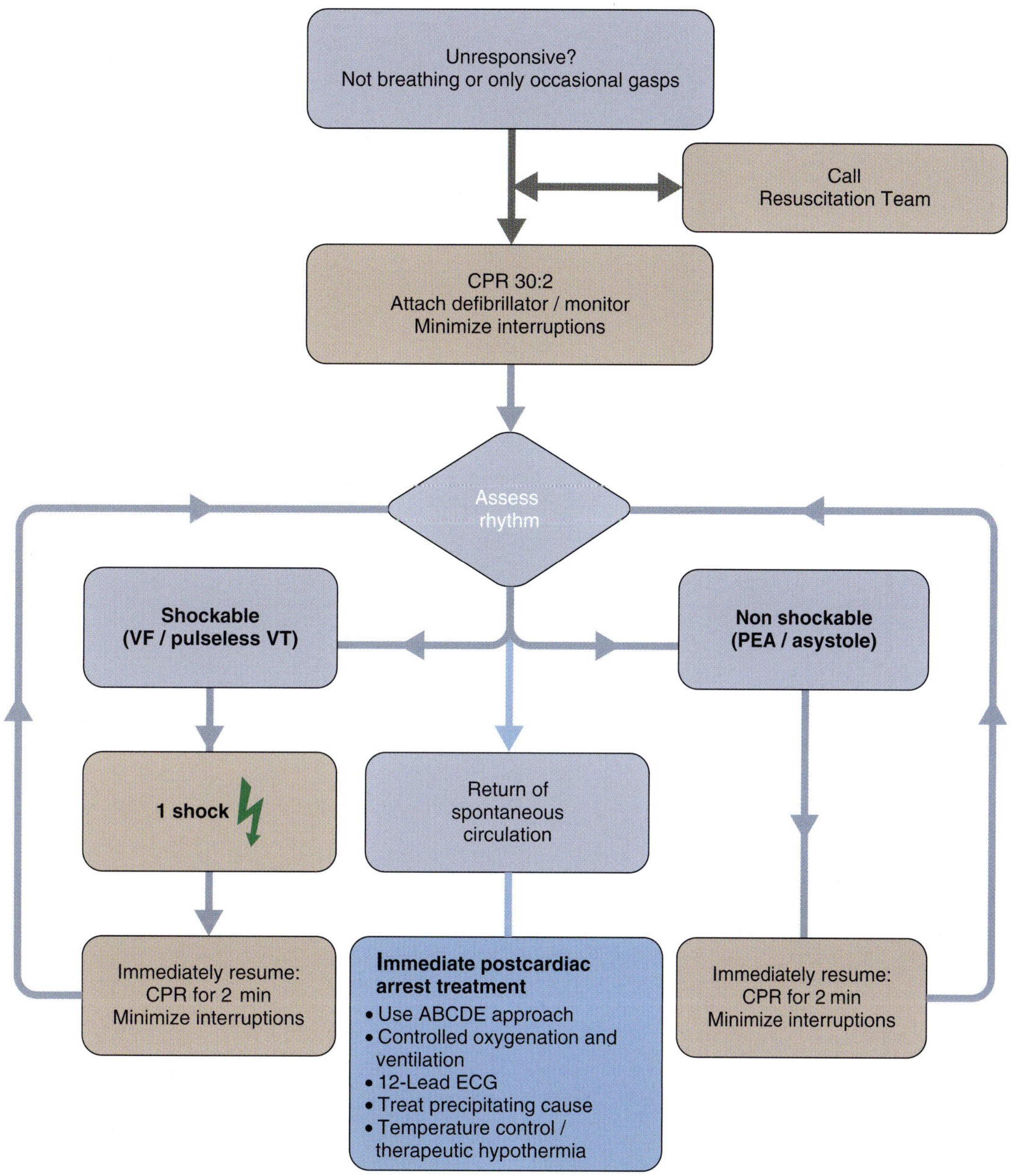

During CPR

- Ensure high-quality CPR: rate, depth, recoil
- Plan actions before interrupting CPR
- Give oxygen
- Consider advanced airway and capnography
- Continuous chest compressions when advanced airway in place
- Vascular access (intravenous, intraosseous)
- Give adrenaline every 3–5 min
- Correct reversible causes

Reversible Causes

- Hypoxia
- Hypovolaemia
- Hypo-/hyperkalemia/metabolic
- Hypothermia

- Thrombosis–coronary or pulmonary
- Tamponade–cardiac
- Toxins
- Tension pneumothorax

Source: Copyright European Resuscitation Council – www.erc.edu – 2014/012.

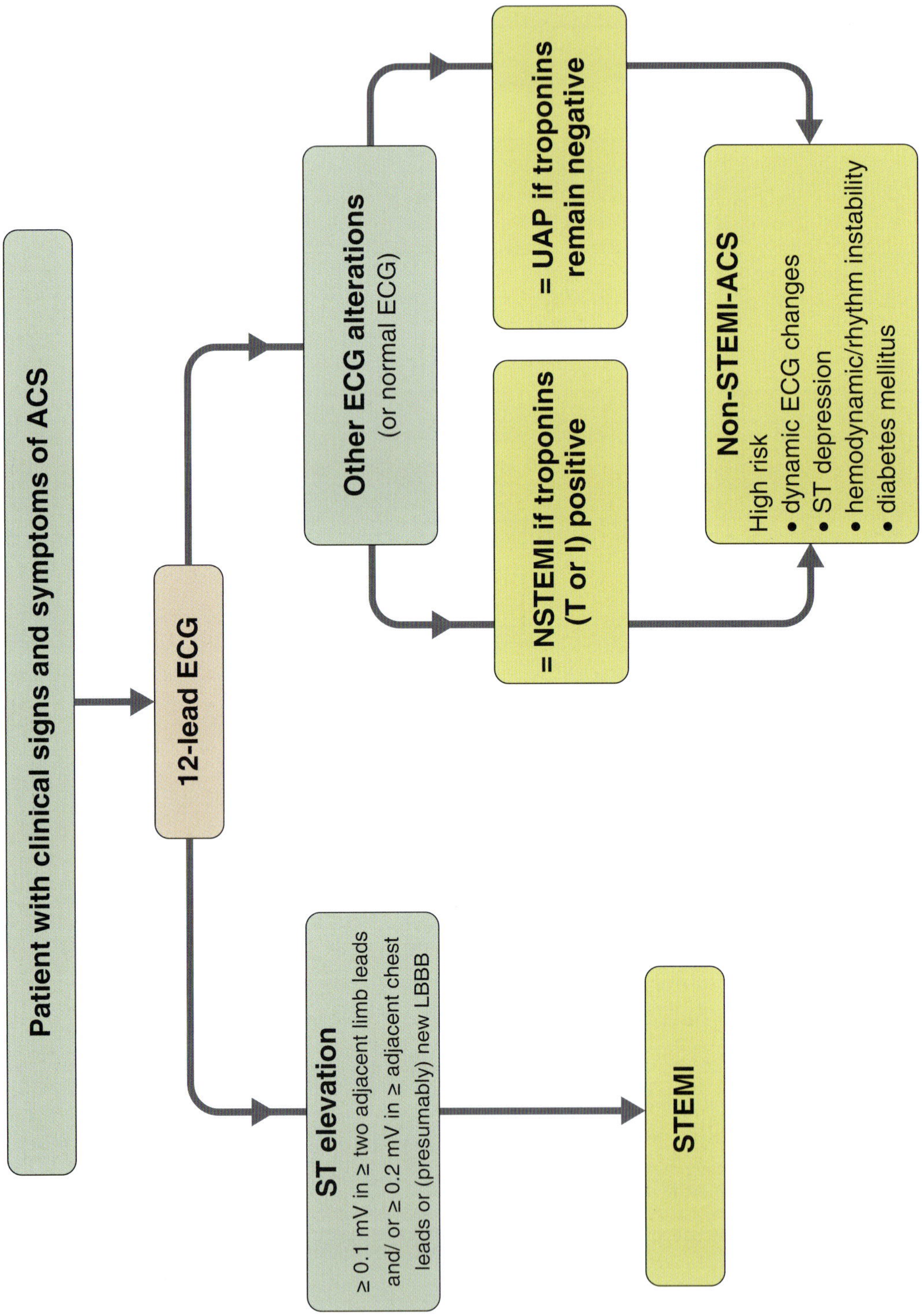

Source: Copyright European Resuscitation Council – www.erc.edu – 2014/012.

The ACS Treatment Algorithm

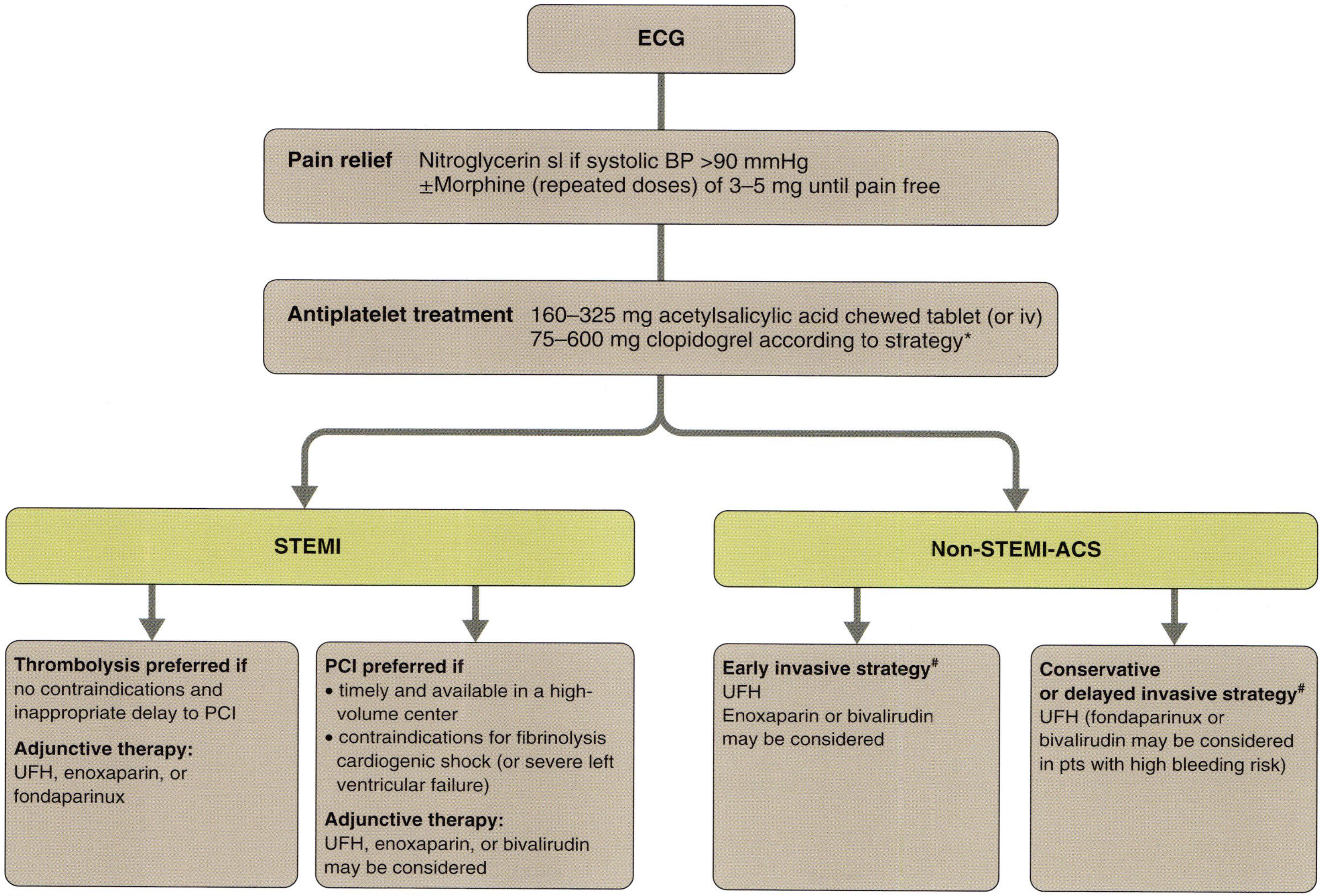

#According to risk stratification.

Source: Copyright European Resuscitation Council – www.erc.edu – 2014/012.

Bradycardia algorithm

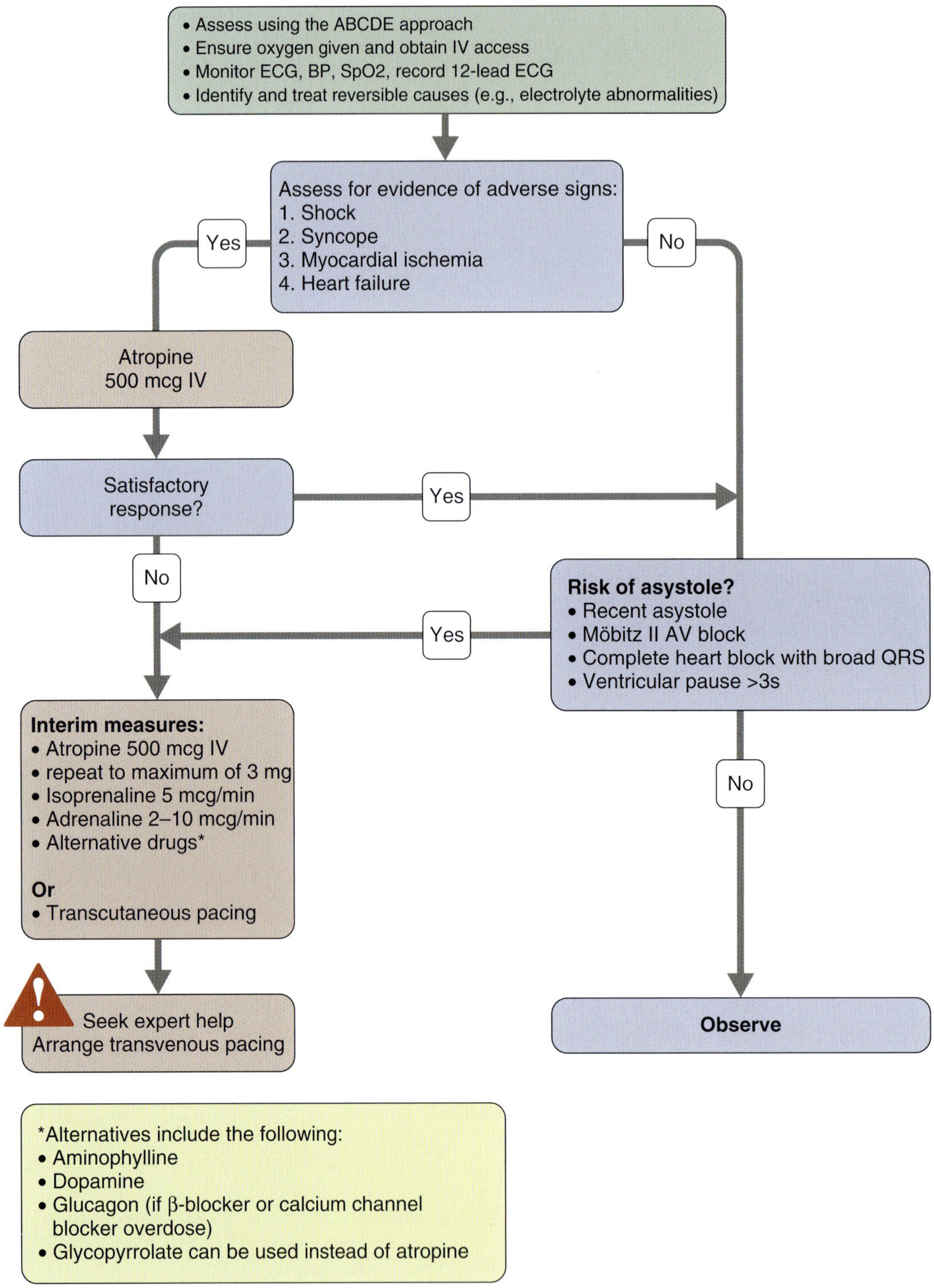

Source: Copyright European Resuscitation Council – www.erc.edu – 2014/012.

Tachycardia algorithm (with pulse)

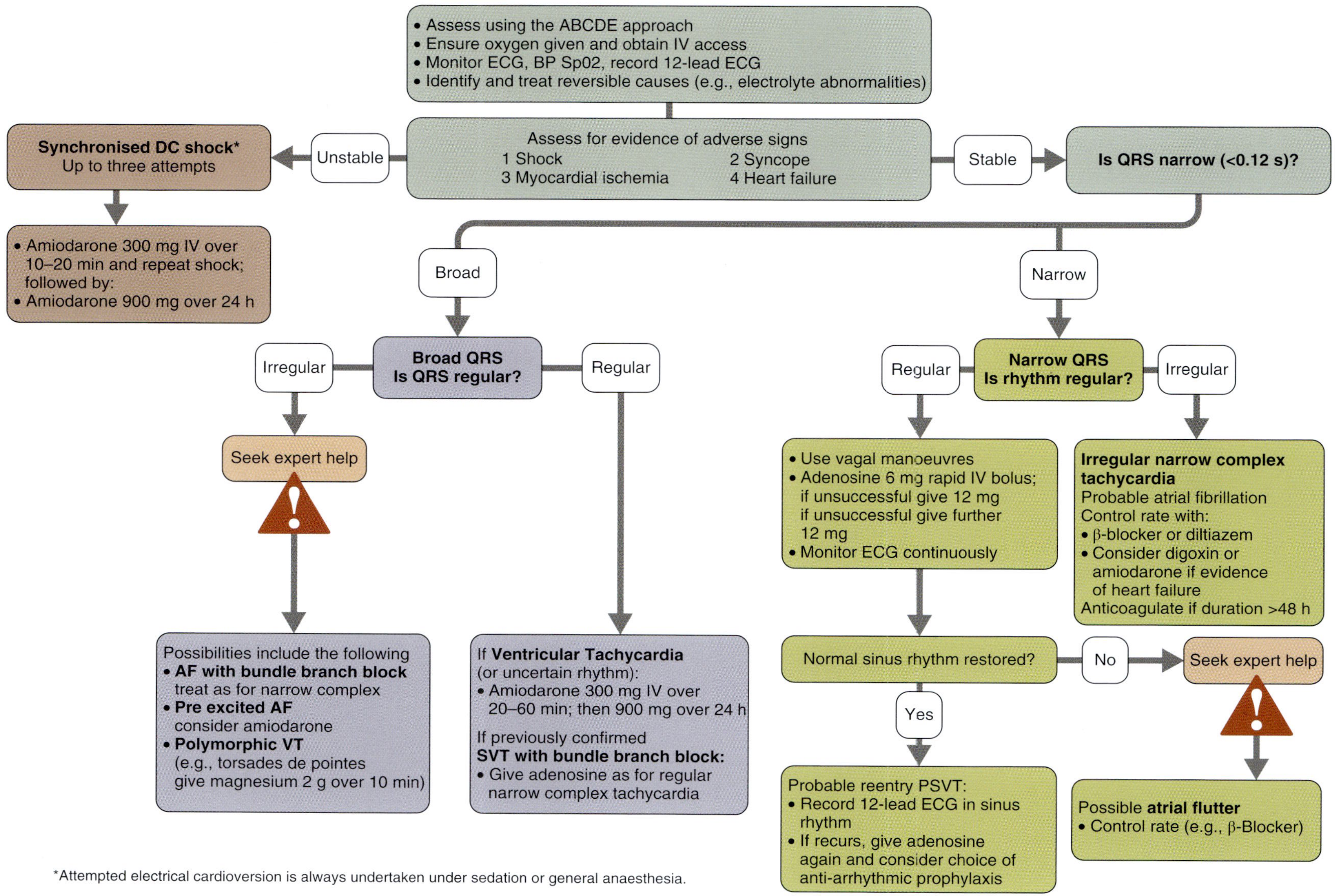

*Attempted electrical cardioversion is always undertaken under sedation or general anaesthesia.

Source: Copyright European Resuscitation Council – www.erc.edu – 2014/012.

Resuscitation Council (UK)

Source: Reproduced with the permission of the Resuscitation Council (UK).

Anaphylactic reaction?

↓

Airway, Breathing, Circulation, Disability, Exposure

↓

Diagnosis - look for:
- Acute onset of illness
- Life-threatening Airway and/or Breathing and/or Circulation problems[1]
- And usually skin changes

↓

- **Call for help**
- Lie patient flat
- Raise patient's legs

↓

Adrenaline[2]

↓

When skills and equipment available:
- Establish airway
- High flow oxygen
- IV fluid challenge[3]
- Chlorphenamine[4]
- Hydrocortisone[5]

Monitor:
- Pulse oximetry
- ECG
- Blood pressure

---

1 Life-threatening problems:

Airway: swelling, hoarseness, stridor
Breathing: rapid breathing, wheeze, fatigue, cyanosis, $SpO_2 < 92\%$, confusion
Circulation: pale, clammy, low blood pressure, faintness, drowsy/coma

2 Adrenaline *(give IM unless experienced with IV adrenaline)*
IM doses of 1:1000 adrenaline (repeat after 5 min if no better)

• Adult	500 micrograms IM (0.5 mL)
• Child more than 12 years:	500 micrograms IM (0.5 mL)
• Child 6 -12 years:	300 micrograms IM (0.3 mL)
• Child less than 6 years:	150 micrograms IM (0.15 mL)

Adrenaline IV to be given **only by experienced specialists**
Titrate: Adults 50 micrograms; Children 1 microgram/kg

3 IV fluid challenge:
Adult - 500 – 1000 mL
Child - crystalloid 20 mL/kg

Stop IV colloid
if this might be the cause of anaphylaxis

	4 Chlorphenamine (IM or slow IV)	5 Hydrocortisone (IM or slow IV)
Adult or child more than 12 years	10 mg	200 mg
Child 6 - 12 years	5 mg	100 mg
Child 6 months to 6 years	2.5 mg	50 mg
Child less than 6 months	250 micrograms/kg	25 mg

Index